CW01637699

PSYCHIATRIC NU

Psychiatric Nursing Skills:

A Patient-Centred Approach

Graham Dexter, RMN, RGN, DipN, RNT, MEd
and
Michael Wash, RMN, RGN, RCNT, RNT

CHAPMAN AND HALL
LONDON • NEW YORK • TOKYO • MELBOURNE • MADRAS

UK	Chapman and Hall, 11 New Fetter Lane, London EC4P 4EE
USA	Chapman and Hall, 29 West 35th Street, New York NY10001
JAPAN	Chapman and Hall Japan, Thomson Publishing Japan, Hirakawacho Nemoto Building, 7F, 1-7-11 Hirakawa-cho, Chiyoda-ku, Tokyo 102
AUSTRALIA	Chapman and Hall Australia, Thomas Nelson Australia, 480 La Trobe Street, PO Box 4725, Melbourne 3000
INDIA	Chapman and Hall India, R. Sheshadri, 32 Second Main Road, CIT East, Madras 600 035

First edition 1986
Reprinted 1987, 1990

Typeset in 10pt Times Roman by
Leaper & Gard Ltd, Bristol, England
Printed and bound in Great Britain by
Mackays of Chatham Ltd, Kent

ISBN 0 412 38050 1

British Library Cataloguing in Publication Data

Dexter, Graham
Psychiatric nursing skills : a patient-centred approach.
1. Psychiatric nursing
I. Title II. Wash, Michael
610.73′68 RC440
ISBN 0 412 38050 1

Library of Congress Cataloging-in-Publication Data

Dexter, Graham.
Psychiatric nursing skills.
Bibliography: p.
Includes index.
1. Psychiatric nursing. 2. Nurse and patient.
I. Wash, Michael. II. Title. [DNLM; 1. Nurse-Patient Relations. 2. Psychiatric Nursing. WY 160 D526p]
RC440.D478 1986 610.73′68 85-13252
ISBN 0 412 38050 1

CONTENTS

Foreword *Mary Connor*
Preface
Acknowledgements
Introduction 1

Part I: Core Skills and Strategies

1. *Personal Skills* 9
Qualities and Attitudes for the Psychiatric Nurse 11
Self-awareness 15
Summary 20
Key Concepts 21
Suggested Further Reading 22

2. *Counselling Skills* 23
Introduction 23
Client-centred 24
Unconditional Positive Regard/Non-judgemental Approach 25
Empathy, Warmth and Genuineness 26
Values 31
Confidentiality 31
Non-verbal Communication 33
Non-verbal Sensitivity 35
Non-verbal Attending 41
Non-verbal Responding 43
Exploratory Responding 44
Progressive Responding 53
Challenging 54
Problem Solving 62
Key Concepts 68
Suggested Further Reading 69

3. *Behavioural Skills* 70
Behaviourism and its Place in Society 70
Ethical Considerations 72
Behavioural Principles 76
Token Economy 86
Desensitisation 88

	Flooding	96
	Positive Conditioning	97
	Assertion Training	100
	Social Skills Training	104
	Key Concepts	109
	Conclusion	109
	Suggested Further Reading	110
4.	*The Psychiatric Nursing Process*	111
	Introduction	111
	Assessment	113
	Planning	127
	Implementation	130
	Evaluation	132
	Key Concepts	134
	Suggested Further Reading	136
Part II:	**Application of Skills**	
5.	*The Depressed Patient*	141
6.	*The Overactive Patient*	159
7.	*The Aggressive Patient*	166
8.	*The Anxious Patient*	174
9.	*The Obsessive Compulsive Patient*	185
10.	*The Hysterical Patient*	195
11.	*The Institutionalised Patient*	203
12.	*The Manipulative Patient*	212
13.	*The Dependent Patient*	219
14.	*The Hallucinated Patient*	228
15.	*The Deluded Patient*	236
16.	*The Child*	243
17.	*The Elderly Confused Patient*	254
18.	*The Dying Patient*	263
19.	*The Bereaved*	277
Part III:	**Extending Knowledge and Skills**	
20.	*Community Skills*	295
	Role of the Community Psychiatric Nurse	296
	Implications for the Community Nurse	296
	Skills of Community Psychiatric Nursing	300
	Key Concepts	304

	Summary	304
	Conclusion	305
	Suggested Further Reading	306
21.	*Human Sexuality*	307
	Introduction	307
	Psychological Aspects of Sexuality	309
	The Sociocultural Aspects of Sexuality	311
	The Physiology of Sexual Encounter	312
	Potential Problems throughout the Life Cycle	315
	Sexuality and the Mentally Handicapped	316
	Sexuality and the Physically Handicapped	317
	Sexuality and the Mentally Ill	317
	Gender Identity and Sexual Expression	321
	Conclusion	324
	Key Concepts	325
	Suggested Further Reading	326
22.	*Creative Skills*	327
	Art	327
	Suggested Further Reading	330
	Dramatherapy	330
	Suggested Further Reading	336
	Music and Dance	337
	Suggested Further Reading	340
23.	*Management Principles and Skills*	341
	Resources	341
	Management Contrasts	347
	Conclusion	359
Appendix I:	Mental Defence Mechanisms	360
Appendix II:	Technique for Reality Orientation	362
References and General Further Reading		364
Index		367

To

Frances, Veronica, Harry and Mary

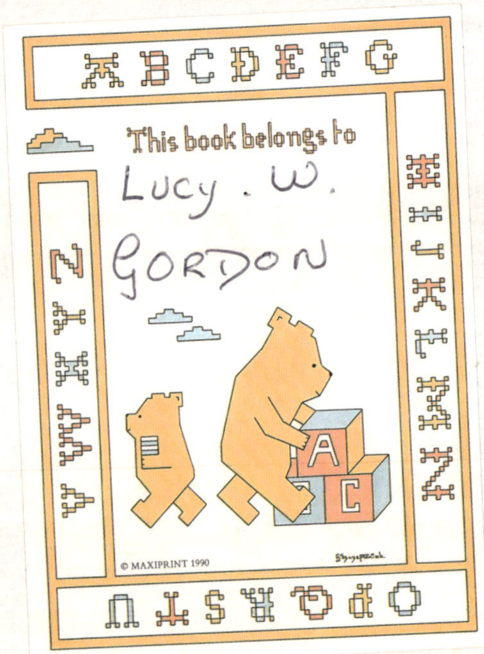

FOREWORD

The 1982 syllabus for the training of the Registered Mental Nurse unashamedly focuses upon the major competencies required of the psychiatric nurse. This book provides a clear statement of the skills required. The authors explore the way in which such skills may be developed from attitudes of genuine concern, warm acceptance and understanding of those in need of psychiatric care.

Because self-awareness is fundamental for the development of interpersonal and helping skills, the authors give the reader an opportunity to reflect personally upon attitudes, values, feelings and behaviours in relation to specific therapeutic approaches. This is done with the help of very realistic case material drawn from their own nursing experiences.

There is a natural progression from basic interactive skills to counselling and problem solving. An eclectic approach ensures that the reader gains information for orientations as diverse as client-centred and behavioural.

Developmental psychology, human sexuality and the social psychology of the family are each areas which merit particular attention in the 1982 syllabus of training. This book provides knowledge and skills in relation to each. The family is considered in relation to the development of the child and in relation to the work of the psychiatric nurse.

An increasing consciousness about the alternative approaches which can contribute to the development of human potential highlights the need for the sound development of skills in therapeutic relationships.

Graham Dexter and Michael Wash have provided a wide-ranging exploration of psychiatric nursing skills. Their ability to draw appropriately from nursing experience gives this book a very realistic flavour. Their message is clear. Patients are persons. Nurses are persons too. The development of the skills presented in this book will empower both nurse and patient, and both will be enabled to be more fully human.

Mary Connor, MA
Senior Lecturer in Guidance and Counselling
College of Ripon and York, St John, York

PREFACE

In this book we have attempted to identify skills which are needed by the psychiatric nurse, and in doing so, identify a body of knowledge unique to the professional psychiatric nurse. The book has been written to demonstrate the basis of a skills approach for both the experienced and the inexperienced nurse to build upon, for we believe that psychiatric nurses, due to both their training and particular mixture of interests, are well equipped to be in the forefront of psychiatry as a developing art and science. We hope that this book in some small way helps this development.

Some of the more recent advances in psychiatric nursing have been reinforced by the publication of a training syllabus for mental nurses (English and Welsh National Boards, 1982). This document highlights the need for a change from a medical model to a social model and from a task-orientated learning experience to a skills approach. We have attempted to reflect this change in emphasis by including such aspects as personal development and self-awareness, human sexuality, the nursing process and counselling skills.

As it is our earnest wish for this book to be widely read, we have tried to make it simple in text and illustrative in case material and dialogue. The case histories we have cited are an amalgam of various experiences and people we have met and are in no way a true reflection of any particular individual; they are constructed to illustrate and facilitate understanding of the concepts involved in the care of particular individuals and any similarity to anyone is purely coincidental.

It is our intention to stimulate interest and pride in the psychiatric nursing profession, knowing that its unique body of knowledge is embodied in the skilled application of an eclectic armoury, i.e. counselling, behavioural and applied psychological techniques.

Finally, we sincerely hope this book reaches not only psychiatric nurses, but all other people interested in helping those in need.

ACKNOWLEDGEMENTS

Firstly we would like to thank Mary Connor, Carl Rogers and Gerard Egan, whose creative thinking and insights have, without question, powerfully influenced not only this book, but our lives.

Additionally we feel that Geoff Stakes, our friend and Senior Tutor, shares with us our sense of achievement in completing this book. Without his help and support our task would have been extremely difficult, if not impossible.

Our thanks for practical support must go to Miss Fiona Darnley, who became much more than just a typist to us. Also to our students, especially from York, from whom we have learned so much, and all the individuals who read the manuscript, in particular Isobel Speight, who gave such objective feedback.

Last, but by no means least, we must give our heartfelt thanks to Jean and Lynne, our supportive, loyal and loving wives.

INTRODUCTION

Whether you are seriously interested in psychiatric nursing or are simply a browser who has selected this volume at random, we hope the contents will be of interest to you and you will continue to read. For this very purpose, we have tried to keep a wide range of contents, from light and stimulating to sobering and thought provoking. We think it appropriate at this point to share with you our views, orientations and attitudes towards psychiatric nursing and finally to reveal the map which may help you negotiate this book.

Firstly, what is psychiatric nursing? Where is it going to, and how do we think it will change? It is our view that psychiatric nursing is currently in a state of transition. Only a decade and a half ago, some psychiatric hospitals were rigid institutions with high walls and predetermined routines which were perceived to be immovable, but this is very different today. The psychiatric nurse's task was traditionally a custodial role, to ensure that the public was protected and isolated from psychiatric patients, and equally that psychiatric patients were protected from themselves. It was in the early to middle 1970s before all the high-walled courtyards were removed and, along with these, some concrete attitudes of the staff also fell. Now in the middle of the 1980s, there are further changes beginning; along with a new syllabus of training for psychiatric nurses, there is a new momentum for all nurses involved in caring for the mentally ill to learn skills which will bring them closer to the patient. The new era for psychiatric nursing should therefore encompass the knowledge which has been built upon by decades of professionals in mental health, and embrace the new optimism of helping patients become more independent and self-directed.

The psychiatric nurse of the future must have the skills of interpersonal relationship formation in much the way a counsellor has, but, much more, she must have a knowledge base of the abnormal mind and be able to adapt her interactions to ensure a skilled approach. Together with this ability she must have at her fingertips an armoury of strategies and techniques from which she can choose, which when directed appropriately will 'help' the patient in every sense of the word. The ability to do this requires sound judgement, based on an awareness of needs which when fulfilled will enable the patient to function as independently as possible. This task is much more difficult for today's psychiatric nurses, for it is no longer simply enough to protect, care for and entertain the patient. The modern nurse has to learn to judge when it is appropriate to withdraw, and help the patient by not helping, and forging new independence.

The authors' main orientation has been within the traditional mental hospital, and consequently much of the material within the book is based on interactions which happen within this setting. This does not mean that the approaches and skills suggested are intended only for those nurses working in hospitals, for it is our belief that these skills are transferable to many settings. Some of the techniques we illustrate are currently practised by nurses with elaborate titles such as 'Nurse Therapist', 'Nurse Practitioner' and 'Nurse Counsellor', and although we use these terms throughout the book, it is not our intention to stress any elitism. Psychiatric nurses with these titles are after all still psychiatric nurses. They have, of course, had additional training and experience in specialised techniques, and therefore have the advantage of an extended role, but this should not deter the learner nurse, staff nurse or charge nurse from acquiring these skills, or having a knowledge of them. When circumstances prevent them from practising with themselves, they may be able to refer patients to nurse specialists who can help. Whatever your current status, experience or situation, it is our hope that this book will help you see further options, motivate you to acquire more skills, and subsequently help your patients more effectively.

Throughout the book, the reader may notice that we have not differentiated between serious mental illness and the less debilitating problems of living. It is true that some authors and clinicians would have classified the chapters in a much more traditional style. However, our intention is to present the material in this book in an uncomplicated way, based on patients being individuals with various problems. It is our hope that by presenting patient problems as separate sub-chapters, you may be able to amalgamate the single symptom and behaviour pattern in any combination to form your own picture of the patient you are nursing, e.g. the depressed, confused, deluded and hallucinated patients, which we attempt to explore individually, may all be part of the more complex picture manifested by the patient you are trying to help at the moment. We hope that the result of this system is that the nurse may come to appreciate that each patient is an individual and may possess problems and needs which are quite different from others and which are perhaps alien to his diagnostic label. For example, 'schizophrenia' is associated with thought disorder and delusions, yet if this occurs in a patient diagnosed as 'phobic', does this mean he is incorrectly diagnosed? The use of diagnostic labels has been avoided within the text, not entirely because we disapprove of labels, but also because they often tend to prejudice, lead to stereotyping, and potentiate stigma. We do not, however, wish to give the impression that they are never useful. They are part of the medical and nursing professions' extended code — a means of short-cutting long descriptions of symptoms. For example, using the word 'tree' is a short cut in language terms — it circumvents having to describe a trunk, bark, branches and leaves. Providing these short cuts are accurate and not stigmatised (i.e. used as value judgements), there are no concrete reasons for not using them, especially when everyone is acquainted with their meaning. Readers spotting medical terms and jargon within the text are asked to forgive us our slips on the grounds that exposure sometimes has the effect of making us less sensitive to their usage.

It is fashionable at the moment to talk of the social, medical, psychoanalytical and behavioural models of psychiatry. Each of these models has a unique theoretical explanation and orientation to mental illness. It has been suggested that this book should state which orientation it leans towards. However, this is a very difficult task, since our own training as psychiatric nurses was centred on a medical model, our theoretical enquiries were mostly psychoanalytical and our post-registration experience has been influenced by the increasing credibility of the behavioural approach. Additionally we are both trainers in counselling, which focuses on an interactional/social model. Consequently, it is not really a question of opting for a particular model, since we do not agree that any one model is necessarily mutually exclusive of any of the others. We hope that psychiatric nurses will become eclectic in their techniques and strategies, knowledgeable in theoretical concepts, and skilful in their interactions. It may be that some of the beliefs and ideas of Freud help in understanding abstract ideas and human behaviour, that learned behaviour or social pressures are useful ways to understand mental illness, but none of these alone explains everything. A psychiatric nurse is someone who cares about, and for, people with mental health problems. Caring, however, is not enough: this attitude must be potentiated with skills and knowledge, and any theory, idea or practice offering to help this proposition should not be ignored.

A significant percentage of the book consists of what can only be described as counselling skills modified and applied to psychiatric manifestation of human behaviour. Psychiatric nurses should not, however, try to be full-time counsellors or believe they are counsellors, for much the same reason as they are not doctors, psychologists, occupational therapists or behaviour therapists. The good psychiatric nurse is partly an amalgam of all these professionals, not of course to such an intensity of specialised degree, but from a broad knowledge base of significant insight. This should not be interpreted as 'Jack of all trades — and master of none', for she is a practitioner in her own right. She is the professional implementor, the functioning component pulling together all these theoretical approaches to plan and return appropriate care for her patient.

To help the reader, the book is set out in three parts, and here is a quick guide to what it contains.

Part I

This part sets out what we believe to be 'core skills and strategies', the essence of skills that are imperative to the sound practice of psychiatric nursing. Chapter 1 focuses upon the psychiatric nurse as a person, her interactive skills of approach, awareness and development. Chapter 2 describes a complete model of counselling, beginning with an orientation of qualities (which we believe apply to psychiatric nurses as perfectly as they do to counsellors) and details basic and advanced skills of counselling from non-verbal communication to challenging skills and problem solving strategies.

Chapter 3 attempts to explain behavioural theory as described by Pavlov and Skinner in a simple and understandable way, using examples and analogies. We hope this approach will potentiate its helpfulness for individuals who may have found other texts more complex and difficult to work through. The chapter ends with discussion of some therapies associated with behavioural theory currently being practised within psychiatric institutions.

Chapter 4 demonstrates how the principles of the nursing process can be applied to psychiatric nursing. It identifies skills and strategies that will be of use to the practising nurse, ensuring that the care that is offered is the care that is needed.

Part II

This section of the book deals with the practical application of the core skills to particular patient behaviour and situations. Case illustrations, theoretical concepts and implications for the nurse are included to enable the reader to visualise a complete picture of the patient, and examples of dialogue are offered to illustrate appropriate skilled responses. The reader is invited to read Part II in any order, as each chapter is separate.

Much of Part II is compiled from our experience with patients throughout our clinical experience and is consequently composed simply of our views and ideas. We hope our ideas are helpful, but would commend their discussion and debate, as we would any stimuli that provoke thought and potentially lead to improving the patient's care.

As many of the chapters in Part II are subjects of entire books by other authors, it is apparent that our discussion of them may at times be cursory in comparison. We have attempted to be as consummate as possible within the publisher's confines, but should the reader be left thinking, 'This is not enough, I want to know more,' or with the feeling of being 'robbed', we apologise in advance and refer you to the section following each chapter, 'Suggested Further Reading'.

Part III

Part III of the book seeks to add a further dimension to psychiatric nursing by extending skills and knowledge in other specialised areas. The chapter on sexuality is included in line with the 1982 syllabus, which focuses upon the study of human sexuality. The material presented may be found in other texts, but is included in this book for psychiatric nurses because we feel it is imperative that self-awareness and a healthy knowledge base are necessary for positive attitudes to be firmly held. It is our view that this clear understanding and insight are necessary in order for psychiatric nurses to help their patients with sexual problems or difficulties. The other three chapters within Part III, 'Community Skills', 'Creative Skills' and 'Management Principles and Skills', are intended to offer some brief insights into complex areas. The ideas of including these areas within the book is to stimulate interest and further reading; they are not an exhaustive in-depth study, but simply an appetiser to an area of complex study.

PART I:

CORE SKILLS AND STRATEGIES

1 PERSONAL SKILLS

Psychiatric nursing is the practice of caring for people who have mental illness, potentiating their independence, and restoring their dignity. In order to fulfil this arduous occupation, the psychiatric nurse must possess a sound knowledge base and the requisite skills of good nursing practice. This ideal nurse must be able to look after the physical needs of the patient, understand the social and psychological function of the individual, both normal and abnormal, and have the necessary ability to direct her skills appropriately.

This first chapter seeks to isolate the basic personal skills, and the attitudes and qualities which make up the ideal psychiatric nurse. We beg the reader to remember whilst reading this chapter that very few experienced nurses will completely measure up to this ideal picture, so there is no need to despair if you do not. It is necessary to paint a portrait of the ideal so that the majority of us who fall short of it may have some goal to work towards.

Some of the skills of psychiatric nursing may be similar to the social skills required for normal interaction, and perhaps quite easily relate to those skills employed by the nurse working in a general hospital. There is at least one significant difference, however. The individual being cared for by the psychiatric nurse may respond quite differently to the average 'man in the street' and the psychiatric nurse must have an abundance of adaptable responses in order to deal with any adverse reaction from the patient.

Responses should be based on sound information or, in an initial meeting, a quick but accurate appraisal of the likely outcomes of any interaction. This skill is the skill of assessment. Assessment and approach skills are the first to be employed in any interaction, and are vitally important.

Assessment of the situation often occurs quickly and spontaneously. There are times, however, when a few seconds' thought, in weighing up the situation before becoming involved yourself, can be useful, both in getting it right and to avoid blunders. For example, would you involve yourself, without hesitation, in the following situations?

— You overhear a group of patients complaining about the staff.
— An irate charge nurse confronting a junior in the office.
— A patient with a severe personality disorder making himself cups of tea after the nurse in charge had said not to.
— A patient, obviously drunk, in the local pub.

We suspect that, if personal involvement occurred in these situations without 'pre-thought' (assessment), the nurse would find considerable difficulty in handling situations of this kind.

Having the ability to *approach* situations is a complex skill in itself. It involves perceiving the person, the environment and the established communication within the situation before one can adjust or adapt personal behaviour to suit the intended interaction The use of appropriate non-verbal communication, e.g. eye contact, posture, gestures, is essential here. (These will be described in detail in Chapter 2.) This alone is not enough as, once in the situation or interaction, the 'personal exchange' may go dreadfully wrong. It is then the degree of sensitivity or intuition concerning the atmosphere that will determine whether or not a change in approach can be subtle enough so as not to endanger the successful outcome of the interaction. For example, how would you feel and cope with the following approaches?

Nurse. Hello, John, it's nice to see you again.
Patient. My name is not John!

Nurse. Come on, Sheila, cheer up, it's not the end of the world!
Patient. It may not be, but I've just heard that my mother has died.

Nurse. How old are you?
Patient. Mind your own business!

It could be argued that the initial assessment in these situations was probably wrong, and consequently the approach was inappropriate. Nevertheless the nurse's ability to cope with these interactions will depend upon her sensitivity, not only to the situation, but to the needs of the patient at the time. The nurse must be able to 'cue' into the patient's feelings in order to act appropriately, thus establishing the foundations of a relationship whereby trust and respect can develop between nurse and patient.

As a psychiatric nurse, you must attempt to behave appropriately within any given interaction. This depends not only upon your assessment of the situation, but also your sensitivity to the patient's needs at the time. Another aspect of assessing is knowing when to interact. It becomes a matter of personal judgement knowing whether to interact at all in certain situations. There are times when people want or need to be on their own; and there are times when interrupting an established set of interactions within any group of people may be less than advantageous. By being sensitive to the situation, the more likely it will be that you will avoid becoming the 'intruder'.

The motives of the nurse become apparent when she is perceived as someone who is sensitive to the situation and the needs of the patient. The patient is able to accept her as a potential helper, someone who has the desire and genuine interest to help and who shows care and understanding. It is clear that interactive skills are the essential foundations on which the potential helper can develop in order to help the patient develop.

What we have just described sounds relatively simple and to some it may seem common sense, but within the behaviours and situations described certain personal qualities and attitudes are inbuilt. The desired qualities and attitudes to be a psychiatric nurse are the same as those to be an 'effective helper'. This involves a certain amount of self-awareness and personal development, both of which we will focus upon in this chapter.

Qualities and Attitudes for the Psychiatric Nurse

One of the prime qualities in a psychiatric nurse is individualism, i.e. those qualities that makes a person unique. Bearing that in mind, we will endeavour to describe what we think are desirable qualities and attitudes that suit this rather demanding profession.

Someone once said to one of us, 'You must be mad working in that loony bin!' The reply at the time was, 'I sometimes wonder myself.' We still wonder today, not that we might be mad, but are we fulfilling a personal need by working in this type of place? Could it be a basic need to help others? One could look further and deeper to explore various theories that may explain this situation. However, we feel that it suffices to say that yes, in some people there does tend to be a desire, drive or motive to help others. Ideally this is not to satisfy a personal need, as psychiatric nursing involves the giving of yourself in order to muster the resources available, thereby being free of selfish motives which may be distracting within the helping process. Many people wish to help others but do not have the 'personal equipment' – such as adequate intelligence, an appetite for reading in order to gather more ideas, having respect for the ideas of others, but also having a sense of reality. The nurse must be a practical person, a person who uses knowledge and skills in a practical way for the benefit of others. She must be a good learner, have an open mind and be willing to listen to anything that may help another to live more effectively. She should be sensible and socially intelligent. The psychiatric nurse should feel comfortable with her own emotions and also the emotions of others in any given situation. A good psychiatric nurse views helping as hard work and a heavy responsibility which may involve entering and influencing the life of another. She should be a good listener, both physically and psychologically, i.e. know what her own body is saying non-verbally as well as verbally, and she should also be sensitive to the patient's non-verbal communication. She must work hard to understand her patient, to be able to see the world through the patient's eyes without emotional entanglement, thus being able to stand back to help in an objective way. The psychiatric nurse is able to accept an individual, without judgement, respecting that person's right to be himself. She genuinely cares, is non-defensive and at all times honest with herself, thus enabling her to help the patient explore feelings, experiences and behaviour in order to identify problems and ways of achieving the solutions to those problems.

A psychiatric nurse is not afraid of giving something of herself, disclosing experiences and feelings if this will enhance the patient's self-understanding. She is not afraid to challenge patients, albeit with care and respect; equally so, she is not afraid to challenge herself (p. 19). Having helped the patient to identify problems, the nurse is then prepared to offer support and guidance to move the patient forward in finding solutions. In doing so she will use any resource that will add to or enhance the effectiveness of the helping process. She will use and master the necessary skills, making them work for her rather than be limited by them. The ideal psychiatric nurse will be living effectively, and by doing so demonstrating this process to the patient. No one is free from problems, but the major difference between the non-effective living person and the person who is living effectively is that the latter is able to utilise self-resource in order to solve or cope with problems, whereas the former finds this extremely difficult.

Many of the skills, attitudes and qualities just described are the ideal. However, they are also realistic in the sense that they can be achieved given the appropriate 'foundation' and training. Once the initial development commences, then the personal growth will continue with skill acquisition and experience.

There are some experiences that even the most skilful person will find disturbing and/or difficult. The psychiatric nurse will experience situations that will require much thought. Certain issues revolving around personal ethics will be explored and hopefully any conflicts resolved during training. These issues may centre on topics like death and dying, the quality of life, the rights of an individual and certain treatments. By being open-minded and willing to learn, the nurse is able to balance realistic attitudes with personal acceptance. Other situations include those for which the nurse is unprepared, e.g. a sudden death, a personal attack, or the sudden realisation of a sense of hopelessness. These and others will require not only personal strength at the time, but an inner strength to recover afterwards.

Psychiatric nursing is a demanding profession. It is both mentally and physically tiring. It requires strength and dedication. If these are given, the sense of satisfaction of not only being able to do the job, but also to be seen to be doing it, is immense. The rewards are not always obvious; they are often intermingled with frustration and resentment. Gratitude is sometimes shown in a peculiar fashion, if at all, and often personal satisfaction is experienced only when some subtle response or improvement is shown by the patient. For example:

Concern had been expressed about Mr Jones. Although he had readily agreed to join in the group, for the past three weeks he had not participated at all. Mr Jones was 83. He had been in hospital for six months and had a history of progressive confusion. Over the past month, he had become less aware of his surroundings, incontinent and non-communicative. The group consisted of fellow patients, all of whom were elderly and experiencing various degrees of confusion. The therapy consisted of reminiscing about the old days, as the memory for past events was often relatively intact, and stories, pictures or music enabled the patients to embark upon a reasonably orientated discussion. However, Mr Jones would not talk and rarely moved. The therapist was considering leaving Mr Jones out of future groups as she thought he had deteriorated beyond help. At the final group meeting, one of the nursing staff interrupted the session, and placed an object on the table in the middle of the group. There was silence, and expressions of surprise, as Mr Jones stared at the object, moved towards it and picked it up. A tentative smile appeared on his face and an overall expression that seemed to be saying, 'Yes, I'm still here, and this I know is part of me.' The object was an old miner's lamp. Mr Jones had been a miner all his working life.

That moment of reality experienced by Mr Jones convinced the therapist that he was not a hopeless case. The response observed by the nurse resulted in tremendous satisfaction for the nurse in her attempt to reach a part of Mr Jones that had not been lost.

Instantaneous peaks of satisfaction such as the one just described are rare. It is said that 'patience is a virtue'. If one relies on waiting for successes in a patient's improvement in life-style, then patience is a virtue the psychiatric nurse must have. It can be said that for the majority of long-stay patients, permanent changes in behaviour are minimal and gradual over the years. Patients often experience setbacks and relapses when it must seem for the nurse like an endless and hopeless struggle to guide the patient towards a better quality of life.

We can see patients we have nursed, helped to dress, shave, bathe and escorted back and forth from the Industrial Therapy Unit living today without that degree of help, surviving with a certain amount of independence enabling them to be considered for holidays, outings and, for the future, part-supervised accommodation. Whether this has been due to a combination of persistent rehabilitation programmes, reduction in the intensity of the illness or more effective medication, the role of the nurse/patient relationship in this progression from dependence to relative freedom cannot be ignored. It is the observation and awareness of this progression to a better quality of life that results in another aspect of personal satisfaction.

To generalise as to where personal satisfaction is experienced is somewhat trivialising the uniqueness of the individual mentioned earlier. Everyone's experience is different; consequently the moments of satisfaction will vary, depending upon the individual nurse and not necessarily upon the experience.

Finally, the psychiatric nurse must be someone special, someone who can attempt to satisfy the needs of others by selflessly utilising her personality in order to give some meaning to the patient's life. This is done mainly by:

- listening with understanding;
- responding with care and respect;
- supporting with trust and confidence;
- reassuring with explanation and honesty;
- physically nursing the helpless with compassion;
- skilfully carrying out procedures;
- overcoming the distaste that would be experienced by most, by concentrating on the feelings of the 'person', and not on the nurse's personal experience.

The skills required of a psychiatric nurse are indeed varied and many. But in order to be proficient in these skills, the psychiatric nurse must be a specialist, a specialist in 'people'.

Self-awareness

Complete the following sentences:

I see myself as
My friends see me as
My family see me as
What I like about myself is
What I dislike about myself is
One thing other people like about me is
One thing other people dislike about me is
One aspect within me I would like to change is
The aspects about me that other people would like to change are

The sentences you have just completed may reflect your present level of self-awareness. By self-awareness we mean self-acknowledgement of one's own feelings and behaviours, accepting and understanding or attempting to understand their presence.

The amount of self-awareness may reflect the congruity of how you see yourself and how others see you.

The following is a verbal account from a first-year nurse, describing how she thinks her first ward experience has been:

I've really enjoyed this allocation, it took me a while to get into it, but after a few weeks, it seemed all my worries were unfounded. I enjoy talking to the patients and I think they enjoy talking to me, even though there have been a couple of dodgy moments, but that's to be expected on this ward. The staff have been really good, the charge nurse I find really thorough, I respect him a lot, and I think he likes me for that. Yes, I've enjoyed this allocation, I think I've done quite well.

On the nurse's ward report were the following comments by the charge nurse:

After a very slow start, Nurse Davis seemed to jump from one extreme to another, i.e. treading carefully at first followed by over confidence and taking the job less than seriously. Her eagerness to relate to certain patients was not welcomed, and even after several guidance sessions, she persisted in her over zealous manner, which resulted in several dramatic episodes which required considerable intervention by the qualified staff. She certainly has a lot to learn.

From these two accounts, there appears to be a considerable difference in opinion in the evaluation of this nurse's experience. The question of which of the two is most accurate is irrelevant, as the main principle here is that the nurse's account of herself is incongruent with how others see her.

The nurse implies in her account that she took everything in her stride, coped well and was liked by the staff. The charge nurse's account implies that she did not take the job seriously and was a hindrance at times.

If the report comes as a shock to Nurse Davis, it is likely that she was not aware of how her behaviour was perceived by others. However, if the report does not surprise her, she may be quite self-aware and her 'incomplete' sentences in this case may read something like:

— I see myself as a keen, conscientious and respectful learner.
— Others see me as overeager, sometimes flippant and a bit of a 'crawler'.

Therefore it is not necessary to see yourself as others see you, but to be aware of both perceptions. However, if the perceptions are different, then you need to ask why. What are the reasons for this discrepancy? If you are conscious of this behaviour and its effect on others, then can't something be done about it? It's not that easy: you can be aware at the level of knowing how your behaviour affects others, but the reasons behind that behaviour require a deeper understanding. How you acquire this deeper understanding stems initially from having this 'role awareness'. Being aware of how you act in the different roles of life and how this behaviour affects the people involved in any particular role play is as far as many people are prepared to search. It takes a certain amount of courage to look at yourself in an honest and purposeful way, for it may result in your finding something that the 'self' does not like. This is in fact usual, but finding something is one thing, while admitting and accepting it another. People will often make excuses for, or deny, negative behaviour they find within themselves, e.g.

> One thing I dislike about myself is that I'm not always honest.
> *Excuse* 'There are sometimes occasions when honesty is not the best policy.'
> *Denial* 'No, this can't be true, I must be honest at all times in this sort of job.'

Psychiatric nurses need to go beyond this superficial 'role awareness' in order to become effective helpers. Within society there exist stereotypes of mental disorders, such as the alcoholic vagrant, the drug abuser, the sex offender and many more individual types of behaviours that people generally find difficult to understand, and consequently wish to leave to people specifically trained to deal with them. As an alternative view to condemning these individuals, the psychiatric nurse must know her own feelings towards them if she intends to help them. If she is negative in any way, then it will hinder her effectiveness as a helper, mainly because personal emotions will prevent her listening objectively, making it difficult to achieve any form of understanding. Negative feelings towards types of behaviour, race or religion are usually based on prejudice. Self-awareness involves not only awareness of how others see you, but also awareness of your own attitudes and values in respect of other people.

Give your personal rating of the following statements, i.e. 0 is 'Don't agree', 4 is 'Agree strongly':

(1)	Homosexuals should not be allowed to teach in primary schools.	0	1	2	3	4
(2)	The Irish tend to be of less than average intelligence.	0	1	2	3	4
(3)	Women tend to be poorer drivers than men.	0	1	2	3	4
(4)	Jews tend to be miserly with their money.	0	1	2	3	4
(5)	Black people tend to be better dancers and sports people.	0	1	2	3	4

Add your score of each individual statement. These particular statements relate to common prejudices that exist in our society today. If you rated the statements honestly and your score is above 0, then you have some element of prejudice within yourself. This may compromise the care that you may give. For example, if you scored at all on statement 1, then you are probably assuming something about homosexual behaviour, whereas, in fact, we cannot assume that a particular form of sexual expression will be detrimental. Even with this knowledge, people with this prejudice will still find it difficult not to rate the statement. This is primarily because knowledge is only one of three components that make up an attitude. All this, however, does not mean that if you are prejudiced it becomes difficult to be a psychiatric nurse. The significant factor here is that you must be aware of your prejudices in order to understand your feelings towards particular people. Once this awareness is established and the feelings accepted as prejudiced feelings, then you can work towards being less prejudiced, especially in situations where it may affect the effectiveness of the helping relationship.

Once you begin to understand your own attitudes and values, you can then begin to realise how important they are to you and how difficult they are to change. This will help you to accept other people's attitudes and values, which are as important to them as yours are important to you. The acceptance of an individual within a therapeutic relationship is essential in order to listen objectively with accurate understanding.

Self-honesty is also a facet of awareness. It enables you to look purposefully at self-behaviour and the reasons behind it. Once the contract to be honest with yourself has been made, then the discoveries can be enlightening. By self-honesty, we mean the admission and acceptance of your own behaviour of feelings, however positive or negative they may be, thus avoiding the use of excuses, rationalisations or denials, e.g.

'The thing I like about myself is the way I readily accept any particular individual.'
'The thing I dislike about myself is my inconsistency in being me, i.e. variation in mood and outlook.'

By being honest and avoiding superficiality, the rest of the incomplete sentences, once filled, become very personal and meaningful statements about yourself.

How often do people look inwards? Is it necessary to do so in order to live effectively? Can being too self-aware actually inhibit you? We believe that before embarking upon entering into the world of another, the 'right' to do so must be earned by looking into your own world first.

The incomplete sentences at the beginning of this section gave you an opportunity to look at yourself. It may be appropriate now, after dwelling on the subject, to look at these sentences again. Once you have made the necessary changes, if any, it may be useful to complete the following sentences, which should guide you further to what we mean by the area of self-awareness.

The things in my life that are going right are
The things in my life that are going wrong are
The occasion when I am most likely to blame other things or people for my behaviour or circumstances is
The situations when I tend to lose control are
My main 'strengths' are
My main 'weaknesses' are
The reasons I am uncomfortable in certain situations are
The reasons why I decided to commence nurse training are

I believe that I look
How I appear to other people is

Self-awareness is not acquired instantaneously, but develops gradually over a period of, for some, months, for others, years. It may be argued that achieving total self-awareness may result in 'stripping' a person of all defences. Everyone requires personal defences to protect themselves from conflicts and anxiety. These defences give time to adjust to certain ways of thinking, feeling or behaviour. We are not proposing that all 'defences' are dropped, but that you should be aware of how behaviour and feelings are affected in any interaction. Some defences may be helpful. They can enable the nurse to feel secure in therapeutic situations, giving an air of confidence which is conveyed to the patient, allowing him to feel able to relax and relate. The nurse who has been honest with herself, and who has experienced self-searching with courage and purposefulness, can feel secure in the fact that she has indeed earned the right to propose herself as a helper. In order to be effective and help the patient to develop, she may have to enter his world and return unscathed.

Summary

We have tried to introduce to you many complex issues involved in human relationships. The ability to interact appropriately is mainly dependent upon your understanding of the person-to-person situation. This includes being sensitive to the patient's needs, showing interest and motivation to understand, and being aware of your own internal 'messages' during any given situation: anxiety, anger, embarrassment and confusion are just some of the feelings you may experience during your interactions with patients. Being aware of these and acknowledging them is the first step towards understanding yourself and thus reducing the likelihood of your feelings compromising the care you give to the patient.

Finally, we recognise that we have described what may be to some the ideal requirements for the psychiatric nurse. It is not necessarily the achievement of these ideals that is the measure of success, but the willingness, motivation and efforts made in striving towards them.

Key Concepts

(1) Interaction skills involve the exchange of behaviours within any given situation. It is essential that the nurse uses these skills appropriately, as many psychiatric patients are either incapable, insensitive or oversensitive in their use and interpretation.
(2) They involve:
   — Assessing the situation.
   — Approaching accordingly.
   — Being sensitive to the reaction.
   — Being aware of her own non-verbal communication and sensitive to the patient's non-verbal communication.
   — Reacting appropriately to the patient's feelings.
(3) Within the behaviours that make up interaction skills are the personal qualities and attitudes to be an effective helper.
(4) A psychiatric nurse is someone who can attempt to satisfy the needs of others by selflessly utilising her personality in order to give some meaning to the patient's life. This is done mainly by listening with understanding, responding with care and respect, supporting with trust and confidence and reassuring with explanation and honesty. She is also someone who can physically nurse the helpless with compassion and skill, and carry out procedures that are essential to maintain or improve the patient's quality of life.
(5) To be able to demonstrate these attributes, the need for self-understanding is necessary, i.e. the nurse must know and accept her own feelings and behaviours, accepting and understanding or attempting to understand their presence.
(6) In order for the psychiatric nurse to help the individuals that society sometimes rejects, she must know her own feelings towards them in order to avoid personal emotions preventing accurate and objective listening, thus making it difficult to achieve any form of empathy.
(7) She needs to be aware of self-prejudices in order to understand her own feelings towards particular people.
(8) Before embarking upon entering into the world of another, the 'right' to do so must be earned by looking into her own world first.
(9) The skills of the psychiatric nurse are acquired alongside the development of personal growth, i.e. self-awareness and the

use of the essential qualities become an integral part of her own personality.

Suggested Further Reading

Argyle, Michael and Trower, Peter *Person to Person: Ways of Communicating,* A Life Cycle Book (Harper and Row, London, 1979)

Burnard, Philip 'Developing Self-Awareness', *Nursing Mirror,* vol. 158 (May 1984), pp. 30-1

2 COUNSELLING SKILLS

Introduction

Counselling is a term that is presently being used in all sorts of situations and circumstances. In some ways this is pleasing, for it shows that there is more interest and recognition for a subject that until quite recently was almost entirely confined to the United States. Unfortunately its wider use in current expression has produced a negative side; the term is used in contexts quite outside its original meaning and, alarmingly, it is frequently linked with disciplinary action.

It is very important, in our opinion, to have a clear idea of what is meant by counselling, and how the skills associated with its practice can help all psychiatric health professionals, if employed intelligently.

The definition of 'counsellor' and 'counselling' as laid out quite simply by the British Association for Counselling best suits our purpose. The Association defines it: 'People become engaged in counselling when a person, occupying regularly or temporarily, the role of counsellor, offers and agrees explicitly to give time, attention and respect to another person, or persons, who will temporarily be in the role of the client.'

The task of counselling is to give the client an opportunity to explore, discover and clarify ways of living resourcefully and towards greater well-being.

The purpose of this chapter is to inform the committed, interested or simply curious, about counselling and its appropriateness in nursing. Our objective is to aid the reader to discover a skilled approach to fulfil the definition, and additionally to identify specifically areas of special interest to psychiatric field workers, especially the psychiatric nurse, and assist her clinical practice.

In addition to the British Association for Counselling's definition, we want to add that certain qualities, and at least basic skills, should be possessed by an individual before she considers herself a 'counsellor' or purports to be practising 'counselling'.

To have an honest intention to help, a desire to promote growth within the patient/client, and a reluctance to offer advice or judgement are in our opinion precursors to effective counselling. Even these alone are insufficient. An understanding and a proficient ability to perform the skills of listening, paraphrasing, reflecting, questioning, clarifying, summarising and challenging are essential. These skills cannot be acquired by simply reading this text, nor by reading any textbook, but are gained by practice. Practising the skills after studying the text requires courage, not just in the personal risk involved, or in commitment to a role, but also the courage required to ask for guidance, to accept constructive criticism, to be self-aware enough to observe yourself and admit your mistakes. The individual who seeks skill acquisition needs to be aware enough to see the dangerous areas and pitfalls when dealing with a client, to avoid harming him. In order to do this you need to be resourceful enough to change direction when feeling out of your depth, and confident enough as an individual to share with the client your feelings, misgivings and uncertainties.

In short, it is our view that you must earn the right to counsel others, by acquiring the skills, owning the qualities, and understanding yourself.

Carl Rogers coined the term 'client-centred therapy', and is considered by many to be the father of counselling. We would like, before continuing with applications and explanations of skills, to consider some of the concepts Rogers and other leading authorities suggest are important in the field of counselling based on client-centred therapy.

Client-centred

This is the linchpin of many counselling models, at least in the initial stages. The idea is based upon the belief that the client is the important person in the relationship, and that he has the resources and ability to help himself if given the opportunity. The counsellor facilitates the client seeing himself more clearly, and does not advise, suggest, persuade or in any way interfere with the client's view of himself. Initially to operate in this manner may mean that previously trained health workers have to shed their preconceived ideas of themselves and their clients, i.e. relationships based on the idea that 'I am the expert — you are the client — you tell me what is wrong and I will tell you what to do.'

Client-centred therapy suggests that the client will, given the correct climate, diagnose, prescribe and treat himself.

It is therefore implicit in the client-centred approach to have a trust in human beings, that all people have inner resources, and above all are motivated to improve.

Unconditional Positive Regard/Non-judgemental Approach

The expression of 'unconditional positive regard' is a fundamental principle of counselling, without which it is difficult to imagine how a therapeutic relationship on the basis of counselling can be maintained. Although the term sounds difficult to understand, the idea is really quite simple. Rogers explains that before a client can really understand himself clearly, he must be able to accept himself. One way of assisting this process is by the counsellor showing that she accepts him — unconditionally. It has been our experience that all the effective and therapeutic psychiatric nurses have this quality to some degree. To have faith, trust and respect for another human being despite his behaviour is probably one of the most difficult things a nurse can be asked to do. She has lived to the age of 18 years at least, during which time she has been bombarded with values and judgements, all playing their part in shaping her personality and character. Parents, friends, the law, society, teachers and colleagues have continually influenced her to believe certain things, to act in certain ways and to think in an 'acceptable' way. Now in this specific therapeutic relationship, she is asked to accept an individual without any kind of judgement, without criticism, and without reservation. Additionally, she is being asked not just to accept, but to respect her client without necessarily knowing what his previous behaviour has been, or who he is, because he is another human being.

To be effective the counsellor has to dispense with her own values, beliefs, prejudices and stereotypes. She must positively, i.e. in a 'friendly' manner, accept and try to understand the other person's values, ideals and beliefs — even if these are totally opposed to her own, and are prejudiced, stereotyped and uncaring.

The advantage this has in the relationship is tremendous, for the client is confronted with another person who does not reject, ridicule or argue with him. He feels that the counsellor is interested, not as so many people are, in themselves, but in him. She is genuinely interested to want to really know him, how he thinks and feels, and still does not judge him. The realisation of this fact engenders in the client the feeling that if someone else is interested, thinks he is worth something, and cares, then perhaps he too should take some time to look at himself more closely.

The practical application of this is, of course, extremely difficult for the inexperienced, and it is our experience that sometimes it is only after a series of successful counselling sessions that the counsellor's fundamental beliefs are changed. Ask yourself these questions and honestly answer them:

(1) Do you believe that most human beings are capable of helping themselves if facilitated by skilled counsellors?
(2) Could you counsel a person convicted of rape, child murder, or some other crime that you find heinous, trying to put his past out of your mind and accepting him with a positive attitude, respecting his values and not judging him for his behaviour?
(3) Do you have enough trust in yourself and your client to be open and honest, and not feel exposed to exploitation by the client?

We would guess your response to at least one of these will be negative, and indeed some of you may have answered 'No' to them all. Indeed, neither of the authors could have honestly answered 'Yes' to them all a few years ago. Despite this, we can assure you that our unanimous answer to them now would be 'Yes'. It is only with the acquisition of counselling skills, practice in counselling situations, and observation of results in effective interactions that our faith in the process has gradually increased to a certain, unshakeable belief.

When you can look back at the three questions and answer them all in the affirmative, we are sure you will be capable of entering into a helping relationship with your client, and expressing unconditional positive regard.

Empathy, Warmth and Genuineness

Another concept accepted almost universally by counsellors is that of the 'core conditions'. Carkhuff and Truax (1979) identify these as empathy, warmth and genuineness. Here we will try to explore briefly what is meant by these terms.

Empathy

Most authorities on counselling agree that this is perhaps the most important quality the counsellor must own. It refers to the ability to understand the client, not superficially, but in an accurate and meaningful way. It requires careful distinguishing from sympathy, and is probably the most misunderstood concept by the inexperienced person interested in counselling. Egan (1975) helps to clarify the idea of empathy by suggesting that it is not an all or nothing quality, and that it can be achieved on different levels.

He suggests two levels of empathy, 'accurate empathy' (primary level) and 'accurate empathy' (advanced level).

Accurate empathy (primary level). The helper must respond to the client in a way that shows she has listened to and understands how the client feels: she must see the client's world from the client's frame of reference; she must communicate her understanding.

Accurate empathy (advanced level). The counsellor is no longer merely responding to the client, but is demanding the client take a deeper look at himself. Egan argues that a counsellor using advanced accurate empathy can use genuineness, respect, understanding and rapport as a power base, where the power is used to 'influence the client to see his problems from a more objective frame of reference'.

Empathy is built up by using skills rather than a quality that a person either has or has not developed. We have noticed, however, that some nurses tend to be extremely quick in establishing advanced accurate empathy, while others need far more time. The time factor is not particularly important, whereas accuracy is absolutely vital. Nurses should not be too eager to compliment themselves on their speedy attainment of empathy. On many occasions we have observed nurses responding to a client's remarks, and receiving swift results by saying something quite profound and very accurate. The client has an overwhelming feeling of relief that at last someone understands, and a great advance in the relationship occurs. Although this is wonderful and no doubt very helpful, all may not be well. For instance, this reaction might have been achieved by a wild and lucky guess, not by accurate observation, skilful listening and thoughtful consideration. Think just how equally and profoundly disastrous it may have been if the nurse had guessed *wrongly.* Our advice in this area is to take the slow accurate route, and not to go for wild stabs in the dark which may have poor overall results.

Probably the most frequent problem in establishing accurate empathy occurs when the counsellor is unable to enter the client's world and understand it from the client's perspective. This difficulty exists because commonly the nurse becomes overwhelmed by her own feelings of sorrow, or perhaps fear, and contaminates or confuses her understanding of the client's world with her own thoughts and emotions.

Sundeen (1976) takes a more systematised view of empathy as a four stage process. Here empathy is broken down into:

(1) Identification.
(2) Incorporation.
(3) Reverberation.
(4) Detachment.

The general idea (simplified) is that the empathic counsellor is able to lose consciousness of self (identification) and become engrossed in the client (incorporation). A process of mental interaction between the feelings of the client and counsellor then follows (reverberation). Finally, the counsellor returns to her own reality (detachment), combining all this and previously gained information into an objective knowledge about the client.

To finish this brief passage on empathy, we leave the final word to Rogers (1967). He describes achieving empathy as 'sensing the feelings and personal meanings which the client is experiencing in each moment, when he can perceive these from "inside", as they seem to the client, and when he can successfully communicate something of that understanding to his client'.

Genuineness

This quality is based on the individual's ability to be himself: he does not have to play a role; he can 'afford' to be transparent; he can own his feelings and express them honestly.

An individual throughout his life may play many roles in different situations and circumstances — father, teacher, friend, husband. As a counsellor he has to be himself, putting away all the prejudices and stereotypes that make us individual personalities, because he needs to be aware that they are just that. Having a sincere belief in human beings and their potential for 'growth' and improvement, he will not have to pretend. He will concentrate all his energies on understanding the client fully and accurately, in the knowledge that he will be challenged about himself. He can honestly share what is appropriate, because he understands himself fully. On the occasions he becomes unhappy with the client, he will say so, and it will probably help him to understand the client better in the long term. However, when the counsellor shares his feelings with the client on these occasions, it will be done skilfully to enable further insight for the client.

For example, Robert, an imaginary client, goes round and round in circles, evading the real issue of his problem. At some point, in order to prevent the counsellor feeling his time is being wasted, and to move the client forward, the counsellor may say something along these lines:

> Robert, I'm not sure we're really getting anywhere — it seems to me that whenever you reach the point of understanding what the problem might be, you steer away from it. Apart from this being rather irritating, I'm not sure we will accomplish much if we carry on like this!

Although this may temporarily inhibit the client, it shows that the counsellor is real — a person too — that he is not prepared simply to go along with everything and anything. In a way, we feel it would devalue the relationship if the counsellor did not occasionally disclose his own feelings. It may be helpful to create a feeling of *mutuality* between client and counsellor, i.e. they both have a shared purpose, they are going somewhere together, they are sharing an experience — an adventure. Genuineness is important. We are sure that not only will it help the client, it will also help the counsellor. Without it we would both have experienced impossible situations when dealing with clients.

An illustration of this occurred quite recently to one of the authors in class. After a particularly harassing morning in the school, and several distraught telephone calls from his wife, he had to participate in a role play to demonstrate listening skills and paraphrasing. After listening to a student disclose a problem for several minutes, he was unable to paraphrase. Eventually addressing the whole class, he admitted that he had not been listening, or hardly. He explained how he had felt during the morning, added that he was extremely embarrassed, and promised to repeat the exercise with more attention. The class was extremely supportive and helpful. Without this genuine disclosure, the paraphrasing exercise would have been disastrous, but as it was, the climate in the class improved distinctly, and a profitable afternoon was spent.

To summarise, genuineness means being 'yourself', not being like anybody else, or trying to live up to or become another sort of person. It involves you as a person being that person in every situation. 'You' as a nurse should be no different to 'you' as a brother, sister or friend. That is to say, fundamentally you do not change your values or attitudes towards people just because of another role. You take on different responsibilities and you may be expected to, and do, behave in certain ways to suit that role, but within that role it is still you. It involves a certain amount of self-awareness, awareness of your own feelings, not presenting a façade. It requires honesty and courage to be allowed to be seen as a real and authentic person.

To hide behind a uniform and to misuse a position of status in order to avoid explanations and difficult situations can be an easy option for people who have not looked at themselves with any degree of honesty. To have any genuineness, you need to know yourself.

Warmth

Warmth is a quality that hardly needs explaining, especially to anyone interested enough in people to read this text. Warmth is so closely connected to the principles of unconditional positive regard that if you have accepted that concept, you already have warmth.

One necessary highlight in this area that perhaps deserves attention is ensuring that your natural warmth is *conveyed* to your client. While earnestly and actively listening to your client, try not to become so tense and anxious about listening that the human expressions of warmth, like smiling, gesturing and posture are lost in the intensity of the moment. Clients need to have your warmth transmitted to them, to encourage them to continue. A smile costs nothing and is seldom misinterpreted, but can mean everything to the client.

'Warmth' is an appealing term: attraction, comfort and safety are associated concerns. To possess it is to be able to demonstrate the acceptance of others as individuals. This acceptance involves adopting non-judgemental attitudes, respecting the feelings and behaviours presented by the client non-defensively, and being open and having a respect for the individual, thus communicating an approachable manner. To emphasise this concept, contrast these qualities with the components of a 'cold person', i.e. one who is rigid in stance and attitude, stern and upright, unsmiling and glaring. From this description, it can be seen that non-verbal communication plays a major part in conveying these qualities. Possession alone is insufficient, and demonstrating these qualities of warmth and genuineness is essential in forming the basis of a therapeutic relationship.

Values

One area we cannot stress enough is the uniqueness of the individual and how important it is to maintain that uniqueness. The client will hold many experiences, people, possessions, beliefs and attitudes as valuable — these are his. Do not try to steal them from him.

A most fundamental and yet frequently met problem in the inexperienced counsellor is her difficulty in preventing her tendency to reinforce or criticise the individual client's values.

The counsellor's values in this context are unimportant, and as such should not interfere with or contaminate the client's values. If, for instance, a client is pregnant and has decided to seek an abortion, it may suggest to the counsellor that the client places a low value on life. This is presumptive and may be completely wrong. However, even if it is so, it should not influence the counsellor's interactions. It would be fundamentally wrong to condemn the client for her values, and no attempt should be made to bring them in line with your own. As in any situation, the counsellor would perhaps want to stay in this particular area of the client's values and try to form some accurate understanding in order that both the client and the counsellor understand the true situation, and if the counsellor is successful in this, logical decisions could be made from the client's point of view.

Confidentiality

Finally, a very important aspect of counselling is confidentiality.

Nurses and health professionals are constantly being reminded of the need to respect confidences, but the implications of this for the counsellor are more difficult. If the counsellor is working independently in a private consultation, confidentiality poses little problem. In most health organisations it is extremely rare for one person to have sole responsibility for care, and to some degree a transfer of information is expected and necessary for the rest of the team to function efficiently. This has caused many problems in nurse counselling, for an implicit trust and a feeling of being able to disclose information of a sensitive nature without fear of the counsellor breaking the confidence are essential for a successful outcome. The counsellor does not simply have to decide whether to break confidence to people outside the normal caring professionals, but also has to decide how much to disclose to her colleagues. Although this is a very sensitive area, and one in which people hold strong views, it is our hope that common sense and professional attitudes will prevail. After much discussion and debate, we consider that the following suggestions may be helpful:

(1) Begin any formal session with a statement of exactly what confidentiality means so that both parties clearly understand its personal implications, e.g.:
   (a) 'I cannot guarantee completely that what you say to me will be in confidence, but what I disclose to the other members of the team will be only in your interests.'
   (b) 'There are certain areas we may discuss that I will feel bound to convey to my colleagues so that they can offer you help as well.'
   (c) 'If I feel during our talks that other staff need to be given some of the information you disclose, I hope you will understand.'
   (d) 'There may be certain facts that I would have to share with other staff: for instance, if you told me you were contemplating suicide.'

These areas should be clearly identified and, if possible, definite policies about such areas discussed and agreed by the team before counselling is undertaken.

(2) If in any difficulty in these areas, be prepared with alternative courses of action, i.e.:

(a) Stop the conversation until the client understands the implications of what he is saying.
(b) Be honest: say you are sorry, but you will have to disclose that.
(c) Seek permission to disclose, even if this requires active persuasion.
(d) Be genuine — say how you are feeling.

To conclude this short introduction to counselling skills, we would like to emphasise that the model we are recommending in this chapter is a *developmental* style, i.e. its basis and essence are a client-centred approach, developing in the later stages towards strategies for helping the client set and achieve goals (see Figure 2.1). The emphasis is on helping the client help himself. The following analogy may clarify this statement.

Life itself may be considered a journey, and from time to time the participant may well hesitate, rest a while, and wonder which direction to take. The direction the person takes must be his choice and his alone, but if someone offers him some spectacles to help him see more clearly, so much the better. Having explored his options, seen much more clearly, and having finally decided to continue in a particular direction, if he should be offered speedier transport and accepts the lift, the journey may be made more easy. The counsellor should seek only to be the spectacles in a true client-centred way. Later, when the model takes on a behavioural approach, the counsellor should offer the speedy method after the goals have been decided by the client, and he needs help in reaching them.

It should be noted that counselling cannot be a compulsory therapy. By its very nature, compulsion would prevent an open and honest interchange. It should not, therefore, be considered the answer or the suitable approach to any client's problems. Perhaps some people do not have any definite goals to be driven towards, but are simply here to enjoy the scenery. If this is true, and it is what they hold valuable, who are we to direct them?

Non-verbal Communication

Non-verbal communication refers to those aspects of communication other than the spoken word. It is not necessary to verbalise words in order to communicate. Thoughts and feelings can be

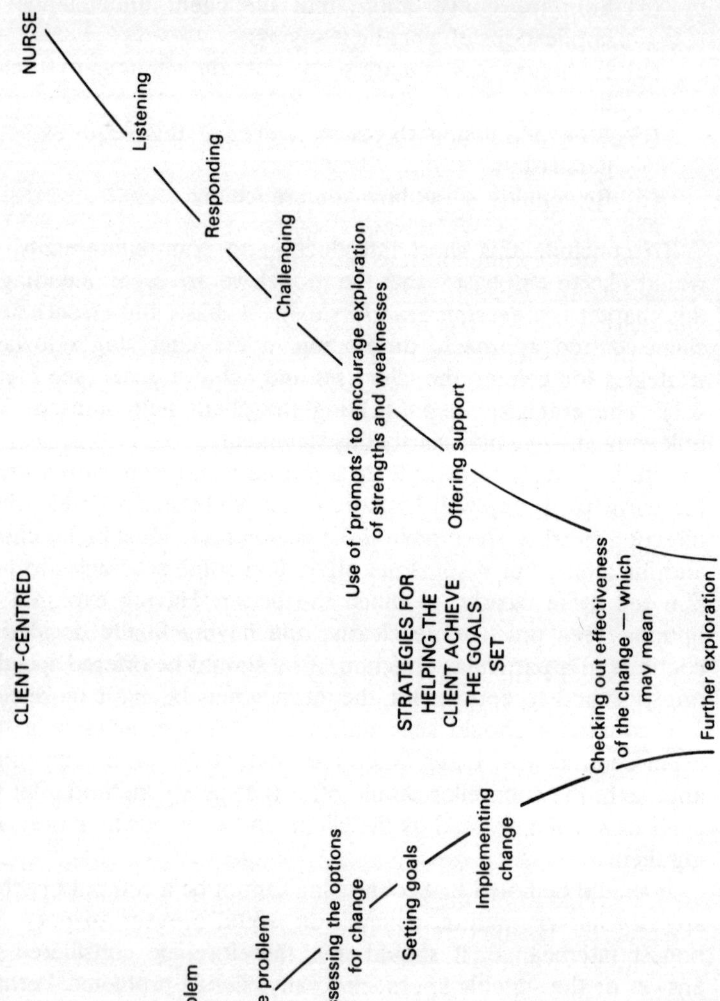

Figure 2.1: Illustrating the Developmental Style of this Counselling Model

effectively transmitted by the slightest gesture or other movement of the body. These gestures and movements often accompany the spoken word, adding to, or even changing, the literal meaning of what is said, or they may occur in isolation. The human being is such a complex set of moving signals that it is extremely difficult to be anywhere without 'saying' something.

The impossibility of not communicating is explored in great detail in a paper by Watzlawick, Beavin and Jackson (1968). It is suggested that communication is constant and continual and non-communication is impossible. However, what is important to the counsellor is that the communication is congruent, i.e. the message sent is the message received, with little room for error or misinterpretation.

In reality, even the intention of saying nothing is still communicating something to those who choose to judge people on appearance alone. The way one walks. talks and gesticulates are all signals given within an environment comprised of people who are complex 'senders' and 'receivers'. It is the degree of complexity in this environment that determines whether or not the message sent will be the message received, or how many distortions will occur.

In order to be an effective counsellor, the nurse requires a depth of understanding that goes beyond superficial requests and information exchange. This understanding is partially gained by the nurse being sensitive to the patient's non-verbal as well as verbal message. The complexity of the individual and the environment in which we live gives rise to the possibility of misinterpreting or ignoring the non-verbal message. Within any human interaction there is potential for the expression of thoughts and feelings to be dramatically misinterpreted. This is particularly so within the caring relationship between the nurse and the psychiatric patient, mainly due to the existence of extremes experienced by the patient in psychological and physical states. The nurse who wishes to understand her patients needs to be sensitive to the meaning of their communication and must use her own non-verbal signals appropriately.

Non-verbal Sensitivity

Sensitivity to non-verbal communication requires an appreciation of the various components that create the wealth of signals we continually convey to each other throughout our lives. These components are:

(1) Face.
(2) Posture and body space.
(3) Gestures.
(4) Touch.
(5) Tone of voice.

1 Face

The human face has a great potential for an immense degree of expression, both of type and intensity, and each part of the face can be observed as a potential communicator. It is extremely difficult to speak without changing facial expression. Some messages are conveyed by nodding, shaking, frowning or simply by using eye contact, mouth and eyebrow movements. The most powerful of these signals involves the eyes. They have been called the 'windows of the soul' and can convey quite clearly the powerful emotions of aggression, fear, concern and love. Observing the state of patients' eyes alone can be very informative. Some examples include:

	Possible emotion
Redness/tearful.	Sadness.
Dull, lack of movement.	Depression.
Lack of eye contact.	Insecurity/unsure/ uncomfortable/depression.
Eye contact/staring/fixed.	Accusing.
Staring with movement.	Excitement.

If the nurse relied upon single observations, it is possible that the interpretation would be wrong, as few non-verbal signals occur in isolation. It is the additional signals that can build up the obvious picture: e.g. red and tearful eyes can be symptomatic of happiness, but the accompanying behaviours confirm the picture of sadness: lack of body movement, head stooped, drooping mouth and speaking in monosyllables with a dull tone.

2 Posture and Body Space

Posture alone can convey certain emotions and attitudes. Try matching the following stick diagrams to the list of terms given:

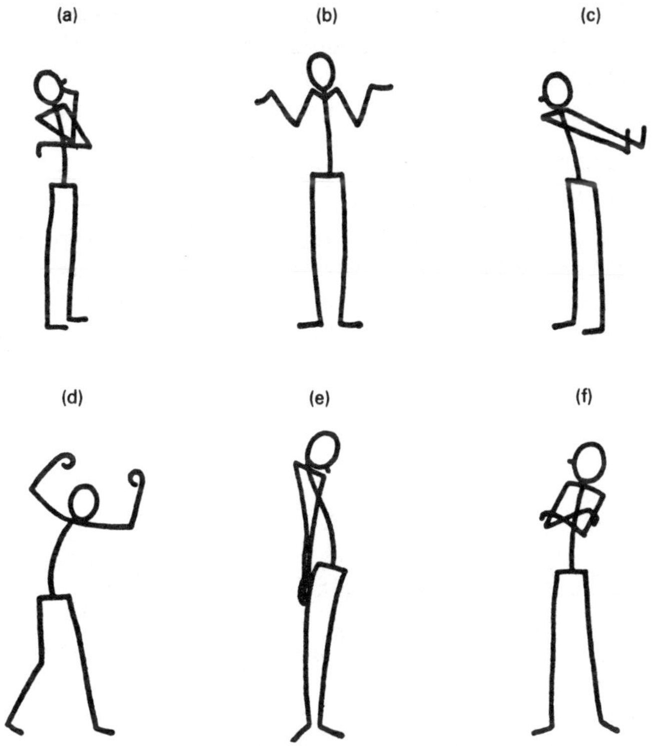

rejecting / dominating / puzzled / shy / angry / indifferent

(From Argyle, 1975).

The distinct positioning of the body, arms and legs seems to be universal for expressing certain emotions and attitudes. Observing the posture of patients could indicate expressions of mood, e.g.

leaning forward head bowed legs and arms closed inwards	could be indicating depression
tense, rocking and generally rigid	anxiety
bizarre, agitated movements	possible reaction to delusions of hallucinations.

Posture alone does not allow an accurate perception of the

patient's feelings. Confirmation of the meaning of any communication from the patient arises out of taking note of all nonverbal signals. Probably the most significant aspect of observing a patient's posture is related to postural change during an interaction. These changes are frequently quite subtle and often occur either by the patient moving towards the nurse or turning away. Moving towards the nurse could indicate that the patient accepts the nurse and is ready to disclose, especially if this approach is made in a relaxed manner. However, if the patient turns or leans away, it could indicate that he is not prepared for the interaction or that he feels uncomfortable talking about the topic in question. If the nurse is sensitive to this, she can act appropriately. If, however, she is not aware of what the patient is communicating, she may inadvertently persist in pursuing an interaction that is one-sided and subsequently spoil her chances of the relationship developing in a therapeutic manner.

Not only is it important to be sensitive to how the body is positioned, but also where it is positioned, especially in relation to others. People, like many animals, seem to have a desire for personal territory or personal space. The behaviour of people on a crowded beach illustrates this, where they mark our 'their' space with towels, deck chairs and windscreens, positioning them in a situation mutually acceptable to all concerned considering the space available. Invasion of this space causes anxiety and discomfort. The same principles apply in a crowded ward, but this time the patient has his locker and a few personal effects instead of beach equipment. A major difference between these two situations is that the patient in the ward experiences many infringements of his space, either by another patient or a nurse who is insensitive to his need. The nurse may sit close to the patient on his bed, or 'barge' into the bathroom, or lean forward with enthusiasm during an interaction. If these situations occur without mutual respect for each other's personal space, withdrawal, defensiveness and resentment could be the response of the patient. It is therefore necessary to avoid taking the nurse/patient relationship for granted and to approach the patient with respect and sensitivity.

3 Gestures

Observation and subsequent sensitivity to hand, head and body movements can be useful aids to assessing the patient's emotional state. A clear example of this is ceaseless hand-wringing or fidgeting observed in anxiety, or the clenched fist seem in anger and tension. Many of the conventional gestures are used in everyday life by all, e.g.

head nod/shake	agree/not agree
shaking fist	anger
rubbing palms	anticipation
beckon	come
extended hand	invitation
shrugging shoulders	do not know/disinterested.

Some long-term patients, due to the course of their illness, will use a gesture rather than the spoken word. The pointing finger, the banging of furniture, the broken cup, the persistent pacing up and down or the tightly folded arms can all be observed as gestures. It is the sensitivity to these within the context of knowing the patient that creates the possibility of the nurse approaching the situation appropriately and consequently increasing the likelihood of understanding the gesture and the reasons for it.

4 Touch

This is probably one of the most primitive and one of the most powerful forms of communication. The amount of touch between individuals varies with culture and type of relationship. Touch is often used in extreme emotional states such as love, anger or distress. On the one hand it can be soothing and reassuring, but, on the other, it can be threatening. It is probably more appropriate to talk about sensitivity to the *non-use* of touch, as people in our society are generally quite inhibited about touching each other. This facet of our culture seems to be accentuated amongst psychiatric patients, making it essential for the nurse to respect and appreciate the patient's readiness to accept, or not accept, various forms of touch. This is especially so when attempting to communicate with patients who may be suspicious or paranoid, for they tend to, on occasions, misinterpret physical contact and may perceive what was intended to be a reassuring touch as one that is threatening, consequently putting the success of the relationship at risk.

Nurses are expected to touch any part of the patient's body, if necessary, and the nurse should therefore appreciate that some people react to touch with anxiety, discomfort and defensiveness, because it becomes an intrusion upon something very private. This appreciation can be attained by examining your own feelings about being touched. These feelings will depend upon how and where you are touched and in what circumstances. Generally, the closer the relationship, the more bodily contact there is. So how much bodily contact is acceptable to patients? Obviously, during physical care of patients the amount of contact given is that directly concerned with the procedure. However, during counselling, the general principle is to use that which comes spontaneously and naturally, e.g. the reassuring hand on or round the shoulder and the holding of hands are frequently used for a variety of reasons, and are very effective if performed in a genuine way.

5 Tone of Voice

This is included in a section on non-verbal communication because how something is said is as important as the literal meaning of the word. In order to receive the spoken word accurately, the nurse must listen to the way something is said as well as the literal meaning of the words spoken. It is possible to perceive how someone is feeling by the way they speak: the tone, the speed, pitch and intensity of the voice are all factors that influence the spoken word. While listening to the patient, it is important to be sensitive to his tone of voice in order to detect true and often hidden feelings, thus confirming or even contradicting the verbal communication. Some psychiatric illnesses include symptoms of thought disorder which cause patients problems in verbal communication. In these situations, listening to the tone and theme rather than the actual content is probably of more value in determining what the patient is trying to say. When listening to a patient, the subtle changes in the tone can often give the nurse an additional clue to how the patient is feeling. If this observation is linked to other aspects of non-verbal communication, while also listening to the content, there is a likelihood of the nurse achieving empathy.

It is important that the nurse focuses upon the whole picture rather than the spoken word alone. One major reason for this is that non-verbal communication can contradict the verbal message, e.g. the patient who responds to the question 'How are you today?'

Verbal reply: 'OK, not bad!'

Non-verbal reply: at the same time as his verbal reply, he shakes

his head, shrugs his shoulders and lifts his hand. A possible interpretation of this could be:
shaking head: 'I'm not all right.'
shrugging shoulders: 'I'm not sure.'
lifting hand: 'Can you help?'

The detailed analysis of this reply is not important. What is important is the nurse's sensitivity to the patient's reply, 'not bad'. Many patients use very little non-verbal expression, particularly the depressed and the long-term dependent patients, and when they do, the changes in expression are subtle, and psychiatric nurses need to be aware of these changes. 'These expressions last about one fifth second and can be seen on slow motion film and by mental nurses but may be missed by many others' (Argyle, 1975).

Individuals do not consciously control every body movement. Many of the gestures that are made are subconscious reactions to thoughts and feelings.

Non-verbal Attending

Not only is it essential to be sensitive to the patient's non-verbal communication, but sensitivity to and awareness of your own body signals is also vital. One major reason for this is that certain psychiatric illnesses are manifested in such a way that the patient may be oversensitive to, or misinterpret, any non-verbal communication. An example of this can be seen in the person experiencing persecutory ideas, who, seeing two nurses talking and gesticulating to each other in the corner, interprets it as referring to him, and rushes up to them shouting abuse and threats. A general awareness of the fact that you are emitting signals continuously and that they may be interpreted from different perspectives may help when nursing this type of patient. However, general awareness is not enough, and nurses must be able to use non-verbal communication effectively within the helping relationship. The appropriate use of non-verbal communication is what we mean by non-verbal attending. Using your body language appropriately in a helping relationship will facilitate the patient's trust and confidence in you. The use of tone of voice, eye contact, touch, facial expression and posture can convey to the patient the qualities of genuineness and warmth.

Attending to the patient in a physical way is saying, 'I'm interested, and listening,' thus forming the basis of a relationship whereby the patient can perceive the nurse as someone who will accept what he has to say, in a non-judgemental manner. Physical attending refers to orientating yourself towards the patient. Egan (1982) summarises this by using the acronym SOLER:

S — facing the patient *'squarely'* as opposed to turning away from the patient is usually considered a posture of involvement.

O — adopting an '*open*' posture as opposed to a closed one. Crossed arms and legs can be a sign of defensiveness and unwillingness to give or receive.

L — *'leaning'* towards the patient usually conveys interest and willingness to be involved. Contrast this with leaning back; here the posture could be interpreted as boredom, at its extreme 'sleep'.

E — maintain appropriate '*eye contact*'. It can be seen when observing people in intense conversation that eye contact is established most of the time. Avoidance of eye contact could signify insecurity, defensiveness and lack of confidence, all of which are non-productive for the nurse as a counsellor. The nurse should be aware that constant unwavering eye contact, i.e. staring, can be interpreted by the patient as threatening. Looking away from the patient occasionally is natural and quite acceptable, but if you catch yourself looking away frequently, this may have something to do with *your* feelings rather than the patient's.

R — *'relax'* within any given therapeutic relationship and many of the behaviours described will come naturally. It also diminishes the likelihood of your fidgeting, which can be distracting for the patient, and often your nervousness will reflect on to the patient, which is hardly conducive to relaxed and thoughtful communication.

This description of appropriate non-verbal behaviour is only a guideline, and should not be viewed as a rigid formula for non-verbal attending. However, it would be unfortunate if the nurse's internal state of warmth and genuineness was contradicted by the nurse's non-verbal communication, causing initial difficulties in the relationship. So it may be useful for the nurse to look at herself and her approach, and ask herself whether, when listening to the patient, she is communicating non-verbally — 'I'm interested' and 'I'm with you.'

The importance of non-verbal attending can be appreciated when you consider that it not only conveys to the patient that you are interested and are listening effectively, but that it also conveys the qualities of warmth and genuineness. Smiling and nodding appropriately, moving in a relaxed and natural way and using touch naturally and spontaneously are all extremely effective. It often enables the patient to relax and feel secure, thus increasing the likelihood of him exploring his problems effectively within a relationship based on trust and confidence.

Non-verbal Responding

Using non-verbal communication can be as effective as a verbal reply if used appropriately. Thus the non-verbal response not only shows the patient that the nurse is listening, but also that the nurse is responding, e.g.

Non-verbal response	*Possible verbal equivalent*
Head nod	'Go on, I understand.'
Smile appropriately	'You're safe, I accept what you are saying.'
Raised eyebrow	'That's particularly interesting.'
Frown	'I'm not sure what you're saying.'
Touch	'Reassure, console, accept.'

You can tell from the tone of voice alone whether a person is 'warm' and accepting, or 'cold' and judgemental. A calm, non-threatening, clear tone of voice will usually have a positive effect on the relationship, as opposed to a harsh, abrupt, loud response.

One non-verbal response that can be considered in this context is the use of silence. This can be very positive if the timing and length are judged appropriately and if it is patient-centred rather than nurse-centred. By this we mean that the silences should be natural ones based on the patient's thought processes, giving him time to think, as opposed to being based on the nurse's need for time to think of something to say, or her anxiety to say something.

The nurse should never feel threatened by a silence. She should be sensitive to the feelings of the patient during silences, judging whether it would be advantageous or not to the patient for her to break the silence and continue the verbal exchange.

It is not uncommon for learners, having studied non-verbal communication, to feel awkward and self-conscious during the initial stages of learning these skills. The question often arises: 'How can I be genuine when I am purposefully engineering my body signals to a position I would not normally adopt? The answer is simply that genuineness is an attitude, which is held firmly and not contradicted by effective use of non-verbal communication. The awkwardness and self-consciousness are natural responses experienced by anyone who sets out to master new skills. Eventually once your awareness of your own non-verbal communication is achieved, it will be possible to correct any negative use. Progress is made from there to using appropriate non-verbal communication naturally, spontaneously and effectively. By studying non-verbal communication, you can increase your awareness of yourself in order to be sensitive to your own and your patient's 'messages' and their subsequent exchange. It is then more likely that the patient will be given every opportunity to express himself and the nurse will have every likelihood of hearing what has been said, *accurately*.

Exploratory Responding

Throughout the counselling process, it is imperative that the nurse '*listens*'. This means not only passively sitting and responding with appropriate non-verbal communication, but also actively listening, i.e. showing the patient that you understand, by your verbal as well as your non-verbal responses. These responses are extremely important, particularly in the initial stages of a relationship, for it is the nurse's ability to empathise with the patient that facilitates the building of trust and confidence, establishing a sound foundation for counselling. The importance of these 'initial responding skills' becomes clear when you consider that this is a very early stage in the helping relationship: the problem or problems have yet to be identified. It is through your use of these skills that the patient can 'explore' his feelings, behaviour and circumstances so that he can see his problems clearly. It is vital, therefore, that the exploratory responding stage is totally patient-centred (p. 24). The skills required at this stage are:

Paraphrasing.
Reflecting.
Clarifying.
Summarising.

Paraphrasing

This involves listening to what the patient says and putting the essential meaning into other words, which are then repeated back to the patient without adding or subtracting anything.

In essence, what this is actually doing is acting as a 'sounding board'. By paraphrasing, the nurse shows the patient that she is listening accurately, and helps the patient hear what he has just said, thus allowing for further thought on the subject if necessary. Repeating the essential meaning back to the patient in a '*tentative*' way allows an element of inaccuracy to be acceptable, and permits the patient to correct the nurse's paraphrased response.

Patient. I find it difficult to concentrate, I'm not sure whether it is the ward, patients or just the way I'm feeling.
Nurse. So your concentration difficulties could be due to several factors or just the way you're feeling at the moment.

This single paraphrase is virtually word for word what the patient said. This is acceptable, especially early on in the relationship. It is important to earn the patient's trust and confidence by showing him that you are listening accurately. However, there are different ways of paraphrasing and, depending upon the nurse's understanding of the patient's position, different ways of paraphrasing would be more or less appropriate. From this last patient's statement, it could be that the nurse detects from the patient's emphasis and non-verbal communication that his feelings are of more, or equal, importance than his stated 'difficulty in concentration'. The repeating or parroting of a word or phrase would allow the patient to expand upon this as appropriate. The nurse could reply in a tentative, questioning way: 'Just the way you're feeling?' This allows the patient to think about the way he feels in order to explore this area if it is important to him at the time. This shows that even early on in the counselling process a paraphrase can be useful in allowing the patient to explore his own feelings, encouraging him to talk freely and expand upon what is important to him.

Other illustrations of paraphrasing:

Patient. I can't stand the way my wife continually harasses me, it makes me so angry.
Nurse. Angry?

Here the nurse repeats just one single word on the basis that she feels this is the area that is probably important to the patient. As it is repeated in a tentative way, it is a 'safe' paraphrase. On the other hand the nurse may paraphrase thus:

Nurse. Harass you?

This would probably allow the counselling to take the direction of exploring his wife's behaviour. This is only acceptable if it is important to the patient to explore this area. Note that this is determined by the patient's choice to pursue this theme. However, you must bear in mind that throughout the counselling process it is the '*here and now*' and its effect on the patient that is the crucial issue when counselling.

Patient. The burden ... I can't cope with it, it seems endless, how is it going to end, what is going to become of me, is there any hope?
Nurse. You think you can't cope with this never ending burden and you're questioning the outcome of it all.

Here the paraphrase involves repeating back to the patient the essence of what he has just said. This is particularly useful in cases where a patient's thoughts are somewhat clouded or confused by extremes of emotion such as anxiety or depression.

Paraphrasing is not just mechanical repetition of what the patient has said, but is the first stage of showing actively that you understand what he has said. This understanding, so far, has focused upon paraphrasing experiences, behaviours and insights, derived from what the patient has stated. However, within any circumstances or behaviour there exist feelings which may not be overtly stated, but are nevertheless in existence. Detection and communication of patients' implicit and explicit emotions are called 'reflecting'.

Reflecting

In order for you to understand the thoughts, attitudes and behaviour of a patient, you must also understand how he feels. Because of the very personal nature of feelings, reflecting is essential in order to achieve mutual understanding of the expressed feeling. What you mean by sad, happy or fearful may be completely different from the meaning for another person. This partly depends upon the context in which these feelings are experienced, and how they are expressed at the time. Reflecting allows the nurse and patient to choose a mutually acceptable 'feeling term' that best conveys the emotion felt at the time (see Table 2.1), e.g.

Nurse. You feel resentful, then, towards your wife?
Patient. Not exactly, it's more that I am disappointed with her.

Here the nurse has detected from what the patient has said a feeling of resentment, and reflected this '*in a tentative way*'. This allowed the patient to focus upon his feelings, helping him look at the situation more clearly and helping the nurse to understand further how the patient feels. Another example is:

Patient. The trouble with me is that every time something goes wrong, I have to resort to the bottle. It just seems that I can't see any alternative. I wonder if it is just me or the situation I find myself in.

We suggest that you try to explain the feelings this patient is expressing. From the written word only, it is difficult and rather presumptuous to do so because there are no accompanying non-verbal clues. However, the feelings we think that this patient may be expressing are related to frustration and confusion. He seems frustrated because of his losing battle against alcohol and he is confused about the cause of his problem. Whether we are right or wrong does not matter; what is important is to reflect back these observations to the patient so that he can think about what he has said, focus upon his feelings and confirm or deny the accuracy of the reflection, e.g.

Table 2.1: Feeling Vocabulary

POSITIVE FEELINGS		
Mild	**Moderate**	**Strong**
relaxed	content	at peace
at ease	carefree	serene
comfortable	secure	fulfilled
untroubled	safe	
patient	independent	determined
smart	intelligent	strong
	capable	sure
	worthy	brilliant
regarded	appealing	affirmed
encouraged	popular	loved
	attractive	adored
	wanted	worshipped
	approved	idolised
sensitive	concerned	pity
sympathetic	protective	
	tender	
regard	trust	admiration
	appreciation	worship
	respect	adoration
	gratefulness	awe
friendly	affectionate	loving
benevolent	caring	in love
warm	like	infatuation
interested	turned on	enchantment
tempted	desirous	ardour
alert	excited	amazed
wide awake	keen	vibrant
aroused	eager	alive
	brave	daring
optimistic	anticipating	zealous
hopeful	enthusiastic	inspired
		intoxicated
good	great	fantastic
amused	jolly	stupendous
pleased	glad	delighted
	happy	elated
NEGATIVE FEELINGS		
Mild	**Moderate**	**Strong**
indifferent	listless	sick
resigned	bored	hopeless
lethargic	apathetic	futile
tired	weak	impotent
fatigued	worn out	exhausted
timid	inhibited	paralysed

shy bashful self-conscious	inadequate ineffectual stuck	useless helpless trapped
disturbed puzzled perplexed	troubled baffled confused mixed up	threatened shocked bewildered horrified
nervous unsure apprehensive	edgy tense worried afraid	in dread terrified petrified frantic
suspicious wary cynical sullen	jealous envious bitter spiteful resentful vengeful	contemptuous disdainful scornful disgusted hatred
moody unhappy disappointed discontented dissatisfied	upset depressed gloomy dismal dejected	crushed destroyed miserable awful disconsolate
unpopular regretful embarrassed dependent	unloved alienated hurt rejected	ashamed worthless hated humiliated
impatient irritated annoyed	indignant angry vexed	outraged furious infuriated

Source: Gerard Egan, *Training the Skilled Helper* (Brooks/Cole, Monterey, California, 1982), Appendix G, pp. 215-18.

Nurse (reflects). So you feel frustrated because of your inability to cope with crises without having to resort to drink.

or It seems that you're in a dilemma and maybe feel confused because you're not sure what the reasons are for your drink problem.

In both these replies the nurse reflects back circumstances that the patient has already stated, and the feelings that he appears to be expressing. Both may be effective in allowing the patient to explore further the area that is particularly important to him. Where the feelings of confusion are more important than the feelings of frustration, the first response may delay the counselling process, as the patient may spend time talking about something that is not the crucial issue, whereas the second response would be a more accurate reflection. The safest reply in this situation, where several feelings have been expressed in one phrase, is to reflect those feelings back to the patient and allow *him* to choose which to elaborate or comment upon, e.g.

Nurse. So you're feeling frustrated because you are unable to cope with crises without drink and confused because you're not sure what the reasons are for your drink problems.

This allows the patient to choose in which direction the counselling should go. One possible direction this may take is:

Patient. That's right. Maybe my frustrations will be reduced if I could understand how I find myself in these situations in the first place.
Nurse. Situations?
Patient. Yes: the situation of stress, the marriage, the job, the kids, it all adds up and drinking my problem away seems to have caused another problem.
Nurse. So your drinking problem seems to be just one on top of many others.

From this short dialogue, it can be seen how the simple paraphrase and the reflecting back of feelings allow the patient to explore his own world in order to achieve and communicate insight into his own problems. It enables the nurse to understand accurately not only the patient's situation, but how he *feels* about it. This accurate understanding is part of what we mean by *empathy* (p. 27). An empathic response combines the skills of paraphrasing and reflecting as seen in the italicised response of the nurse to the patient with a drink problem. It involves the element of *feelings* and the *possible reasons* for those feelings.

In order to practise the skills of paraphrasing and reflecting effectively, thus achieving empathy, they need to be closely related to the quality of 'unconditional positive regard' (p. 25). If this is not present within the nurse, listening will be inaccurate due to the fact that the nurse's own feelings and attitudes are serious 'barriers'.

Clarifying

There are times when listening to what a patient is saying is difficult because of all the detailed complications of feelings and circumstances conveyed to the nurse, often in one uninterrupted sentence. In this situation and in any other circumstances where confusion may occur, the nurse must convey her genuineness, be honest, and admit that she is confused.

Patient. We used to understand each other, have a respect for each other, now we don't seem to talk to each other. It doesn't seem fair that she should punish me like this.

Nurse. I'm not quite sure what you're saying. You seem to be saying there's no communication between you and also that she is punishing you.

This admission by the nurse allows the patient to focus back on what he has said in order to communicate more accurately, thus helping not only the nurse's understanding, but the patient's as well. The example given was a specific request to clarify something that was ambiguous. Often a patient will say several things in an attempt to explain the situation and, in doing so, will convey quite conflicting experiences.

Patient. I can't understand it, what happened just amazes me, it was fantastic yet it's so soul destroying that the stimulation and satisfaction I achieved at the time barely seem worth it now.

Nurse. Am I right in saying that the experience was a positive one at the time, but now you're wondering whether it was worth it?

It can be seen from the last two examples that clarifying can be just an extension of paraphrasing and reflecting. The main difference is that the nurse picks out the part that is confusing and asks directly whether her understanding is correct. This portrayal of honesty and subsequent genuineness will often be reciprocated by the patient. If the nurse happens to say anything that he finds confusing, because the nurse has previously admitted difficulties in initially understanding, the patient will also find it easier to admit confusion.

Another use of clarification occurs when a patient states several factors that at the time seem equally important to him.

Patient. It's not just the financial aspects that are involved, I mean, I can't ignore the marriage, the kids, and my involvement with this other man, they are all part of it, not to mention me being here.

Nurse. You have mentioned many factors that are affecting you at this present time. I'm wondering which one of these is the one that you may wish to talk about further.

Allowing the patient to choose increases the likelihood that the counselling will progress to a crucial area affecting him in the 'here and now'. On the other hand, he could choose an area that he feels safe in and is able to talk about. In this situation, further skills are required, e.g. challenging (p. 54). Notice that the nurse is not asking the patient which of the factors is most important to him. This would involve much more exploration before he could decide, as it requires him to disclose his value orientation. Thus it can be seen that the skill of clarifying gives an opportunity to correct any inaccurate understanding on the part of either the patient or the nurse.

Summarising

This involves bringing together the main issues and feelings that the patient has conveyed to the nurse so far. It is a skill that involves very accurate listening and empathy, for it could have a negative effect on the counselling process if, in her summary, the nurse were to leave out what the patient thought was a major issue. If the summary is accurate, it conveys to the patient that the nurse understands. Summarising to convey understanding is one reason why it is an extremely useful skill to use at the beginning and end of any counselling session. It helps form a basis on which to proceed at the beginning of any session, it checks progress and avoids the temptation to go round in circles. At the end of any session it acts as a stopping point, but one that can be picked up next time. In doing this it often acts as a form of reassurance to the patient, that the nurse understands, progress has been made and that it will be picked up again later. It is useful not only at the end or beginning of a session, but also during, especially when there is a temptation to 'back track' or dwell on certain issues that have already been covered. Summarising during counselling often helps to focus upon scattered thoughts and feelings. It is often useful here to ask the patient whether he is able to say 'where we have got so far'. This involves the patient checking back on his thoughts, feelings and behaviours and communicating the crucial facts to the nurse, which can be very useful in a situation where the nurse suspects that the patient is having difficulty in bringing together his feelings and circumstances and may *too* readily accept the nurse's summary. Asking the patient to summarise too often, however, may reduce the nurse's credibility to demonstrate the skill in question, so must not be used too frequently.

'Let me see if I've got this right so far' summarising can be a useful skill at the beginning, during and after a counselling session. It involves bringing together ideas and feelings in order to focus upon scattered issues or to check progress so far. In doing this it checks understanding and often acts as a form of reassurance: 'Would you say that sums it up?' or 'Have I left anything out?'

Notice again the tentative statement is stressed: 'Have I got this right?' 'Is there anything else?' This is very important in order for the counselling at this stage to remain 'patient-centred', i.e. the counselling does not follow the direction of the nurse's ideas, but purely the patient's perspective. It says to the patient also that 'I am trying to listen and I accept that it is possible for me to leave something out or get something wrong.'

After a summary, especially during or at the beginning of a counselling session, a reminder of the helping contract established can be very useful. This is often stated in terms of:

Nurse. Where do you see us progressing from here?

Reader. Well, it may be useful for me to look at some of the 'key concepts' involved with this chapter so far (see p. 68 — concepts 1-8).

Progressive Responding

The preliminary skills previously described, and the development of the necessary qualities discussed in the introduction, combine to ensure that the nurse is able to create a closeness, a rapport, an empathic relationship. When this is achieved, the nurse may be able to help the patient to find solutions to his problems.

Progressive responding is the final stage of our counselling model. The previous skills of exploratory responding should have helped the patient begin to understand what problems he may have and generally to see himself much more clearly. Now it is necessary for the nurse to help 'change' occur. It is essential to understand that these skills should not be used *until* an empathic relationship has been developed, or the nurse may be in grave danger of advising, directing or prescribing for the patient from her own perspectives.

The imaginative reader may have already discovered the limitations of the skills so far. They are, of course, extremely potent for engendering self-awareness, and this in itself may be all that is necessary to stimulate change. Some patients may become aware of themselves, and decide that they want to change, but are unable to find effective methods of doing so. Some patients may have developed such sophisticated defences that, although they see problems in their situation, they are unable to connect them with themselves and continue to disown responsibility for them. In this type of situation, the nurse who is able to use only preliminary skills may begin to feel frustrated as the relationship of trust and self-awareness becomes deeper and greater, but without seeming to resolve any of the difficulties.

It is our belief that in order to move forward from this situation, to facilitate change in patients that seem entrenched in their helplessness, and in order to effectively help, more advanced skills may be needed. These are the skills of problem solving from a client-centred approach.

It is our contention that problem solving from the patient's frame of reference is chiefly facilitated by the use of skilled and effective *challenging*.

Challenging

What is Challenging?

Connor, Dexter and Wash (1984) had this to say about it:

> In order to identify problems, the nurse may need to helpfully challenge the patient. Challenging is one of the most important skills used when responding, and particularly at this stage of problem identification.
>
> Sometimes the nurse will notice that there are certain discrepancies in what the patient is saying. These need to be challenged. The patient may seem to be evading the problem, perhaps by blaming other people for his predicament. If this is

reflected back to the patient in a positive way it will help him to challenge himself about the way he is responding to his own situation.

Challenging is a very powerful way of helping people, but because of its power it can be either helpful or harmful. Attempts at trying to shock patients into changing their attitudes may have the negative result of anger and resentment.

Good challenging helps the patient to think carefully and positively and it often helps the patient to see exactly where he wants to make changes in his life.

Sometimes, very sensitive areas of thoughts, feeling or behaviour, require great courage from the patient. In such situations, the patient sometimes finds it easier to escape from reality. It is the responsibility of the nurse to be sensitive to this and to encourage the patient to face his problems rather than turn away from them. Challenging can re-motivate the patient, persuade him not to give up, and help him find what strengths he needs in order to face a problem.

The skill of challenging is the skill of giving honest feedback to a patient in a sensitive way, with the intention of introducing new ideas or new ways of looking at a situation. An effective nurse tries to enable the patient to begin to challenge himself in a way that encourages positive and realistic goals to be set before trying to change specific behaviour.

The authors go on to suggest that challenges can be graded from very good challenge to bad negative challenge, with consequent feelings engendered.

Type of challenge	*Effect on patient*
(1) Very good challenge	Patient feels enlightened.
(2) Good challenge.	Thought-provoking.
(3) Average challenge.	Confused.
(4) Negative challenge.	Resentful.
(5) Bad negative challenge.	Very resentful.

Case Illustration

Maggie is talking to a nurse about her problems related to alcohol. The dialogue here may help you to see how challenging may help the patient fulfil the prerequisites of problem solving (the initial steps).

Maggie. There doesn't seem much point staying sober around here, nobody listens to me until I'm drunk – then at least I get an injection to help me calm down.

Nurse (challenges discrepancy and the genuineness of the remark). You say staying sober is pointless as no one listens to you unless you're drunk (paraphrase) and yet you also seem to be saying that when you're drunk you become excited and you need calming down with an injection (reflection and paraphrase). I'm a bit confused about this, are you saying the drink makes you excited, and you want to be calm, or am I right in suspecting what you really mean is you think no one listens to you? (clarification)

This example illustrates that the skilled nurse may be able to use various skills as a response, all showing empathy, but each one having a different depth, and subsequently the patient's reaction may differ accordingly. It seeks to challenge the patient to look more closely at what she means.

The next example illustrates the nurse attempting to enable Maggie to identify the *real* or main problem by challenging. Note the contrasting style of challenging and decide which one is the most helpful.

Maggie. My husband is having an affair, I know he is, he's a rat, no wonder I drink such a lot.

Nurse. It's nothing to do with your husband, so maybe he *is* being unfaithful, perhaps he's fed up with living with a drunk. If you stopped drinking maybe he'd be more faithful.

or (Carefully, tentatively and with genuine puzzlement) You appear to be very angry with your husband, but I'm wondering exactly how much you can blame *him* for what's happening to *you*?

We hope it can be seen in the second example that the nurse allows the patient to challenge *herself* about the real problem. The first nurse can only be presumptive, she cannot know which event came first, neither should she assume the drinking is the main problem. The second nurse allows a more open-ended challenge, which may result in the patient not only looking closely at which of her own statements contains the major problems, but also which is her fault or problem which can then be *owned* and dealt with effectively.

Staying for a while with Maggie's problem, it may be helpful to see that once the problem is identified and owned, it can be expressed more clearly and the next step attempted, i.e. 'I see what you mean, my problem is that I deal with my feelings about my husband by drinking, but what can I do to stop him behaving like he does?'

Nurse. I think you are now saying it's your feelings that are the main problem, but I still sense you are planning on trying to change your husband. I wonder if that's very realistic, for instance, if your husband heard you say that what would he say?

Maggie. Well, he'd probably say it's my life and I'm going to enjoy it, if that makes you unhappy, I'm sorry but I have to be me.

Nurse. I'm wondering if 'stopping him behaving like he does' is very realistic, then?

Maggie. But what else can I do?

Nurse. Perhaps you could try to imagine how you would like to see yourself in three months' time as realistically as possible, and work towards that in small steps.

Although this appears to be directive, in fact the nurse is suggesting a structure, almost like offering a journey rather than prescribing a destination. From this position the nurse can help structure the journey but should not push in any particular direction. For instance, the nurse may challenge the patient when his goals are vague and unspecific, i.e. 'I want to be better.' The nurse is correct to challenge also when the patient is being unrealistic, or the methods chosen are ineffective or inappropriate. Care should be taken not to direct but to challenge in a way that allows time for the patient to reflect carefully. These following examples of challenges, we believe, emphasise this point:

Patient not owning problem and being vague

Patient. Life has really kicked me around.

Nurse challenge. You seem to be saying you have no control over 'life'. Perhaps we ought to talk specifically about what it is in life that kicks you around.

Patient has unrealistic goals

Maggie. I'm going to discharge myself today, go out and get myself a job.

Nurse. It's great to see you so energetic, Maggie. Have you any specific ideas about this job?

Patient may have chosen ineffective or inappropriate methods to reach her goal

Maggie. I'm sick of feeling so frustrated and angry with him, I'm just going to slap him in the face when he visits tonight.

Nurse. You feel very angry because you believe him to be the root of your frustration. Are you saying hitting him will help you reach your goals?

Maggie. I'll just kill myself.

Nurse. Killing yourself may be a solution to this particular frustration, but how is that going to help you reach the goal we discussed earlier?

Principal Skills of Challenging

1. Summarising. This skill centres around the counsellor's ability to pick out common themes, recurring issues, and feed them back in an accurate, non-judgemental way. Elucidating feelings associated with each idea and without adding or subtracting material may enable the client to see contradictory ideas and emotions and challenge himself to sort these out.

2. Confrontation. This is an invitation for the patient to confront himself with discrepancies he holds within himself. For example, he says he wants to give up drinking but he hides alcohol in his locker, or states, 'I get bad chest infections but I continue to smoke.' The nurse here simply feeds back this information in one sentence, when previously it was separated by other material. It is, however, much better if strengths are challenged rather than weakenesses, i.e. 'You have told me how difficult life is for you — you are unemployed, your wife has left you, you are in financial difficulties — and yet you are still able to smile about it. I think you have many untapped resources if only you could reach them.'

Games and smokescreens may need to be confronted, as these are often used by patients to keep the roundabout turning and prevent the nurse helping. When the climate of the relationship is secure, these games and smokescreens are easy to confront, i.e. 'I'm really trying to understand how you are feeling, but it seems to me that every time you talk to me about your mother you become uncomfortable and change the subject.' 'You seem to feel tired or bored with these sessions whenever I sense we're really starting to get somewhere.' 'I hear you saying something you feel very uncomfortable with, but at that point you make a joke and laugh, I'm not really sure I understand you.'

3. *Immediacy.* This skill is to do with having an appreciation of what is happening between nurse and patient at times throughout interactions, and is characterised by nurse statements such as 'I sense you are feeling disappointed with me.' 'I seem to have upset you when I said that.' 'You're annoyed because I got that wrong,' and by patients' statements such as 'I don't think I really meant that. I think I said it because I thought you'd like it.' 'I'm having problems concentrating because I want to tell you how much I appreciate you trying to help me.'

These potentially highly emotional interactions need to be explored before the business of counselling can continue. They require to be confronted by both parties so that purposeful client-centred therapy can continue.

4. *Data-based hunches.* These are made from a position of deep understanding of the patient and, as suggested, are based on data. They begin with an empathic response such as 'You seem to be feeling puzzled about that' and continue with the hunch 'and I sense that you may be feeling angry over the way you've been treated'. This has to be data-based because not only may it be insulting to be considered so transparent, but without data you may be a long way from the truth. Consider this patient response to this last statement:

Patient. Why do you say angry?
Nurse. Well, because when I see that puzzled look appear I also notice you clench your fists and your lips tighten

as opposed to:

Nurse. Oh, just a lucky guess, I suppose

or more mystical:

Nurse. I just feel these things.

The response should also be tentative, as there is probably no greater sin in counselling than telling someone what they are feeling, except perhaps not allowing them to feel at all. For example:

Patient. I just can't cope, I feel terrible.
Nurse. Oh, I'm sure you can, it's not that bad.

5. *Self-disclosure.* This is useful to show the client that you too are a real authentic person with feelings and experiences. It encourages disclosure from the client, and may as a side benefit offer new perspectives to the client. It must not be distracting or a way of offering advice. It challenges by inviting comparisons between the counsellor and client's emotions, behaviours and coping strategies.

Patient. I feel so hurt and rejected since my husband divorced me. I really don't know what to do.
Nurse. Listening to you say that makes me think back to my divorce; I felt a little like that, but mostly I was very angry, it eventually occurred to me that being angry wasn't very constructive. Do you see yourself in any of this?

Unacceptable self-disclosure
Nurse. You should worry, if you had my overdraft, you really would be in trouble

or

Nurse. Yes, my husband left me last year, he was a nice man and I want to cry when I think about it

or

Nurse. What a coincidence, I'm ... a ... as well.

The latter examples are not appropriate because, even if honest, they are too distracting, turning the counsellor into the client, and really reducing the proceedings to mutual sympathy and destroying the counsellor's credibility. After all, how can a patient put trust in someone who's in a worse mess than themselves?

6. *Information giving.* Finally, the skill of giving information to

patients is one with which most nurses are familiar. It is, however, important to give information tactfully, clearly and at the right time.

For instance, John discloses that he is very distressed because he believes he has syphilis. He bases this belief on the fact that he has a painful sore on his penis. There are many possible responses but let us examine four typical ones.

(1) 'Don't be silly, syphilitic sores are never painful, it can't be.' Confidently reassuring, but humiliating and broke a golden rule by denying John's feelings.
(2) 'Well, why don't you go to the doctor and get it treated?' Sensible advice, but shows no empathy and only selfish regard — i.e. I don't want to know, show a doctor.
(3) 'Oh dear, how dreadful, I hope it's not. That would be difficult for you to explain to your wife.' Sympathy from the nurse's values and perception does little other than make the patient more aware of how the nurse sees the problem and may not focus upon the concerns of the patient.
(4) 'You're obviously very upset about this, John, but I'm wondering how much you know about syphilis. I believe it's not usual for sores to be painful. I sense that just worrying about it is not really helping.' This begins with an empathic response and offers information that may be useful to confront John's feelings and behaviour. The final challenge is a data-based hunch which motivates John to consider other opinions. Note that the nurse does not prescribe action but simply helps precipitate it.

Challenging Skills Rules

(1) Only challenge when an empathic bond exists, and the relationship *could* stand an unskilled challenge should things go wrong.
(2) Challenging should be an invitation for the patient to look at himself more closely, not an excuse for the nurse to attack or punish the patient.
(3) Using challenges to shock, or as a disguise for prescribing, is not skilful and will usually succeed only in creating resentment.
(4) Challenges are most effective when sandwiched between empathic responses, e.g. 'You're feeling puzzled and uncertain because you can't decide what to change in your lifestyle. → On

the other hand you've said if you continue to smoke and drink you may not have time to change. ← I see you're feeling anxious because of what I just said.'

(5) If in doubt, use an empathic response, not a challenge.

Problem Solving

It is necessary initially to look at the route to effective problem solving and the individual steps in the process. We have identified four major stages and 21 necessary steps which may help the patient find and reach his goals.

Assessment

The patient needs to:

(1) Know which are his *real* problems.
(2) See his problems as his *own*, e.g. 'My problem is my wife' is not owned.
(3) Have control of it personally, e.g. 'My death is not controllable, but the way I prepare for it is.'
(4) Be motivated towards its solution.
(5) Identify main problem and auxiliary problems.
(6) Express his problems in a specific form (rather than in vague terms).

Planning

The patient needs to:

(7) Identify the overall goal, know where he is going.
(8) Have an appreciation of steps towards the goal (subordinate goals).
(9) Be committed to reaching the goal.
(10) Feel it is his goal.
(11) Express it as a worthwhile and realistic goal.
(12) Identify what will help him, and what will hinder him reaching his goal.
(13) Have a time scale to work within, and know when it is achieved.

Implementation

The patient needs to:

(14) Understand the method of reaching the goal.
(15) Succeed by achieving one step at a time.
(16) Choose each step carefully, ensuring it is reasonable.
(17) Feel rewarded by each step.

Evaluation

The patient needs to:

(18) See what has been achieved.
(19) Know what remains to be done.
(20) Understand the changes that have taken place.
(21) Be able to assess the overall results.

To achieve these objectives throughout the stages of problem solving will require all the nurse's counselling skills, but predominantly challenging skills will be invaluable.

It is suggested by Egan (1982) that one particular method of helping people make decisions and solve problems is to consider the problems and the goals as diametrically opposite. He suggests that goals and problems can be thought of as the two extremes of a forcefield (forcefield analysis) and that the forces involved are facilitating and restraining forces. Connor, Dexter and Wash (1984) term this as hindering and helping factors. Our amalgam of this simple but useful device is shown in Figure 2.2.

Egan suggests that if the helping (facilitating) factors are strengthened, and the hindering (restraining) factors are weakened, the goal can be more easily reached. The idea essentially is that the facilitating factors are a group of resources which, when fully used, may make up a solution. The restraining factors are a group of influences, either people, places, things or behaviours, that are stumbling blocks and are counter-productive to reaching the goal.

It can be seen from Figure 2.2 that specific prompts can be used to help the patient see these ideas more clearly. After dividing helpers and hinderers into internal and external resources, the patient can be prompted with open questions: what emotions, thoughts, people, places, methods and objects will help or hinder

Figure 2.2: Helping and Hindering Factors

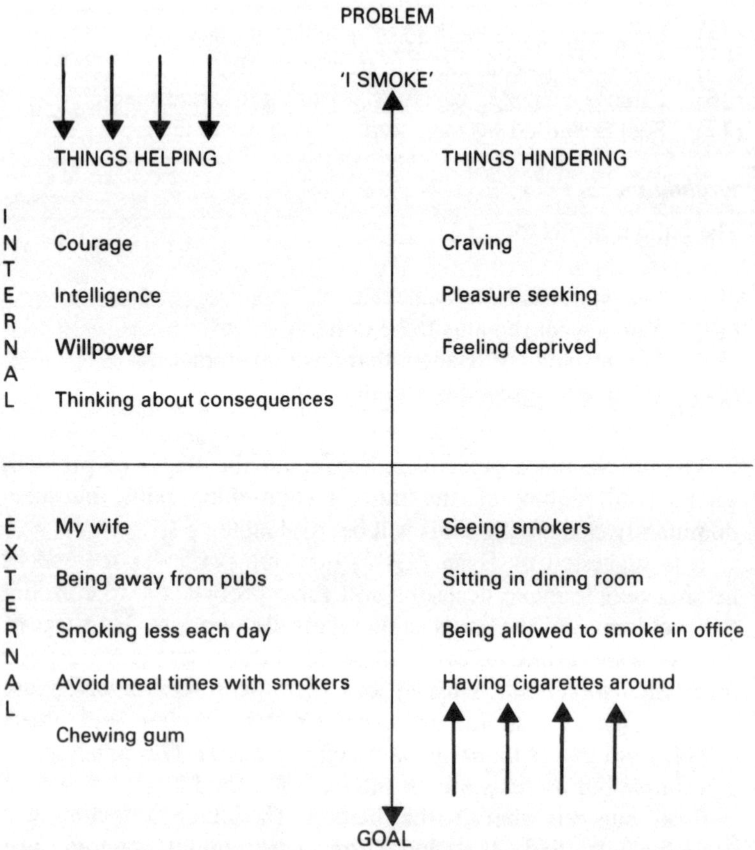

'BY NEXT MONTH I WILL SMOKE A MAXIMUM OF 5 CIGARETTES A DAY.

BY CHRISTMAS I WILL BE A NON-SMOKER.'

NB Owned

Realistic

Worth while

Specific

Achievable

Within time scale

him achieving his goal? This prompting will help the patient generate ideas. The first lists of helpful and hindering factors are not censored, challenged or in any way influenced, as these are purely the patient's total 'brainstormed' ideas, which may be inappropriate, unrealistic or just plain silly. Nevertheless, the patient should be allowed to choose freely from the list which he feels are the most appropriate, effective and reasonable — as shown in the second list.

Egan's original idea holds great promise in helping the patient explore his ideas and behaviours in an organised and structured way, and reveals obvious strategies for solving problems from the patient's own value orientation.

It is then simply a matter of helping the patient see ways in which he may weaken the hindering things and strengthen the helping influences. For example, the first hindering factor was 'craving'. If the patient is asked how many things he can think of that will weaken his craving and then selects the strategies that he thinks will work — then they probably will. Conversely, if we take the first helping factor in the external section ('my wife') and ask him to explain what strategies will potentiate his wife's influence, he will be able to see how he can elicit his wife's aid most effectively.

By looking at these influences in a detailed and structured way, the patient starts to appreciate what is going on in his life. He can at last see what has been holding him back from doing the things he has wanted to do, and finally find realistic strategies to succeed instead of continuing to fail. The skilled nurse may at this point be able to inform the patient about how behaviours are reinforced, so that he can see how his undesired behaviours have previously been fixed by rewards (see 'Behavioural Principles', p. 76). Maggie's example here would be 'I've been rewarding myself for avoiding facing my feelings — I've been drinking, which has relieved my anxieties (negative reinforcement) which has reinforced my drinking habit further, and snowballed into preventing me seeing what's really happening.' This type of insight is not only helpful from a historical perspective, but the understanding of the principle may enable her to avoid future traps. It is extremely important at this point to stress that this approach of trying to 'teach' the patient about behavioural influences in his life is *totally* different from telling him what to do behaviourally, devising behavioural strategies or analysing him. Skilled information giving is required, not prescribing behaviours for individuals. We acknowledge that this is extremely difficult to do, especially with psychotic or mentally handicapped patients. Counselling is not the panacea for all ills, and for the small number of patients who are incapable of self-direction counselling may not be the most creative approach to the solution of their problems.

Steps 18 to 21 could be considered almost self-explanatory, but using appropriate skills of challenge remains a priority. Simply because there has been an effect or a change does not mean it is cherished. An action programme devised by the patient may not have succeeded or may have simply uncovered more problems. Often reaching the final stage simply means starting again from the beginning. It has been suggested that by far the commonest reasons for not effecting a solution are these:

(1) The strategies devised by the patient have not been followed.
(2) The problem was not the real problem.
(3) The goal was not achievable, realistic or worth while.
(4) The motivation for change was insufficient.

These areas are therefore most important to challenge in evaluation or much time can be expended following plans that are destined to fail. Far better to return to basics at this point than to pursue an unhelpful direction.

To refer back to the stages of problem solving, you may now be able to reflect on how challenging may be useful in each stage.

Assessment

The patient needs to express specific, owned, real, controllable problems and sub-problems, and be committed to their solutions, e.g. 'I smoke cigarettes' (main real problem) 'because I am under stress and I am bored' (sub-problems) 'and I really wish I could stop.'

Planning

The patient needs to express a specific, owned, realistic, worthwhile, stepped and measurable goal that he is determined to reach in a set period of time, e.g. 'I will give up smoking cigarettes at a rate of one cigarette a day and I will be a non-smoker by December 12th.'

Implementation

The patient needs to examine the resources available to him, both internal and external, including people, places and things that will strengthen his strategies and help him to reach his goal. Conversely, he needs to examine the people, places and things that will hinder the process, and devise ways of weakening their effect, e.g. 'I am aware that to give up smoking I need to limit my craving, and spend less time at the pub. My wife will help me in the former, so I will spend as much time with her as possible. Being bored will increase my craving so I will endeavour to occupy myself with a new hobby.'

'I spend more time at the pub when I really fancy a drink, so I will weaken this effect by having some cans of beer at home.'

Evaluation

The patient needs to express:

'I am now a non-smoker.'
'I have succeeded in stopping smoking.'
'I like what I feel.'
'I like what I have become.'
'I am pleased.'
'Other things that have happened are ...'
'I've only partly succeeded in ...'
'I wish I could ...'
'My next step is ...'

Nurses commonly complain that patients they want to help cannot or will not be helped. It is our contention that this model of counselling skills, although by no means original, may in some way help the nurse to see new perspectives in helping. It is not our wish that the nurse should be strait-jacketed by our ideas in this chapter, but simply that they may offer an alternative approach for the care of some patients. The skilled nurse may well combine many skills she already possesses to potentiate what is presented here. We would commend this, as it is not our wish to discourage any initiative that will ultimately help your patients.

Key Concepts

(1) 'People become engaged in counselling when a person, occupying regularly or temporarily, the role of counsellor, offers and agrees explicitly to give time, attention and respect to another person, or persons, who will temporarily be in the role of the client.'

(2) An effective counsellor must have an honest intention to help, a desire to promote growth within the patient/client, and a reluctance to offer advice or judgement.

(3) An understanding and a proficient ability to perform the skills of listening, paraphrasing, reflecting, questioning, clarifying, summarising and challenging are essential.

(4) It is our view that you must earn the right to counsel others, by acquiring the skills, owning the qualities, and understanding yourself.

(5) To be effective the counsellor has to dispense with her own values, beliefs, prejudices and stereotypes, in order to accept and try to understand the other person's values, ideals and beliefs, even if these are totally opposed to her own.

(6) The qualities of empathy, warmth and genuineness are essential prerequisites to the client/counsellor relationship.

(7) By being sensitive to your own, and the client's, non-verbal behaviours, you are likely to demonstrate to the client interest and warmth, thus increasing the likelihood of enhancing the relationship.

(8) Exploration of the client's problems requires the counsellor to demonstrate understanding and the need to allow the client to express freely his thoughts, feelings and behaviours. The skills that help the client do this are paraphrasing, reflecting, clarifying and summarising.

(9) Sometimes the client finds it difficult to see his problems clearly because the realisation and acceptance of the problems may provoke some anxiety. When this occurs, challenging skills are needed to move the client forward.

(10) Once the client has identified and owned the problem, the counsellor may help the client brainstorm useful ways in which the client can set and achieve his goals.

(11) Assessment of helping and hindering factors is a useful way of looking at factors that will help and prevent the client

achieving the goal.

(12) By offering support and encouraging feedback, the counsellor can help the client evaluate the outcome of his attempt to change, thus offering an opportunity for further exploration.

Suggested Further Reading

Armstrong, Shirley W. and Rouslin, Sheila *Group Psychotherapy in Nursing Practice* (Collier-Macmillan, London, 1963)

Carkhuff, Robert R. and Anthony, William A. *The Skills of Helping* (Human Resource Development Press, Amherst, Massachusetts, 1983)

Dean, Harry and Dean, Margaret *Counselling in a Troubled Society* (Quartermaine House, Sunbury, Middlesex, 1981)

Egan, Gerard *The Skilled Helper: A Model for Systematic Helping and Interpersonal Relating* (Brooks/Cole Publishing, Monterey, California, 1975, 2nd end, 1982)

French, P. *Social Skills for Nursing Practice* (Croom Helm, London, 1983)

Hardin, S.B. and Halasis, A.L. 'Non-Verbal Communication of Patients and High and Low Empathy Nurses (Study)', *Journal of Psycho-social Nursing and Mental Health Services*, vol. 21, no. 1 (January 1983), pp. 14-20

Ivey, Allen, E. and Simek-Downing, Lynn *Counselling and Psychotherapy Skills, Theories and Practice* (Prentice-Hall, London, 1980)

Kalish, B. 'What is Empathy?' *Americal Journal of Nursing*, vol. 73, no. 9 (1973)

Kennedy, Eugene *On Becoming a Counsellor: A Basic Guide for Non-Professional Counsellors* (Gill and Macmillan, Dublin, 1977)

Munroe, E., Manthei, R.J. and Small, J.J. *Counselling: a Skills Approach* (Methuen, Wellington, New Zealand, 1980)

Nurse, Gaynor *Counselling and the Nurse: An Introduction*, 2nd edn (HM and M Publishers/John Wiley, Chichester, 1980)

Pratt, John W. and Mason, Allen *The Caring Touch* (HM and M Publishers, London, 1981)

Priestley, Phillip, McGuire, James, Flegg, David, Hemsley, Valerie and Welham, David *Social Skills and Personal Problem Solving. A Handbook of Methods* (Tavistock, London, 1978)

Proctor, Brigid *Counselling Shop: An Introduction to the Theories and Techniques of Ten Approaches to Counselling* (Burnett Books, London, 1978)

Rogers, Carl *Client-Centred Therapy*, reprinted 1981 (Constable, London, 1951)

______ *On Becoming a Person: A Therapist's View of Psychotherapy* (Constable, London, 1967)

Speight, Isobel 'Communicating with Psychiatric Patients' in W. Bridge and Clark J. Macleod, *Communication in Nursing Care* (HM and M Publishers/John Wiley, Chichester, 1981)

Stewart, William *Counselling in Nursing: A Problem Solving Approach* (Harper and Row, London, 1983)

Tschudin, Verena *Counselling Skills for Nurses* (Baillière Tindall, London, 1982)

3 BEHAVIOURAL SKILLS

Behaviourism and its Place in Society

Firstly it may be necessary to say that although most nurses and allied professionals view behaviourism with a range of emotions from reverence to dread, it is in fact a basic component of our everyday lives. It is a school of thought which offers a distinctly different perspective, and, when used thoughtfully, can be of immense help to the psychiatric nurse.

There should be no magical or mysterious power associated with behaviourism; only the uneducated or disinterested need to feel at a loss with it. It is hoped that you, upon reaching the end of the chapter, will be able to practise its simple principles, feel comfortable in its use, and assimilate it in your repertoire of skills.

The human being is essentially a complex creature, comprising skills, knowledge and emotions, each of which has been learned. It is the way in which this learning has occurred that the behaviourist is interested.

Essentially all humans seek pleasure. This may not necessarily be in an overt form, but may take many diverse expressions. It may simply be in watching an interesting film, enjoying the praise of others, or, more subtly, the satisfying feeling of taking a difficult task to a competent completion. Equally, however, a person avoids the unpleasant, or punishing, situation. These may include physiological occurrences, i.e. pain, discomfort, anxiety or the more subtle situation giving rise to feelings of uselessness, hurt or failure.

From a very early stage of development, a child quickly learns that most behaviour will be followed by a predetermined consequence. For instance, crying will result in being picked up and soothed by Mother, and touching a naked flame is followed by pain. This direct method of learning may set up patterns of behaviour that will follow the individual throughout his life.

Even more intricate patterns of behaviour may be learned in this way: take, for example, attitudes and thoughts. A schoolboy will quickly learn which attitudes and expressed thoughts will be rewarded — in a family where racial prejudice is evident, the child learns that racial statements such as 'I hate blacks' will be rewarded by father saying, 'I don't blame you, so do I.' If the first statement is accompanied by attention and a smile, it is far more likely to strengthen that attitude than if it was followed by a swift kick.

Within a family or social group, issues of prejudice or interest will be fostered by the already formed attitudes of the significant members of that group. This pattern is followed from the isolated family group to the larger institution of schools, and finally in the individual's working life.

It could be argued that if this in fact is the case, why do children grow up with attitudes and values different to their parents'? Essentially very few significant variations do occur until circumstances separate the individual from the reward, or the reward loses its meaning, i.e. approval of father is no longer highly prized, and therefore it is no longer rewarding or another view or attitude is being rewarded much more effectively. This can be seen to happen when an influential figure disagrees with previously set attitudes; most commonly these are teachers, friends and lovers.

At this point a few examples of learned behaviour may help us to understand just how many of our behaviours may well have been learned in this fashion.

John (aged 11) was found naked one day in the garden shed playing mothers and fathers with Julie (aged 9). His father severely rebuked him and beat him. Subsequently when John experimented sexually with his friend Gordon, he was not punished. This may lead, should similar events continue to occur, John into adulthood with secure feelings in homosexual relationships, and severe anxiety in heterosexual ones.

George found great social esteem from his friends because he was skilful at football, yet felt unrewarded by his 'B' grades in arithmetic — subsequently his arithmetic grades became worse and he spent more time practising his football skills. It is obvious that, from a very early stage, George is far more likely to become a sportsman than a mathematician.

The above examples are simple illustrations and should not be taken as serious attempts to explain complex human behaviour, but none the less they do serve to show that some rewards/punishments may influence some behaviour. It could be argued that people's lives can be directed and prescribed from a very early stage by the amount of reward they receive. Conversely, they can be controlled by the degree of punishment to which they are subjected.

The previous examples could be said to be almost natural or coincidental influences, and that to a degree is true. However, what of the rules of society? Certain prescribed ways of behaviour in various cultures are not only expected and taught in this way, but contrived by statutes, i.e. the law dictates certain behaviours.

The vast majority of people, termed 'law abiders', conform to rules and obey. Generally this is to avoid punishment, but may otherwise well be because society rewards the law abider.

The industrious and caring person in society is rewarded by the social group, not only by money, but by elevating him to the ranks of high esteem. Doctors and nurses, for instance, are generally highly respected and admired people. This social reward may explain why tiresome and irksome duties are still completed despite meagre monetary reward.

If all this can be accepted as in essence true, it opens up many possibilities for the psychiatric nurse. It shows that if behaviours have been 'learned' in this way, then they can be 'unlearned'. Conversely, new behaviours can be learned and past behaviours removed. This in practice is the foundation of behaviourism as a therapeutic model. It is important that in all this we are not carried away in an enthusiasm to help, but, as professionals, we must never lose sight of the fact that we are dealing with people.

Ethical Considerations

There is no doubt in our minds that the use of behavioural theory is one of the most potent forces the psychiatric nurse can employ. Whether this is for the benefit or to the detriment of the patient depends largely on the knowledge and skill of the person running the programme.

The first issue that arises before any attempt is made at changing an individual's behaviour is one of consent. Behaviour can certainly be changed without an individual's consent, but how easy this is, and how certain you can be of positive outcomes, are doubtful. Certainly in our experience, the more consenting and consequently more motivated the patient is, the more effective the treatment.

When in fact can a programme begin without the patient's consent? It seems reasonable that the two main circumstances are:

(1) When the behaviour is dangerous to the patient, i.e.
   — overdosing;
   — headbanging;
   — similar physically hazardous behaviours.
(2) When the patient is unable to give 'informed consent', i.e. he is unable to understand or appreciate a choice proposed and the concerned professionals agree that a change in behaviour will enhance the patient's 'quality of life'.

Even if it is decided to go ahead with a behavioural programme, there remain several ethical or moral issues which will need to be carefully considered:

(1) Who decides what are desired and undesired behaviours in any given individual?
(2) Would it be right to change religious, cultural or social behaviours of patients which they may value?
(3) Should sexual or political attitudes be changed in patients when these are implicit in their values?
(4) Specifically, certain categories of patient raise special problems. What right do we have to change behaviours of patients who are suffering from, for example:
   — personality disorders;
   — suicidal risk;
   — institutionalisation,
   — anorexia;
   — psychoses;
   — mental handicap?
(5) What restraints should there be when dealing with children?

All these questions are honest ones which have to be answered by the individual team, on an individual case basis. It would clearly be irresponsible of us to try to generalise in each category those which should or should not be treated by behavioural methods. On the other hand, general principles and guidelines can be suggested.

In the first instance, what is desired or undesired should not be decided by one person. When considering behaviour change, it should be evaluated objectively. The values and beliefs of the patient should not be set aside simply because they are not held by the evaluator. For example, staying in bed until noon may not be very valuable to the therapist, but it may well be something prized and treasured by the patient.

The nurse may be prejudiced against particular forms of sexual expression, e.g. homosexuality, masturbation or adultery. This should not mean that for that patient they are not valuable, or do not add to his quality of life — they are not automatic areas for behaviour change.

This particularly sensitive area becomes more difficult when considering the patient who is admitted compulsorily from the courts for something such as child molesting. Should his behaviour, however illegal, be changed without his consent?

It would be our view that as the behaviour is not hazardous (within the institution) and usually the patient is able to give 'informed consent', then clearly he should not be compulsorily treated by behavioural means.

Occasionally a patient may insist or demand treatment. This equally may raise problems. Even if the treatment is thought to be inappropriate by the team, have they the right to withhold it? There must be room for flexibility and negotiation in all these areas, but in all cases careful and thoughtful consideration *must* be a precursor to treatment.

In areas of religion, culture and political beliefs, it would appear that most therapists agree that it would be unethical to interfere. However, there have recently been cases reported of religious and political 'brainwashing' which may require, or at least benefit from, some behavioural therapies. The question here is, do the two wrongs make a right? In the first instance, the brainwashing broke the rule of consent, but would not treatment for his present state equally break the rule again?

Patients with 'personality disorders' are often people who have different values to the society in which they live. If this is causing problems for them in their everyday lives, or is continually bringing them into conflict with authority, then possibly behaviour therapy would be beneficial. It is, however, our belief that consent is still required.

The suicidal and the anorexic patient may be considered together. In both these cases it would seem clear that if intervention is not pursued, the patient may well die. If this is the case, it seems reasonable that any treatment that seeks to raise the potential for recovery is certainly worth careful thought. Once the patient dies, he obviously loses his ability to choose and his ability to change his mind — and the preservation of this prerogative would seem to be one worthy of any effort expended, even perhaps without the patient's consent.

A case in point would be the deeply depressed patient, for it could be argued that whilst in this state his judgement is seriously impaired, and therefore informed consent is not a realistic premiss. The one exception to this that immediately springs to mind is the terminally ill patient. A patient in severe pain or suffering should certainly be given every opportunity for help, whether by counselling or any other methods available. However, to create a behavioural programme simply to extend his life without consent would require exceptional circumstances and a lot of explanation.

The institutionalised patient, the psychotic and the mentally handicapped generally fall into the category of those unable to give informed consent. However, they should be given every opportunity to discuss with the psychiatric nurse any programme before its implementation. Let us not delude ourselves, these patients too can appreciate even subtle changes in the care offered to them, and an explanation, even if not fully understood, may well be gratefully received, and avoid unnecessary distress.

The treatment of children is a special case that needs the full consultation and agreement of parents or guardians. Each case should be accurately monitored, preferably by an independent observer, to ensure a child's behaviour is not changed out of context to his or her stage of development. Adult values and behaviour should not be imposed on a child, neither should his or her formative development be out of step with the social and cultural facets of the home and family. The child is after all going to return to the family and friends he or she left (if hospitalised) and the values and benefits held by peer groups should remain intact so that he or she can reintegrate back into the community on discharge.

Other ethical rules need to be established when using behaviour therapy. For instance, if punishment is to be used, how severe should it be? As a member of a caring profession, the nurse must be clear where she stands. It is our view that each individual will have her own values, and will place limitations on what she feels able to engage in — even in the best planned behavioural theory. Each individual should decide, without pressure from any source, what she is prepared to do.

Generally the individual in any team who is prepared to go to the least lengths in areas of punishment should determine where the maximum boundaries should be drawn. To clarify this, if Nurse X says she is prepared to deny Johnny his meals for two days in order to facilitate him eating at the table, and Nurse X says she would only be prepared to deny him for six hours, then six hours should be the maximum boundary. Any decision such as this should be made by a team, and the lowest common denominator is generally the safest and most ethical.

What types of punishments are acceptable? Shocks, pain and social isolation are direct punishments. Removal of freedom, food, cigarettes and basic human rights of privacy and individual expression may be others. But how far can the professional go?

Boundaries are very difficult to set, but again each individual should think carefully and see whether she can answer these questions in the positive:

(1) Would the programme be acceptable if I was the patient?
(2) If the patient was my relative or friend, would I *easily* agree?
(3) Is the programme potentially hazardous; has it been carefully considered and explained to my satisfaction?

If this is so, most probably the programme is acceptable.

What are acceptable as rewards? Thought has to be given to how morally acceptable are such rewards as alcohol, drugs, sexual gratification and artificial social rewards. Each of these has built-in dangers and the individual should question how, when and why these are to be given and, more seriously, what the long-term effects are likely to be.

The three areas previously examined for punishments remain applicable to rewards, and may be used as a guideline to assess suitability.

It must be said that very rarely should programmes be 'severe' enough to provoke any reservations in the caring individual. However, in order that enthusiastic individuals do not become over-zealous, vigilant observation of programmes must be maintained. It is for this reason that 'ethical considerations' have been included in this text.

Behavioural Principles

Behaviour therapy is based broadly on the work of Pavlov, a

psychologist experimenting in physiological responses in animals, and Skinner, who also worked with animals, but generalised his work into human psychology.

Pavlov

Classical Conditioning. The essential idea is that there are various stimuli in the environment that evoke reactions in response. If artificial stimuli are presented at the same time as the original, then there is a linking or association to such an extent that eventually the false or artificial stimuli will evoke the same reaction (Figure 3.1).

In a more practical (psychiatric) setting, the person who has a fetish may well have been classically conditioned (Figure 3.2).

One type of treatment for alcoholics uses the principles of classical conditioning in aversion therapy. Here an electric shock causes an unpleasant feeling. When drinking alcohol is linked with the shock, then a gradual association is formed between alcohol and the unpleasant feeling (Figure 3.3).

So the work of Pavlov shows us that it is possible to create a response by linking a previously established stimulus-reaction together with a new one. From a practical psychiatric nursing point of view, this has quite a powerful potential.

The Work of B.F. Skinner

Operant Conditioning. The basic idea of operant conditioning centres on the observation that by presenting something rewarding or appealing following a behaviour, that behaviour is strengthened or increased. Conversely, if a behaviour is followed by something of an unpleasant nature, that behaviour is weakened or reduced. Although the conditioning process can be demonstrated and proved scientifically in a laboratory using animals, its implications and ramifications when practically applied to human subjects are immense.

Human behaviour is so complex and its motivation so diverse that much intricate and specialised work has been done to enable its application to the 'treatment' of human subjects. Much of the work of clinical psychologists and nurses or therapists in the field of mental illness is based on what has come to be known as the 'behavioural approach'. Hence in its simplest form we have 'behaviour modification' and in its more complex form 'behaviour therapy'.

Figure 3.1: The Classical Conditioning Process

SMELL OF FOOD (termed 'unconditioned stimulus')	evokes →	SALIVATION (termed 'unconditioned response')
SMELL OF FOOD + RINGING A BELL	evoke →	SALIVATION
	This results in ↓	
RINGING A BELL (now termed '*conditioned stimulus*')	→ evokes	SALIVATION (now termed '*conditioned response*')

Figure 3.2: Plastic Mac Fetish

KISSING YOUNG LADY (unconditioned stimulus)	evokes →	SEXUAL AROUSAL (unconditioned response)
KISSING YOUNG LADY + WEARING PLASTIC MAC	evoke →	SEXUAL AROUSAL
	This may eventually lead to:	
WEARING PLASTIC MAC (conditioned stimulus)	→ evokes	SEXUAL AROUSAL (conditioned response)

Figure 3.3: The Classical Conditioning Process in Aversion Therapy

SHOCK	evokes →	UNPLEASANT FEELING
SHOCK + ALCOHOL	evoke →	UNPLEASANT FEELING
Then ↓		
ALCOHOL	evokes →	UNPLEASANT FEELING

Behaviour Modification and Behaviour Therapy

There appears to be some confusion in some people's minds about the difference between these two expressions. Our understanding of the difference is quite simple. *Behaviour modification* is generally accepted as referring to the principles of learning theory, and the various behaviour change strategies most widely used. These would include positive and negative reinforcement, extinction, modelling and shaping (see Poteet, 1978; Gentry, 1975). It could be argued that behaviour modification is concerned largely with Skinner's work, whereas behaviour therapy has a much broader definition.

We consider *behaviour therapy* as a term including any technique designed to change behaviour for the patient's benefit. This would include much of Skinner's work and Pavlov's ideas, and perhaps even some of the therapies included within humanistic psychology theories. Behavioural counselling (Krumboltz and Thoresen, 1969) may be seen as a typical example of this. Using behavioural principles in a rather more eclectic way to effect a behaviour change for the patient's benefit would be our wider definition of behaviour therapy (see Wolfe and Lazarus, 1966; Barker, 1982).

To summarise, behaviour therapy is a general term which includes many therapies, and incorporates behaviour modification principles directed towards therapy. We take Barker's meaning of therapy here to mean 'an offer of help' (Barker, 1982, p. 11). Consequently we prefer the term behaviour therapy as this implies a therapeutic design or intent that behaviour modification may not.

Basic Principles

The following is intended as a basic guide to the principles and techniques of behaviour change with which the nurse should be familiar. Focusing upon operant conditioning, behaviour change can be broadly separated into two main areas: A. Increasing or strengthening. B. Decreasing or weakening.

A. *Increasing and strengthening behaviour* can be achieved by two methods — positive reinforcement and negative reinforcement.

Positive reinforcement. This occurs when a behaviour is followed by a response or event that the individual finds rewarding to such an extent that it will increase the likelihood of the behaviour being repeated.

It can be seen then that a positive reinforcer may be anything the person finds rewarding or pleasant and tends to increase/strengthen a behaviour. A technical definition of positive reinforcer: 'a pleasant stimulus presented to a subject following a response in order to strengthen that response' (Houston, Bee and Rimm, 1983).

A positive reinforcer may be different for each individual —

perhaps a chocolate for a child, a smile for an adult, indeed a masochist may find a slap in the face rewarding. Examples:

(1) A little boy cuddled by his mother when he smiles is likely to produce an increase in smiling.
(2) A school child praised for hard work is likely to work harder.
(3) If you are given £20 for predicting the winner of the 2.30 at Kempton Park, your 'predicting' betting behaviour is likely to increase.

Therefore, the positive reinforcers were:

(1) A cuddle.
(2) Praise.
(3) Money.

Negative reinforcement. This refers to increasing or strengthening a behaviour by *removing* an unpleasant occurrence or stimuli, following a response. So in colloquial terms it is in fact the 'relief' from the negative reinforcer (the stimulus) that rewards the preceding behaviour.

A technical definition of negative reinforcer is: 'an unpleasant stimulus taken away from a subject following a response in order to strengthen that response' (Houston, Bee and Rimm, 1983). Examples:

(1)(a) If a rat is placed in a box of which the floor has a mild electric current, it discovers that jumping up removes the unpleasant stimuli and consequently its jumping up behaviour increases.
(b) If the whole box is electrified and the rat discovers by pressing a lever inside the box that the current is removed, then lever pressing behaviour increases.

Now to put this into human terms, which is far more complex:

(2) When a baby cries, its mother may find it unpleasant, but when the baby is picked up it stops crying. Here the mother is being rewarded by relief from the crying and subsequently her 'picking baby up' behaviour may well increase.
(3) If an addict to diamorphine begins to experience withdrawal

symptoms, nausea, sweating and stomach cramps, he will find this an unpleasant experience (aversive stimulus). He finds 'relief' from this unpleasant experience by injecting himself intravenously with more diamorphine. Therefore the removal of these symptoms occurs when he increases injecting the drug. His behaviour is said to be *negatively reinforced.* By removing an unpleasant feeling, his preceding behaviour (injecting) has strengthened.

(4) Persistent headaches may lead to increased aspirin taking.
(5) Anxiety removed by diazepam may lead to increased ingestion of the drug.

In these examples the negative reinforcer was something aversive removed which subsequently increased a behaviour.

The negative reinforcers were:

(1) Electric current.
(2) Baby crying.
(3) Withdrawal symptoms.
(4) Headache.
(5) Anxiety.

The strengthened or reinforced behaviours were:

(1) Jumping and lever pressing.
(2) Picking up baby.
(3) Increasing dose of diamorphine.
(4) Aspirin taking.
(5) Diazepam taking.

B. *Decreasing or weakening behaviour.* There are two methods of decreasing or weakening behaviour: punishment and extinction.

Punishment. In its technical sense, this means the removal of something the individual finds pleasant, or the presentation of something the individual finds unpleasant. The use of either of these is designed *to follow* a behaviour and thus weaken or reduce its occurrence.

(1) A schoolboy is eating his lunch, which he is obviously enjoying, but at the same time is 'messing about'. He is removed

from his meal or his meal is removed from him until his 'messing about' stops. This is punishment by removal of a pleasant stimulus.

(2) As the boyfriend's hand reaches the top of the young lady's leg, he receives a resounding slap across the face. In most cases this will lead to a reduction in the preceding behaviour. This is punishment by presentation of an unpleasant stimulus.

It may be helpful to consider at this point the difference between punishment and negative reinforcement. A punishment is an aversive stimulus which follows a behaviour and is designed to *stop* that behaviour. A negative reinforcer is an aversive stimulus which when removed *increases* the behaviour which immediately preceded its removal. It is seen then that punishment and a negative reinforcer are both aversive stimuli — unpleasant. But punishment is *applied* to *stop* or weaken behaviour, and a negative reinforcer is *removed* to *increase* or strengthen behaviour.

Extinction. The second method of weakening a behaviour is called extinction. Here the idea is to ensure that the undesired behaviour is not rewarded. No reinforcement is given or taken away; the behaviour is totally ignored. This applies the principle that if a behaviour is not rewarded, it ceases to occur.

One important aspect that should not be overlooked, however, is that when this procedure is followed, there is almost inevitably a dramatic increase in the behaviour you are trying to reduce. This is technically referred to as '*extinction burst*'. This is because the behaviour in the past has always a elicited a reward of some nature. Now there is no reward being given, the behaviour initially increases in a frantic attempt to gain the usual reward.

In practical terms, extinction, if it is carried through consistently, will work. However, there are several problems associated with this technique for psychiatric nurses:

(1) If the behaviour you are trying to reduce offers a hazard to the patient, it is impossible, morally and perhaps legally, to ignore it. For example, if a patient has previously been rewarded with attention when taking an overdose, or slashing his wrists, it remains impossible simply to ignore him.
(2) On a conventional ward there are many staff who perhaps would find ignoring a patient's adverse behaviour difficult, if

not impossible. This would mean in practice that extinction would not be complete. In fact his behaviour would be spasmodically rewarded (intermittent reinforcement) and this would maintain, quite effectively, his adverse behaviour.

(3) It would be almost impossible to control the environment to such an extent in a conventional ward to ensure that extinction was complete. Other patients, visitors and uninformed colleagues invariably interfere with this type of programme.

A simple illustration of extinction and what has been referred to as intermittent reinforcement is the example of the fruit machine. A person putting money into a fruit machine does so in the hope that he will be rewarded with a win. If he continues to put money in and has no success whatsoever, he would soon discontinue the practice — extinction would occur.

Generally, the individual does win reasonably often, initially. This produces positive reinforcement and leads to the person playing the machine more and more frequently. Each win is so powerfully rewarding that even if he receives little reward, he will continue to play. He will in fact continue to play even when the machine pays out very infrequently as long as he is rewarded 'intermittently', and when long periods of non-payment occur, his playing will increase frantically to achieve any kind of payout — 'extinction burst'. At this point, non-payout will have to occur for some considerable time before he will stop playing the fruit machine at all — extinction.

As can be observed from any social club or public bar, the fruit machine is extremely powerful; it appears to have no boundaries to its addictive power. Intellect, social, religious or cultural influences appear to have little effect on it — such is the power of positive intermittent reinforcement.

How then can these principles be applied in the conventional ward? How can extinction be useful?

In many ways behavioural principles should not be applied in singular form. The nurse must look to the general ideas and adapt and improvise them appropriately. As an example, let us see how an 'attention seeking patient' could be helped through the use of the principles we have looked at so far.

Jim Middleton is a patient originally admitted with bizarre behaviour, hallucinations and delusions. These symptoms have long since disappeared, but there now remain the residual effects of staying in hospital for twenty years. He does not take care of his personal hygiene, he refuses to eat with other patients, and he constantly takes off his clothes and lies naked on the floor.

Firstly it is important to observe his behaviour, to see what rewards he is receiving for his present state. It may be seen that:

(1) Nurses help him dress, wash and shave.
(2) He is allowed to eat alone in a comfortable chair, with the television or radio on.
(3) When he undresses, a nurse invariably scolds him, but then assists him dress and return to his chair.

The examples show that his behaviour is basically being reinforced by the nurses' attention, and by being treated differently from the other patients. Additionally, it may be that he is rewarded by the television, radio and sitting in an easy chair, and by the caring attitude, albeit chastising, of the nurses assisting him when he lies naked on the floor.

Perhaps also if we look at the nurses' behaviour, it could be said that they too have behaved in such a way because they have been negatively reinforced. Having a patient go without meals, lie on the floor without clothes, or live in an unhygienic condition may initiate feelings of anxiety, unpleasant feelings of unworthiness and inadequacy within them. The relief of these feelings by 'caring' for the patient then reinforces their behaviour by removing these feelings and allows them positive reinforcement of satisfaction of a 'job well done'.

With a knowledge of the principles operating within the ward, the skilled nurse may be able, reasonably quickly, to remedy this unhappy situation. A simple programme for Jim may be as follows.

Positive reinforcement. Jim will be rewarded with praise when he arises from bed — whatever state he is in. He would be left in bed until such time as he did arise.

At any time when his behaviour showed improvement, e.g. dressing, washing and shaving himself, he would be rewarded with either praise and attention, or something more tangible — e.g. cigarettes or sweets. To avoid reinforcing undesired behaviour, he would not be allowed to eat, other than a very basic calorie enriched drink, unless he came to the table with the other patients.

Punishment (removal of pleasant rewards). Television, radio and his easy chair should be withheld from him whenever possible, without precipitating an aggressive incident, and used wherever possible as a reward for positive behaviour.

Extinction. Wherever possible, Jim's negative behaviour is ignored. All social reinforcement, smiles, hellos and other acknowledgements of his presence would be unforthcoming whilst his behaviour was negative. However, when it is necessary to intervene, assistance should be given in the minimum socially reinforcing way, without smiling or social contact. Jim should only be helped to a stage where he is no longer a hazard to himself, and during the period where he is being ignored the nurse should continually observe for any behaviour that could be rewarded.

Negative reinforcement. Jim's hunger and need for social acknowledgement would be powerful negative reinforcers, which would be removed at any period of positive behaviour.

The skilled nurse must be able to observe continually for factors Jim finds rewarding and use these to help reinforce desired behaviours. Although many problems within this programme may occur, if the nurse can understand what has gone wrong and adjust the programme accordingly, then eventually desired behaviour will emerge. By the simple principle of not rewarding undesired behaviours, and continuously rewarding those that are, the behaviour generally will improve.

Finally, two principles that are very important in behavioural work are shaping and modelling.

Shaping

Shaping is a technique that is analogous to sculpting clay. By gradual progression, the clay takes shape into the final intended result, as does behaviour moulded by reinforcing responses that occur progressively nearer the final desired behaviour. The principles of shaping rely on rewarding any initial behaviour that even remotely resembles the final desired outcome. In order to continue receiving rewards, the behaviour must progress, so successive approximations are always rewarded. It should be noted, however, that the reward must be withdrawn once each further stage is reached, or the reward risks fixing behaviour at that stage.

In Jim's case this would mean that once he had been

encouraged to dress himself properly, he would be rewarded only intermittently for achieving this, and rewards would be concentrated on the next stage, washing and shaving.

Modelling

This is powerful when associated with shaping. Rather than waiting for the behaviour to occur spontaneously, the nurse may 'model' or demonstrate what she considers the desired behaviour to be, and rewards the subject when he imitates it. Through rehearsal this method can be very powerful, especially when a good rapport is in evidence, and the subject is receiving some intrinsic reward for pleasing the nurse.

It is hoped that you now have an overall appreciation of some of the most important principles of behaviour change. The remainder of this chapter is concerned largely with some examples of specific therapies which incorporate these principles in directed and specific ways towards helping the patient. It is our intention that, with a better understanding of both principles and specific therapies on behavioural lines, the psychiatric nurse can add to her repertoire of skills to become a more effective helper.

The therapies selected are not intended to be an exhaustive description of all behavioural therapies available. There are many more less familiar and obscure ones that we do not feel able to describe. For this reason, suggested reading is given to fill any gaps and to provide direction should you be stimulated to research further.

The samples of therapies offered here have been selected on the basis that we believe these are currently the most likely to be practised, and it is probable that some nurses will become involved with them in the early parts of their careers. We believe they represent a fairly wide distribution of the behavioural skills that may be required of the psychiatric nurse in modern practice today.

Token Economy

Token economy is essentially the use of artificial reinforcers which strength behaviours because they acquire the power of their exchange value, i.e. one token buys one cigarette. In much the same way as money is a reward and an incentive to most people in society, the token — usually a worthless piece of plastic — represents a saveable item that can be exchanged for anything the patient may find rewarding.

In practical terms, wards or hostels that use this system of behaviour modification have a shop which deals in tokens. Consequently the token can be exchanged for anything in the shop. Additionally, certain privileges may be paid for by tokens, such as a day off, an outing, leave, cinema, a late night out or a 'lie in' in the morning. Its usefulness becomes clear to the observant in that once the 'pleasure' link has been made between the symbol (token) and the purchase of a reward with the token, they become instant reinforcers of any behaviour the institution wishes to strengthen. The withholding or removal of tokens becomes a punishment and can be used to weaken any behaviour that is not desired.

Its simple management becomes a valuable asset to the psychiatric nurse, as she may build a programme that 'shapes' a patient's behaviour by allocating 'targets' for the patient to reach. These targets are measured in tokens. For example, 'If you can save ten tokens by Saturday, you can go swimming instead of doing your normal ward work.'

One major problem in dealing with psychiatric patients using behavioural principles is what is referred to as *satiation*. This is when the reward offered becomes unrewarding. For example, a patient is offered a cigarette for shaving himself, when in fact he has a thousand cigarettes in his locker. It would be pointless using food as a reward when the patient has just consumed a large and pleasant meal. The patient is in a state of satisfaction, so offering rewards such as these will not strengthen his behaviour.

Avoiding satiation is necessary for token economy to be most beneficial. As the reward is artificially conditioned, the token will represent a reward that can be exchanged for anything the patient truly wants or needs. It is unlikely in an organised system that the patient will ever reach a point of satiation using tokens.

Table 3.1 shows an example of what a token economy scheme might be. The advantage of this is that the token reward can be adjusted when the patient starts to find the task easier, and can then gradually be incorporated into his general behaviour with social rather than token reinforcement.

An example of this would be: Jim refuses to get up. While he stays in bed he receives no reinforcement (no token); when he does get up he receives ten tokens. This is because he will get the most reward for what he finds most difficult.

Table 3.1: An Example of What a Token Economy Scheme Might be

Time	Behaviour	Reward Token
08.00	Gets up	1
	Washed	1
	Showered	1
	Dressed	1
08.30	Eats breakfast using cutlery correctly	1
09.00	Helps clear tables	2
09.30	Goes to O/T	1
10.00	Participates in work	3
10.30	Helps give out coffee	2
11.00	Participates in work	3
11.30	Returns to ward and lays the tables	3
12.00	Socialises with other patients	1
13.00	Returns to work	1
14.00	Participates in gardening	Up to 10
16.00	Returns to ward	
17.00	Sets tables	
	Bath	Number of tokens
	Wash clothes	decided by nurse as
	Iron	appropriate
	Cook supper	

Subsequently Jim gets up more and more easily, so he is given three tokens and social encouragement for getting up and seven for having a wash. This readjustment and sequencing can continue until the complete repertoire is built up, and Jim's behaviour is positively fixed. This process is in fact a shaping programme, with a gradual reduction of reward as opposed to an abrupt end of reward when a stage further is reached.

It can be seen, then, that token economy may be very useful in helping motivate the long-stay patient, especially in his initial stages of rehabilitation, and has a potential, if skilfully used, to aid more complex social behaviours in the more advanced programme.

Desensitisation

Desensitisation is the behavioural treatment for patients with phobias. A phobia will be expressed as some form of behaviour. Whether this is in the form of actions or thoughts, it is invariably shown in physiological terms, e.g. palpitations, sweating, pallor, nausea. For example, a person phobic towards rats will avoid places where he is likely to come in contact with them, he will think about them with dread, and should contact be unavoidable, will certainly react physically to them, breaking out in a cold sweat, increasing pulse and respiration.

The use of desensitisation, like all behavioural treatments, should be carefully considered. A patient with a phobia can sometimes be desensitised by a skilled nurse or therapist. However, that does not mean to say that all the patient's symptoms will disappear. The reasons for the development of the phobia may not have changed during therapy, and consequently other symptoms may arise and be just as debilitating following successful treatment by desensitisation. This phenomenon is referred to as 'symptom substitution'. To offset this occurring, it is often desirable to begin other therapies simultaneously with desensitisation. For example, a patient who has developed a phobic reaction to leaving his house may have a deeper mental problem that will require treatment by psychotherapy or counselling, as well as a simple desensitisation programme for the overt fear reaction to going out. If then a 'double barrelled' treatment programme is started, the chances of symptom substitution developing are greatly reduced.

Anthony developed a fear close to panic whenever he went outside his house. At first he forced himself to leave and go to work, but his anxieties did not subside and he found it impossible to concentrate once he had arrived at work. As he worked as an accountant and needed to concentrate for long periods, his superiors at work soon became unhappy with his performance so he took sick leave and sought medical help. After a month of unsuccessful treatment with minor tranquillisers, it was decided to seek help from a behavioural approach.

It was apparent at this stage that Anthony had a frank agoraphobia and in order for him to return quickly to work, he would benefit from a behavioural programme of desensitisation. However, it was also clear that he was not suffering from a simple fear of the outside; his phobia had developed due to many complex factors involving unresolved personal conflicts.

Before desensitisation began, much time was spent with Anthony to uncover some of the psychological problems he was experiencing. For example, during discussions many things were discovered about him, the most significant being:

(1) The cause of his mother's death the previous year had remained unresolved.
(2) His wife, who had never worked before, had begun to talk about finding a job.
(3) His teenage children were demanding more independence and making preparations to leave home.

It was clear to the nurse that urgent treatment must start by assisting Anthony's return to work, because while he was able to avoid the fear of going out, this negatively reinforced him being housebound. It was also apparent that his last few days at work had been extremely unpleasant, which he had found punishing. While he was ill his wife would not consider finding a job, and similarly his children would not want to leave home; this he found rewarding.

A Behavioural Explanation of Anthony's Phobia Formation

As previously discussed in the section on behavioural principles, certain factors operated in Anthony's phobia formation, these being:

Punishment (serves to extinguish behaviours) i.e.
Going to work — followed by superiors complaining about his performance (punishment).

Result
↓
Weakens the desire to go to work.

Negative reinforcement (relief from an aversive stimulus → strengthens preceding behaviour).
Anthony's anxiety and unease when starting off for work were removed when he decided not to go.

Result
↓
Decision to 'not go to work' is strengthened.

Positive reinforcement (rewarding situations).

While Anthony has this 'illness', his wife discontinues her plans to find a job (positively reinforcing his illness). Similarly the children say they will stay at home until he gets better again (positive reinforcement for Anthony to remain ill).

The nurse's main job is clearly to desensitise the main focus of fear, and continue counselling Anthony in order to help him uncover the underlying problems and deal with them.

From the above, it may well appear that if the reasons for the phobia's development are removed, all will be well, so counselling and psychotherapy may appear to be the better solution.

In fact counselling was begun with Anthony two weeks before desensitisation, but even if this has been completely successful, the patient is still left with a learned behaviour. He has in fact been conditioned to respond physiologically to certain situations and circumstances, just as the simple rat phobic has learned to respond with fear to the sight of a rat. Similarly, Anthony, even when fully aware of the causes of his phobia through counselling, was still left with fear responses to leaving the house. Desensitisation therapy was required to break down these responses and replace them with more appropriate behaviours.

The Programme

Firstly Anthony was asked to explain his fears, how he felt in various situations, and to place these in a hierarchy of fear (see Table 3.2). It may be helpful to study the table before reading on. Note the end column which shows how the body is reacting. It is the body that acts as a reinforcer for Anthony's behaviour. When he relieves these symptoms, he negatively reinforces his behaviour.

Symptom (aversive stimuli)	Behaviour	Effect
Heart palpitations →	Returns home →	Feels calmer
	↖	↓
		Strengthens his behaviour (by negative reinforcement).

This is called 'avoidance behaviour' and is the reason the phobia has been so well and truly fixed. If this pattern can be broken down, the conditioned behaviours can be replaced by more valuable ones.

The hierarchy helps the nurse because it allows her to understand exactly how the patient is feeling, simply by asking him to pin-point at any time where he is on a scale from one to eight. By explaining to the patient what is happening, and reassuring him constantly, she can 'talk' the rating down, and therefore break down this avoidance behaviour. To explain this a little more

Table 3.2: Anthony's Hierarchy of Fear

	Situation	Feelings	Physiological Responses
1.	Knowing I'm staying at home	Calm	Normal
2.	Looking out of the window	Uneasy	Pulse rate slightly raised
3.	Going to the door	Anxious	Pulse rate up, B/P raised, palms of hands perspire
4.	Opening the door	Very anxious	Breathing becomes increased, over breathing develops
5.	Stepping outside	Feeling of panic	Breathing rate increases, sweating generalised, palpitations begin
6.	At the gate	Faint, nausea	Symptoms increase, physical feelings of weakness, muscles refuse to work
7.	At the bus stop	Uncontrolled panic, impulse to run	Indecision is enabling anxiety symptoms to continue, fainting is now a possibility due to extensive over breathing
8.	Arrival of bus	Complete confusion, panic building to terror	Physical symptoms of anxiety cannot be maintained further, all symptoms have reached a crescendo, adrenaline in the system will either be utilised in running or be broken down in the body.

graphically, let's see exactly how the nurse begins.

Firstly Anthony will be taught how to relax, using simple breathing exercises and muscle relaxation. For this the patient is asked to sit in a relaxed position and breathe deeply but slowly. Then, as he breathes in, he is asked to tense the muscles in his legs and arms and clench his fists, as he breathes out he says, 'I am feeling calmer' and simultaneously relaxes his tensed muscles. This technique takes only a few minutes to teach, but is invaluable in the process of desensitisation for several reasons.

(1) It aids an adequate supply of oxygen to the body, and prevents over breathing. This will affect the secondary physiological reactions that occur in panic attacks such as confusion, palpitations, nausea and faintness.
(2) It relaxes the muscles so that blood flow is not restricted, and reduces the shakiness.
(3) Verbalising 'I feel calmer' is reinforced when the body responds in a desirable way and allows the patient to feel in control.

The nurse can now move on to take Anthony through his phobic journey, constantly asking him how he is feeling. He can now appropriately use relaxation to prevent him avoiding the situation until he is completely desensitised.

Finally, let's look at a brief dialogue between the nurse and patient at his garden gate.

Nurse. OK, Tony, you've made it to the gate, you're doing great, tell me how you feel now.
Anthony. Awful, I want to go back in.
Nurse. Well, awful doesn't tell me a lot, how do you rate it on your scale?
Anthony. Around six.
Nurse. Right. You're breathing too quickly, remember what we did before, breathe in and tense, breathe out and relax and repeat, 'I feel calmer.'
Anthony. I feel calmer ... I feel calmer ... I feel calmer.
Nurse. Carry on, you're doing fine, just a little slower.
Anthony. I feel calmer ... I feel calmer.
Nurse. Fine, how are you feeling now?

Anthony. Much better, around three on the scale.

Nurse. Good, that's great, we'll carry on for a few more minutes, then, when you're really relaxed, we'll finish for today and tomorrow we'll go a little further.

This process is continued until all avoidance behaviour is broken down and Anthony feels quite relaxed at all stages of his journey. The nurse accompanies him until he is quite sure that he can succeed on his own. Failure at any one of the steps can be very traumatic, so the main aim is to make the steps meaningful but not insurmountable. Therefore the patient has additional reinforcement for the achievement, but no negative reinforcement for avoiding the task.

If for some reason the nurse miscalculates the difficulty of the task, and the patient is unable to continue the exercise and, say, runs inside, this will create a potentially destructive situation. It can to some extent be offset by ensuring that the verbal reassurance given when back inside the house is directed not at how relieved he is feeling, but how well he has progressed. The reinforcement is therefore directed at his achievement of some goals, rather than his failure.

Alternative Theoretical Considerations

Within this approach to phobic patients, we have focused strongly upon the operant learning theory of phobic formation, i.e. that the fear is rewarded by events following its avoidance. We have also intimated that rather complex mental processes may have contributed to this phobia formation. Additional theoretical considerations, which may help the nurse when evaluating the phobic patient's behaviour, and in turn help the patient understand how the fear was originally created, are given by Mowrer (1960). This theory combines a classical conditioning situation with subsequent operant reinforcement. For example:

Pain Unconditioned stimulus	evokes →	Fear Unconditioned response
Pain + Dog (dog bite) Unconditioned stimulus + Conditioned stimulus	evoke →	Fear Unconditioned response + Conditioned response

Dog	evokes →	Fear
Conditioned stimulus		Conditioned response

This explains in Pavlovian terms why once you have been bitten by one dog you become afraid of all dogs. During his experiments with conditioning, Pavlov also discovered that this pairing phenomenon (i.e. the unconditioned with the conditioned stimulus and the unconditioned with the conditioned response) would not continue indefinitely. He showed in his experiments that the conditioned response became weaker and gradually extinguished (*extinction* in classical conditioning terms) if the original unconditioned stimulus did not recur:

Sight of dog	evokes →	Fear
Conditioned stimulus		Conditioned response
Second sight of dog	evokes →	Reduced fear
Third sight of dog	evokes →	Further reduced fear

Consequently, failure of the original pain to recur allows for the conditioned response (fear) to reduce gradually. Pavlov's trials showed individual differences between subjects in how long extinction took, and also that even after some time had elapsed and extinction was thought to be total, an isolated single response was possible.

If this is the case, then how can phobias be maintained? It is evident that not every dog or even every tenth dog is likely to bite the conditioned person, so how is it that the conditioned response does not extinguish? Mowrer (1960) proposes that someone afraid of a dog will actively seek to avoid dogs, and that subsequently the negative reinforcement (relief of potential anxiety situations) maintains this avoidance behaviour. This is called the 'two factory theory'.

Another theory which may support the maintenance of phobic reaction is that of Ellis (1962). This theory suggests from a cognitive perspective that once a fear exists, the individual may perpetuate it by 'self talk' which supports the fear. The subject says to himself, 'I must not go to the park, there will be dogs there, and they will bite me,' or 'Dogs are dangerous,' 'I'm scared of dogs,' 'Dogs always bite me.' More significant perhaps is the possibility that when faced with a dog his thoughts may become the stimulus creating a fear response — 'Oh my God, there's a dog, it's going to bite me — I'll get rabies and die.' Running away from this situation may serve only to be a powerful negative reinforcement for subsequent avoidance of other dogs, and perpetuate the phobia.

Whichever theory is correct, and it is not unlikely that they all have relevant insights, it can be seen that desensitisation may be beneficial in most cases. Gradual exposure to the focus of the phobia would serve to extinguish any conditioned response, using positive reinforcement, and reducing the efficacy of negative reinforcement in avoidance would helpfully reverse any learned behaviour pattern; and any cognitive reinforcement should be reversed by the evidence of experience. ('The dog didn't bite me, dogs aren't dangerous, I've no reason to be scared of dogs.') The latter idea of breaking down negative or unhealthy mental 'self talk' by the evidence of experience is well exemplified by the following therapy.

Flooding

The procedure is based on the premiss that the physiological responses of anxiety and panic cannot be maintained for prolonged periods, and that by being confronted by his fears the patient will, by necessity, overcome them.

In practice this is quite true. If it is impossible to avoid a phobic focus, the importance of the fear will dissipate relatively quickly. In other words, the patient who is phobic to dogs may be confronted with a room full of them and be offered no escape. Similarly, the agoraphobic patient may be taken into a town centre and made to stay until his fear is reduced.

However, it would be unusual for a patient with a dog phobia or agoraphobia to be treated by flooding. Neither would appear to require such potentially traumatising treatment, as both seem to respond to more gradual desensitisation. The main advantage flooding has over desensitisation is that it has a significant time advantage, which may be a major consideration in some disorders such as examination or travel phobias. Providing the procedure and likely effects are fully explained, and full consent is obtained, flooding may be a useful technique for such cases. However, we believe it would be irresponsible for us to leave flooding without adding some notes of caution. It should be remembered that faced with no escape from a flooding situation the patient's state of arousal may be very high, which would certainly result in an increased blood pressure and heart rate. Failure to ensure that the patient's health is able to maintain these cardiovascular changes would, in our opinion, be no less than professionally negligent. Should the patient collapse or faint for any reason irrespective of any possible physiological problems, flooding will have failed, as the patient has achieved an escape. Finally, the nurse involved in the procedure should assure herself that the patient will not suffer any psychological trauma as a result of this treatment.

Positive Conditioning

Positive conditioning is a behavioural technique based on Pavlov's work, which extends the foundation work of desensitisation. For example, if you have a patient who is phobic to rats, it is possible to achieve by desensitisation a state where the patient is no longer afraid of them — has a neutral attitude towards them. This is a desired result perhaps with rats, but what of the patient who seeks help because she is having difficulty of a sexual nature? If, after desensitisation, the patient is left with a neutral attitude to sexual behaviour, is this enough? Clearly the patient is still not returned to full function. This is where positive conditioning can be used appropriately to take over where desensitisation stops.

Sally, a 22-year-old married woman, was diagnosed as frigid. She had been married for a year when finally in desperation she went to her GP for help.

Sally had experienced pain during intercourse since her marriage. This had at first inhibited her sexual arousal, and led to her making excuses to her husband for not making love. On the occasions when sexual intercourse had taken place, her anxiety and tension had led to an even more painful experience. Eventually Sally completely avoided all sexual contact, and the mere thought of sex precipitated an acute anxiety attack.

After physical examination, it was decided that Sally required surgical intervention to relieve the pain she experienced during sex. Due to the urgency of the problem, this was expedited with very little delay, but subsequently Sally remained unable to return to lovemaking with her husband.

After several months of unsuccessful attempts to restore a normal marital relationship, Sally became increasingly depressed and was finally admitted to a psychiatric hospital with the symptoms of anxiety and depression. After a period of assessment, the diagnosis was thought to be depression associated with sexual phobia. Sally was in agreement with a course of desensitisation and responded very well to the treatment. She was taught how to relax and control her fear through breathing exercises. She was able to verbalise her anxieties and gradually conquer her fears of the sex act. During her short stay in hospital, she had three periods of weekend leave and on the last of these occasions was successful in having sexual intercourse with her husband.

Although her husband was delighted with the results of the therapy, Sally felt after a few months that she should be feeling more pleasure during sexual activity rather than the *non* feelings she expressed. It was at an out-patient follow-up that she told these feelings to the nurse/therapist, and in consultation with her doctor it was agreed to try to *positively condition* her towards a more pleasurable sexual experience: *positive conditioning.*

The Procedure

The theory of positive conditioning is simply to enable the patient to associate feelings of pleasure from one specific situation to transfer to another.

Sally was asked to choose some suitably relaxing music, which she found easy to listen, to, but not too distracting. The nurse asked Sally to relax and listen to the music, which at this point was playing at a very low volume, then to think of some pleasant experience she had in the past, and recall this to her. The subject of this 'pleasure experience' can be anything from a quiet conversation with someone she knew to lying on a beach in the sun.

Sally was then asked to intensify this feeling of pleasure in her thoughts, perhaps thinking of a particular experience that was even more pleasing. At this point the music was turned up slightly louder. Finally, Sally was asked to think of the most pleasing thing about this experience — intensifying the feelings of pleasure even further, and the music volume was increased accordingly.

This process was continued many times until the music itself could initiate these pleasures feelings without Sally having to recollect the pleasant experiences. The process may take as short a time as one half-hour session, or as many as 20. However, it should be continued until the nurse is sure the association exists.

Once the association is made, other artefacts may be introduced into the process. Sally repeated the process with the music, lying in a bed with her favourite nightdress/néglígé, perfume, sheets, continental quilt, etc. This also facilitated an association of pleasure with the articles and music. Once this association was firmly made, the process was ready to go into the final stage.

Sally underwent the treatment and her husband was acquainted with the procedure and was understanding enough to co-operate with it. Sally and her husband made love with all the articles previously conditioned, the music, perfume, nightie, sheets, etc., and gradually, over a period of months, the association of pleasure with the music etc. extended into the lovemaking itself. Within six months the normal pleasure responses of sexual intercourse were available to Sally with or without the accompaniments.

When a case history such as this is related, it often appears far fetched or slightly ridiculous. However, for the sceptics amongst you, may we remind you that this technique is not limited to therapy. The so called 'great lovers' of the past have employed most of the techniques in this therapy, by attempting to associate themselves with good food, music, wine, setting the seduction scene in pleasure arousing settings — soft lighting, soft furnishings, satin sheets, etc.

All these techniques are essentially Pavlovian:

Stimulus		Response
Food/perfume etc.	⟶	Pleasure
Food/perfume + ? Rudolf Valentino	⟶	Pleasure
Rudolf Valentino	⟶	Pleasure

The example of Sally's case was a special one, and will probably only be seen in out-patients' clinics and special centres. The procedure is usually under the supervision of clinical psychologists or a consultant psychiatrist specifically involved in psycho-sexual treatments. However, the general principles of positive conditioning hold true in various psychiatric situations. It is up to the psychiatric nurse to make herself familiar with these techniques and apply them within the resources available to her in appropriate situations. The principles involved are probably how some of our own behavioural responses have been conditioned in us, and they are potentially very powerful if used effectively.

Assertion Training

Assertion training is essentially taught through positive reinforcement, shaping and modelling. Many patients in psychiatric hospitals lack assertion skills, from the depressed patient in the recovering stages to the institutionalised patients of many years' standing.

Hospitals and institutions generally have a detrimental effect on the individual's desire to be an independent person. Many patients have learned to be subservient, to be told what to do. It is for these people, and many in the community, that assertion training can be a very helpful tool.

Before the process is explained, it is important to note that assertion training does not mean aggression. There are certain people assertion training would not benefit, for whom in fact it would be ill advised. Assertion training is definitely contraindicated in patients with latent aggressive drives, psychotic patients and potentially suicidal patients.

Ideally assertion training should be part of a course in social skills training, but certainly it is a necessary precursor for the timid, shy and inarticulate person before social skills training begins.

The purpose of assertion training is not to produce an aggressive, overbearing and truculent individual. It is simply to allow the individual to be more free to express his desires, feelings and thoughts in a clear and socially skilled way, without the accompanying anxiety that so many of us feel.

We wonder how many of you may have experienced the horrible feelings, the flushed features and sweating palms, when circumstances have prevailed where it has been necessary to complain? When it has really been important to state your case? How many times have you 'let things go' because it would be too traumatic or too much 'hassle' to say what you really feel?

It is, of course, your intellect that will determine in any given situation how to react, but additionally, how many time have your emotions ruled, restricted or inhibited your responses? Yet again, it can be seen how negative reinforcement by avoiding situations has in fact strengthened a reluctance to assert yourself. Similar to phobias, it is seen that avoiding the focus is very rewarding and breaking this down can only be achieved by positively rewarding the desired behaviour.

A few years ago, a colleague of one of the authors attended a behavioural course in assertion training. He was at the commencement of the course a rather polite, gentle and socially skilled individual. Roughly half-way through the course, during a dinner together, there appeared to be a total change in him. He was loud, rude and totally unskilled with waiters and the author to the extent that he was nearly left to finish his meal alone. He was, of course, suffering from an over exposure of therapy, which occurs quite frequently in short courses. It took him about a month gradually to assimilate his assertion skills into context on returning home. This graphic example serves to demonstrate that assertion training should be done slowly and surely, and preferably in conjunction with a social skills training course.

The Procedure

It should be remembered that each programme should be tailor-made for each individual. This can be done by observation and discussion with the patient. By noting situations that occur where a more assertive behaviour would be worth while and relating this to the patient, it is possible to pre-organise the individual for training, and increase motivation for change.

Individual or group exercises will enhance the desired outcomes at an early stage. Simple exercises modelled first by the nurse can be very useful as a basic step. Here are a few examples that, as can be seen, progress:

(1) *Eye contact exercise*
A group of patients sit in a circle and each patient in turn faces to his right and makes eye contact with the patient next to him, and states, 'I am (Joe Smith), what should I call you?' The patient responds by returning eye contact and saying 'Hello, Joe, my name is Fred Jones.' This continues in a circle with the nurse giving social reinforcement for each pair.

(2) *Eye contact + increasing volume*
The above exercise is repeated but the volume of speech is subsequently increased with each round.

(3) *Touch + eye contact + volume*
The second exercise is repeated, this time with each patient making physical contact with the other. (Usually appropriate contact is hand to shoulder.)

Variations of these can be made, i.e. passing objects around the circle, stating loudly what the object is. Or patients can hold hands in a circle saying 'Charge', firstly in a quiet voice and progressing to loud, and finally standing on a chair, still holding hands, but with them raised in the air shouting 'charge' at the tops of their voices.

The object of these exercises is gradually to allow the patient to becme less embarrassed in farcical situations and generally to disinhibit himself. The exercises should be made to fit the climate of the group. In each exercise the nurse's role is to model each step and reward the individual when successful.

Once this basic level is achieved, the nurse will design further more intricate exercises, tailored to the individual's needs.

Following the 'Charge' exercise, for instance, a refusal exercise may follow. Each patient requests (politely) something or some task from his partner, and the response should be:

'No, I don't wish to do that.'
'No, I don't wish to give you that.'
'I'm sorry, but I wish to keep that myself.'

Once the nurse feels sure that each patient is able to control his own wishes, and verbalise them confidently, more advanced and realistic exercises can be devised.

There are many practical applications of assertion skills training. Three practical and real programmes in which one of the authors was involved may be of interest.

Case One

Stephen, a personal friend, was very timid, and found great difficulty in embarrassing situations, which he had learned to avoid. He found it difficult to take faulty goods back to shops, and quite recently had had great difficulty in purchasing contraceptives. He had gone into chemists' shops and purchased innumerable supplies of aspirins, toothpaste and other articles, but had not been able to say, 'A packet of Durex, please.'

After applying a few basic exercises in communicating, he felt more confident. The advanced exercises devised for him were as follows. With the author present he purchased a pack of plain cigarettes, and shortly afterwards returned to the shop and exchanged them for filter tips. This was rewarded with praise, explaining that in fact most people are only too pleased to help if approached in a reasonable way. In fact it is important to make sure that each exercise is completed and does not go wrong, so, unbeknown to Stephen, the event had been pre-organised with the shopkeeper.

Once Stephen's confidence was built, it was easy for him to progress. Similar exercises were invented for him, including negotiating a change of dates for a holiday, exchanging smoking for non-smoking seats in the local theatre and culminating in him asking, in a crowded toilet in a pub, whether anyone had a 50 pence piece in exchange for five tens, and additionally announcing that he required it for the Durex machine.

Following this training Stephen changed quite remarkably, finding new confidence and interest in his job and acquaintances. Within six months, he had been promoted to under manager, which he intimated was mostly due to the therapy he had received.

Case Two

During psychotherapy Susan disclosed that one of her problems within her marriage was a lack of physical satisfaction during lovemaking with her husband. The problem stemmed mainly from her inability to discuss sexual matters frankly with him.

Using a modelling and rehearsal technique, employing an empty chair, she was able to use vocabulary that she had felt inhibited about previously. With constant reinforcement she soon became confident enough to disclose openly to the chair how she felt.

Before she was discharged this problem was discussed with her husband, who promised he would co-operate and help Susan explain how she felt with him as she had previously done in rehearsal. Susan's permission was, of course, sought before this, as it was an item of strict confidentiality.

Subsequently, Susan's sexual relationship with her husband improved and, along with it, her confidence increased and some of her mental problems disappeared.

Case Three

Mike, a student nurse, complained that he was unable to communicate to his seniors certain reservations he had about ward policy and his role in the ward. It was apparent that he would not be able to confront the charge nurse immediately in an open and honest way, nor would it be wise.

For him, then, a simple shaping programme was devised, with a student nurse colleague as the supportive therapist. Mike was to list the ideas and suggestions he wanted to make, and the constructive criticism he thought would be helpful. At each opportunity that arose, over a period of weeks, he and his colleague approached the charge nurse in private and discussed, in gradually increasing time periods, the less important to the most serious suggestions and criticisms. The student colleague was to make fewer and fewer contributions during the course of the programme, but was to continue the reassurance and support (see Table 3.3).

By the end of the allocation, Mike was surprised at how much he had been able to achieve with the charge nurse. Although he had not been able to change all the things he had hoped, he now felt more prepared to verbalise his ideas to other senior nurses in subsequent allocations.

It can be seen then that assertion training can be very effective not only for the patients, but for yourself if thought out well and with a little imagination, using behavioural principles applied intelligently.

Social Skills Training

A knowledge of social skills training is extremely important for professionals working in the mental illness field. Many patients who have been in hospital for long periods, or acute patients who find relationship formation difficult, may greatly benefit from this training.

For many patients in hospital, the need for social skill in any interaction has been removed, or its importance neglected. Patients tend to be given their daily requirements of food, warmth, entertainment and cigarettes without question, and certainly without a demand for 'please and thank you'. These requirements have become the patient's right without question or argument, and consequently the social graces have become redundant.

When one of the authors was last involved with social skills training with eight long-stay patients, most of whom had been in hospital over 20 years, he was quite startled to discover that none of them knew each other's names. Despite the fact that several slept in the same dormitory and sat together at meal times, none of them was aware of each other's existence. For them life

Table 3.3: A Possible Programme for Increasing Communication

Interview	Time	Topic	Student Input
Interview 1	2 minutes	Ward reports	Verbal support for whole interview
Interview 2	5 minutes	Days off	Verbal support as appropriate
Interview 3	7 minutes	Patients' meals	Non-verbal support throughout interview
Interview 4	10 minutes	Personal clothing	Non-verbal support 1st half of the interview
Interview 5	12 minutes	Trips out for patients	Non-verbal support 2nd half of the interview
Interview 6	15 minutes	Drug administration	Simply in attendance
Interview 7	18 minutes	Doctor's rounds	
Interview 8	20 minutes	Holidays for patients	Non-attendance but support afterwards

had become so monotonous, uninteresting and inflexible that a normal social interaction had been reduced to a blind meaningless togetherness, without acknowledgement or contact with their company of peers.

Some years ago, as a student nurse, one of us remembers his Principal Tutor define mental illness as a 'breakdown of interpersonal relationships'. Without seeking causes, or anything more technical, we have always tended to agree with him. If this statement is true, and it is accepted that social skills are a cornerstone of interpersonal relationships, it can be seen that social skills training is essential in most manifestations of mental illness.

The Procedure

Social skills training largely uses the principles of shaping and modelling. It is also hoped that when primary stages are reached, the intrinsic satisfaction and reward will self-perpetuate the learning or relearning process. Success will breed success, or, as in this case, a smile will breed more smiles.

How can the average nurse begin in social skills training? What should she do? How can exercises be formulated? In fact for the nurse, social skills training should be one of the most easily implemented schedules. The reasons for this are as follows:

(1) Most nurses are very socially skilled and present 'good' models for patients to follow.
(2) By examining their own social skills, it is only a single step to generalise these into simple exercises for the patient to engage in.
(3) The nurse is the most powerful person to reinforce social skills in the patient, as they are in constant contact 24 hours a day.
(4) The nurse is in control of very powerful reinforcement situations during the day, i.e. meal times, activities, cigarettes, recreation, hygiene and dressing.

It should be within all nurses' capabilities to list the components of their social skills, and by reinforcing them in the patients, to teach a high degree of proficiency.

A typical list may be:

Greetings: (non-verbal) smiles, nods, handshakes, waves; (verbal) 'Hi,' 'Hello,' 'Nice to see you,' etc.
Names: rehearsal and memory of significant people in everyday contact.
Interest: remembering the significant interests of people around you. Mental notes of particular people's hobbies, pastimes — in order to make interesting conversation.
Conversation skills: appropriate listening, eye contact, encouragement and remarks. Appropriate responses at time intervals.
Hygiene: general and oral hygiene and an awareness of the effects of its absence.
Body space: appropriate space requirements for the rank, culture and type of relationship, i.e. acquaintance/friend/lover. This should also include appropriate use of touch.
Dress: differentiating types of dress customary for various situations and environments. This should include colour matching and choice of colours for congruence of occasion, e.g. black or dark for funerals, light, bright for weddings.
Eating: use and knowledge of conventional standards. Conversation during meals and ordering or preparation of meals.
Money: knowledge of currency, values and budgeting.

Social skills may be taught individually or in groups. Essentially, individually constructed exercises should be tailored to the stage of skills the patient is presently operating. In long-stay wards, often the entire population may need to begin at a very basic stage and progress via modelling exercises and shaping programmes.

An Illustrative Case

Four long-stay patients who had been in hospital on the same ward agreed to work with a nurse purely on social skills, progressing to a daily living programme with a view to discharge together in a group home.

(1) The patients were introduced to each other and rehearsed each other's names by throwing a cushion around in a circle saying their own name and the name of the person catching it. The nurse is included in this, and this continues as a warm-up exercise daily in each formal session.

Each patient is asked to discuss with the others his particular interests or concerns and then each patient is asked to say what he could remember of each of his companion's interests. This also continues daily until each has a better understanding of the other, then is intermittently repeated throughout the training.

(2) Meal times are arranged so that the four patients are seated together. The nurse will eat and make social contact throughout the meal, thus modelling a skilled interaction. Subsequently the nurse encourages and praises similar imitative interactions on future occasions.

(3) Gradual progression through the basic skills continued via two and three hour sessions of role playing, conversational skills, smiling, body posture and responding appropriately in various situations, e.g. a supermarket, public house, restaurant.

When these had been achieved in role play, the sessions were extended into the real situations with the nurse present giving support and encouragement.

(4) The patients were asked at any time during the training to comment on each other's oral and personal hygiene, thus helping the others to become more aware of the detrimental effects this has on social interactions. The nurse also contributed to this by comments followed immediately by helping the patient come to a solution, i.e. shower/bath/oral hygiene and positively reinforcing the result.

(5) Organised shopping expeditions for food and meal preparation were taken in turn by each patient and followed by social reinforcement. Patients were encouraged to verbalise their praise of each other's abilities, and also to make constructive criticisms in a socially acceptable way.

(6) Choice of personal clothing was linked with particular events and excursions so immediate social reinforcement was available appropriately in each situation.

(7) Finally, before discharge, a trial period of four weeks on a set budget was agreed with the nurse supervising daily in a hospital 'half way house'.

The outcome of this short course (approximately three months) was remarkable. The four patients were discharged and are still supervised by a community psychiatric nurse and social worker. These particular patients have now been discharged for three years and are fully integrated back into a suburban society. Although still requiring support and one patient being readmitted for two weeks, they have remained stable and are well accepted by their neighbours and the general community.

Key Concepts

(1) Behaviourism has a significant role to play in people's everyday lives. Understanding behavioural science can be tremendously helpful to psychiatric nurses, and secure a better quality of life for the patients they seek to help. Skinner and Pavlov's experimental work has proved beyond reasonable doubt that behaviour is largely dependent on stimuli within our environment, responses to that stimuli and the consequences following that response.

(2) From the experimental work done by Skinner and others, behaviour modification principles can be extrapolated and applied to humans in real life situations, i.e.
   (a) Weakening behaviour by punishment and extinction.
   (b) Strengthening behaviour by positive and negative reinforcement.
   (c) Developing behaviour by modelling and shaping.

(3) Using a more eclectic approach, and incorporating the principles of both operant and classical conditioning, a wide range of treatment programmes can be created to help the psychiatric patient. This rather broader use of behavioural principles is termed behaviour therapy.

(4) Before commencing any behavioural treatments, the nurse should consider the ethical and moral issues involved, i.e.
   who — is the client? (child, psychotic patient, etc.)
   — gave permission/consent?
   — decided what is desirable change?
   what — behaviours are being changed?
   — methods are to be employed?
   why — is it necessary?

   Are all these questions being answered in an ethically supportable manner? How would you feel if you were the patient?

Conclusion

This chapter seeks to explain some difficult concepts of

behavioural science in a rather simplistic way. We hope that ending the chapter with some programmes may by analogy help focus some of the principles of behaviourism, and aid the nurse to gain deeper insight. Since behavioural programmes were introduced into psychiatric nursing, perhaps as recently as two decades ago, much ingenuity and imagination have gone into making them work for psychiatric patients. Many patients who may have remained in hospital are now discharged and living effectively in the community due to the help they received from behavioural strategies employed by conscientious, knowledgeable and caring nurses. It is our hope that this chapter may stimulate interest in and produce a greater potential source of help for psychiatric patients.

Suggested Further Reading

Barker, Philip *Behaviour Therapy Nursing* (Croom Helm, London, 1982)
Barker, Philip and Fraser, Douglas (eds.) *The Nurse as Therapist: A Behavioural Model* (Croom Helm, London, 1985)
Berni, Rosemarian and Fordyce, Wilbert E. *Behaviour Modification and the Nursing Process*, 2nd edn (Mosby, St Louis, 1977)
Blackman, Derek *Operant Conditioning: An Experimental Analysis of Behaviour* (Methuen, London, 1974)
Carlson, Carolyn E. and Blackwell, Betty *Behavioural Concepts and Nursing Intervention* (Lippincott, Philadelphia, 1978)
Eysenck, H.J. *Behaviour Therapy and the Neuroses* (Pergamon Press, London, 1960)
Gentry, W. Doyle (ed.) *Applied Behaviour Modification* (Mosby, St Louis, 1975)
Mackay, Dougal *Clinical Psychology: Theory and Therapy*, Essential Psychology Series F3 (Methuen, London, 1975)
Marks, Isaac M. *Fears and Phobias* (Heinemann, London, 1969)
Mathews, Andrew M. and Johnston, Derek W. *Agoraphobia: Nature and Treatment* (Tavistock, London, 1981)
Schaefer, Helmuth H. and Martin, Patrick L. *Behavioural Therapy* (McGraw-Hill, London, 1969)

4 THE PSYCHIATRIC NURSING PROCESS

Introduction

When a patient is admitted, he is often in a condition where his needs are obvious, e.g. the unsteady patient requires assistance when walking, the dehydrated patient requires fluid, the overactive patient requires rest. Frequently, after careful assessment, these needs are met by the nurse. The information gathered by a single nurse on first meeting the patient is invaluable, not only to the nurse in question, but for other nurses in the team. A psychiatric nurse is trained to use observational skills in order to build up a profile of an individual. It is this skill of observation, often combined with effective listening and questioning, which allows the nurse to identify more than the obvious needs, and ensure that *all* the needs of the patient are met.

To facilitiate this course of action effectively, a *systematic problem solving approach* is useful. This approach is described in four stages:

— Assessment
— Planning.
— Implementation
— Evaluation.

Although this approach will be described as four separate stages, they are, in fact, dependent upon each other and often occur simultaneously for different aspects of nursing care, e.g.

Two policemen accompanied Mr Miles into the ward office. He was in a neglected state and appeared agitated. The staff nurse, taken aback by this sudden interruption, turned and said, 'Hello, what's all this about then?'

Mr Miles reacted, using verbal abuse directed towards the staff nurse, the other staff and this 'so called bloody prison disguised as a hospital'.

It took the considerable skill of the charge nurse to distract and reassure Mr Miles and, by offering a cup of tea, she succeeded in taking him to a quiet part of the ward where the foundation of a nurse/patient relationship could be established.

These interactions illustrate that, because of the insensitivity of the staff nurse and his subsequent response, the charge nurse had to use her skill in order to defuse a potentially awkward moment.

Analysing this in the framework of the nursing process, the stages can be illustrated by applying them to the immediate needs of Mr Miles:

Assessment: The patient is in an agitated, anxious state. He seems to have been neglecting himself recently, is overactive and highly sensitive.
Planning: To defuse the situation, distract the patient and channel his energies to something more positive.
Implementation: Using a calm approach, distract the patient.
Evaluation: This approach is successful from an interpersonal point of view and for this particular incident.

This would satisfy the immediate needs of Mr Miles.

Once these needs have been met, longer-term goals will be set by further assessment and subsequent planning involving the patient, to agree these goals of care. Further plans would include:

— encouraging adequate nutrition;
— facilitating the maintenance of personal hygiene.

Further assessment, planning and evaluation would take place as the relationship progresses, and the patient becomes more involved in agreeing his own care goals. The information that this nurse has gathered within the first few hours with the patient is invaluable to the current and future nursing care of the patient. It becomes necessary therefore to communicate these observations to the rest of the staff in order to maintain continuity of care. The nursing process facilitates this communication effectively by allowing the nurse to note systematically his observations in such a way that the patient's problems and subsequent needs are identified. These needs, once placed in priority, agreed by the patient, and written into his nursing care plan, can be acted upon by the whole team, thus allowing the patient to be nursed skilfully and with an adequate knowledge base. The record of the ongoing assessment and care plan which states the problems, the nursing care which is expected to resolve them and the date of review ensure continuity of care by other nurses who add up-to-date information, and provides a 'baseline' for effective evaluation. Where evaluation leads to the conclusion that progress has not been made, another form of approach can be tried. Aspects of this overview will become clearer when each stage is considered in detail.

Assessment

Assessment is a continual process of gathering information in order to establish the needs of the patient. The information, once accumulated and organised, provides a basis for evaluating the patient's progress. It aids the understanding of the patient if performed skilfully, and engenders trust and confidence in the nurse. Assessment of the patient is the basis of structured nursing care, allowing planning and implementation of an individualised nursing care plan. It requires the nurse to have all the skills described so far, mainly interpersonal, listening and questioning skills and, in addition, *observational skills.* Before embarking upon a description of 'assessment', it seems appropriate to consider the skill of observation.

Observation involves being sensitive to the relevant facets of patient behaviour that may be useful in aiding the patient's recovery, and which must be communicated accurately and objectively.

Increased sensitivity and awareness of the sort of things psychiatric nurses should be observing arise out of relevant studying and experience.

The following list will serve as a useful guide to the observation that the nurse may make on any patient:

(a) General appearance.
(b) Speech.
(c) Behaviour patterns.
(d) Mood.
(e) Activities.
(f) Eating/dietary habits.
(g) Sleep patterns.
(h) Interests/hobbies.
(i) Attitude.
(j) Insight and judgement.
(k) Memory and orientation.

The above list serves as a general guide to the different aspects of behaviour and thinking the nurse may observe and perceive. The skilled nurse is one who can observe and decide on the relevant and significant facets of behaviour and record them accurately. When recording, it is important to distinguish between observations made and conclusions drawn from them. Only actual behaviour should be recorded, without the presumptive explanation of it.

The physical state of the individual should be noted as well as his general appearance and behaviour. This enhances the overall picture of the patient, and increases the likelihood of identifying all his needs. Table 4.1 may help highlight the various observations the nurse may make.

The nurse decides on the relevant facts and communicates these as objective observations so that the care team can identify particular problems. Other reasons for observation are:

— to ascertain signs and symptoms on which a diagnosis can be made.
— to note improvements or deterioration in the patient's condition in response to treatment, including drug side effects, or to changes in environment.
— to be aware of any new physical or mental illness developing.
— to recognise signs that suggest the patient is likely to behave in such a way as to harm himself, or others.
— to assess those factors in the patient's personality that can be exploited in aiding his recovery.

The information gained from the charge nurse formed the first steps towards assessment. The patient, however, is only one source of information. Table 4.2 summarises other sources.

The reasons for assessment are as follows.

(1) *It ensures specific problems are identified.* The obvious needs of the patient are most likely to be met by any caring professional. However, if it was left at this superficial level, many issues and often fundamental problems would be left unidentified. Mrs Little, for example, was admitted presenting symptoms of severe depression. Her history indicated a progressive deterioration over the past six months. On admission her needs were those commonly experienced by depressed patients relating to basic physiological needs, observation and acceptance. It was because

Table 4.1: Some Physical Observations that may be Useful

Part of the Body	**Possible Observation**
Hair	General condition Infested Wig
Eyes	Red/sore Tearful Glasses/contact lenses
Nose	Signs of infection Breathing problems
Ears	Clean Wax
Mouth	Expression Infection Dehydration (tongue) Teeth Self-care Cyanosis
Arms and hands	Puncture marks Bruises Neglect Movement Tense Sweaty palms Nails Position
Body	Posture Deformity Shape
Legs	Illness/deformity (bone) Oedema/swelling Mobility safe or not Type of walk Position/tense
Feet	Blisters Deformity Shoes
General	Skin — rashes — red — dry Dress — clean — unkempt

Table 4.2: Sources of Information

We obtain information from	By	In order to	Thus identifying
The patient			
Other nurses		Acquire a	
Relatives	Observing		Patients'
Friends		nursing	
Past records			
General practitioner	Questioning	history and	problems
Psychiatrist			
Social worker		patient	
Psychologist	Listening		and needs
Chaplain/priest		profile	

the nurse used her listening and questioning skills that she discovered that Mrs Little's husband had died over a year ago, and her daughter had recently moved away. These facts could have been missed, facts that are of paramount importance to the patient and should be known if any therapeutic relationship is to be established.

(2) *It helps establish what is normal for the patient.* This is important in order to avoid expecting a person to fall in line with the organisation of the ward. Mr Brown, for example, is not used to eating an evening meal, usually goes to bed around eight at night, and rises early. Reported observations of Mr Brown's behaviour could be interpreted as poor appetite, withdrawn in the evening, with early morning waking (see p. 147). It seems important for observation based on the knowledge of what is usual for that particular patient to be made, thus avoiding misinterpreting quite normal behaviour for some clinical manifestation of a particular illness.

(3) *It serves as a basis for evaluating the patient's progress and the effectiveness of nursing care.* Initial assessment will all too often build a profile of a patient in desperate need. The profile will show as time progresses whether or not the patient is improving or deteriorating, and whether the nursing care is appropriate, effective or otherwise. Without this 'baseline', monitoring progress becomes difficult, as there is very little to measure against.

(4) *It facilitates understanding, thus enhancing the nurse/patient relationship.* The empathic understanding (see p. 27) the nurse achieves is dependent upon the understanding of that patient's

behaviour, feelings and experiences. This understanding is partly achieved by using the skills of listening (see p. 41). The profile established and the subsequent records kept will enhance the chances of the *nursing team*, as opposed to one individual, achieving some degree of empathy. It creates a total view of the patient rather than a fragmented one.

So far it has been established that assessment involves information gathering. We have explained:

— How the information is gathered.
— When the information is gathered, i.e. continually.
— Why the information is gathered.
— Where or from whom to acquire the information.

What remains is related to the practical application: what is specifically assessed, and how is it recorded? There are many assessment forms available, all designed to help the nurse cover all relevant areas associated with the 'patient profile'. The differences are usually due to the variation in specialities, i.e. the information required from an elderly person will have a different emphasis to a younger person whose stay in hospital may be much shorter (acute) (see Figures 4.1 and 4.2). From these two forms, it can be seen that the assessment of the elderly is more physically orientated than the assessment of the younger patient. We believe that the assessment should continue to be tailor-made to the emphasis of care in any given area, e.g. elderly, child, rehabilitation. General considerations common to all areas should be included. A model of nursing that may be helpful when compiling these is that of the activities of living by Roper, Logan and Tierney (1981). These cover the whole spectrum of life functions and encompass the:

physical
psychological } needs of the individual
social

They are:

— maintaining a safe environment;
— communicating;
— breathing;

— eating and drinking;
— eliminating;
— personal cleansing and dressing;
— controlling body temperatures;
— mobilising;
— working and playing;
— expressing sexuality;
— sleeping;
— dying.

By considering each aspect and relating it appropriately to the patient, a complete assessment is ensured. Using appropriate listening and questioning skills *relevant* information can be gained from each area *if appropriate at the time of assessment.*

Some useful exercises to do now would be to:

(a) Analyse the two assessment forms and question:
  — are all the activities of living included?
  — if not, why not? Are they all appropriate?
(b) Write down some questions that would:
  — be appropriate to each activity of living.
  — would gain significant information from the patient.

The activities of living are very useful as a guideline toward total patient assessment. They do, however, require further expansion in order to ensure that all relevant details are covered. Another list, which could act as a guideline on a nursing history sheet, seems more specific and appropriate to psychiatry (see Table 4.3).

None of the lists presented so far attempts to place activities in any order of priority. The priority of care is established very early on, and is dependent upon the specific needs of the patient at that time. Maslow (1970) described the human hierarchy of needs (see Figure 4.3), which serves as a useful guideline for nurses in caring for patients in relation to these priorities. Maslow's theory essentially states that the lower needs are the basic needs of living, and until those are satisfied to a level whereby functional living is possible, very little, if any, motivation can be aimed at satisfying the higher needs. In practice, this means that a patient who is in severe pain is not going to mind if the nurse does not involve him

Table 4.3: Nursing History Sheet

Patient's name
and other admission details:

Psychological	*Physical*
Mood/affect	Eating/diets
Memory	Sleeping/resting
Intellect	Weight
Perception	Hygiene
Speech content and quality	Dress
Communication	Elimination
Psychotic traits	Health/exercise
Neurotic traits	Alcohol/tobacco/drugs
Personality and presentation	Sex
	Mobility
Social	Sight
Family/partner	
Friends/relationships	Hearing
Accommodation	
Work	*Patient's view of admission/referral*
Finances	
Legal problems	*Immediate nursing problem*
Social life	
Hobbies/interests and partners	
Spiritual	

Source: J. Heath, G. Law and I. Cross (1982).

in choosing which pair of pyjamas to wear. The nursing priority in this case is to relieve that patient of pain. This principle can be related to all areas of care, but most are not as clear cut as the example given. Rather than a decision being made on what needs should be catered for first, it is usually a question of emphasis, finding out which need should be concentrated on most, at the same time not neglecting the higher needs which, of course, become progressively more important as the lower needs are satisfied.

Once sufficient information has been gathered to enable the nurse to identify the individual patient's nursing problem, and the obvious priorities are established (often these must be seen to without delay, especially those that are life threatening or whereby a patient is a danger to himself or others), then steps can be taken to communicate these accurately in some form of care plan. This usually involves transferring information recorded on an assessment form onto a care plan form in the guise of a nursing problem. As

Figure 4.1: Information Sheet

PERSONAL INFORMATION	MEDICAL/PARAMEDICAL INFORMATION	SOCIAL & ECONOMIC INFORMATION Delete where appropriate
NAME: Mr/Mrs/Ms	CONSULTANT:	ACCOMMODATION IN COMMUNITY:
ADDRESS:	REGISTRAR:	HOSTEL, PART III, RENTED ACCOMMODATION
TEL: M/S/SEP	GENERAL PRACTITIONER:	House, Bungalow, Flat
D.O.B.:	ADDRESS:	FURNISHED/UNFURNISHED
RELIGION: Relationship	TEL:	CENTRAL HEATING Yes/No
OCCUPATION	COMMUNITY SW:	LIVES WITH SELF — RELATIVES — FRIENDS
NEXT OF KIN:	TEL:	FINANCIAL STATUS:
NAME:	CPN:	Income Wage Pension Interest Benefits Other:
ADDRESS:	TEL:	Who takes care of these:
TEL: Relationship	DAY HOSPITAL:	Self Relatives Friend Solicitor Hospital Court of Protection Other:
OTHERS INVOLVED:	TEL:	
NAME:	OTHER DISCIPLINES INVOLVED AFTER ADMISSION:	Please specify
ADDRESS::	Social Worker:	NAME:
TEL: Relationship	Occupational Therapist:	ADDRESS:

NAME: ADDRESS: TEL: Relationship	Physiotherapist: Psychologist:	TEL:
TIME OF PRESENT ADMISSION:	OTHER RELEVANT INFORMATION:	ADDITIONAL SOCIAL INFORMATION:
REASON FOR PRESENT ADMISSION:		HOBBIES/INTERESTS:
	NURSING HISTORY SHEET (Please delete inappropriate words and/or remarks)	
PSYCHIATRIC PROFILE: MOOD:	PHYSICAL DISABILITY/DISORDERS PHYSICAL DISORDER: TREATMENT:	PHYSICAL DISABILITIES/DISORDERS continued PERSONAL HYGIENE: General Hygiene Remarks: Very Tidy Tidy Untidy Good Fair Poor Assistance needed

Figure 4.1: continued

THOUGHT CONTENT:

ORIENTATION:

BEHAVIOUR:

OTHER OBSERVATIONS:

APPEARANCE:
Normal Dehydrated Obese
Frail Thin
Remarks:

SKIN CONDITION:
Wounds Rash Abrasions
Decubitus Ulcers Oedema
Jaundice Bruises
Remarks:

TEETH:
Good Poor Dentures Upper
Lower

HEARING:
Good Poor Fair Wears Aid
Left Right

SIGHT:
Left Eye: Good Fair Poor Blind
Right Eye: Good Fair Poor Blind
Spectacles: Yes/No
Permanent Reading Only

DIET:
Appetite: Good Fair Poor Fluctuates
Special Diet:
Dislikes:
Sugar: Yes/No

FLUID INTAKE:
Good Fair Poor Fluctuates
Dislikes:
Sugar: Yes/No

TOILET HABITS:
Bladder: Continent Incontinent
Nocturia Dysuria Stress
Bowels: Continent Incontinent Fluctuates
Regular Constipation
Use of appliances: Yes/No
Remarks:

	SLEEP PATTERN: Needs Daytime Naps Yes/No Good Short Periods Long Periods Restful Restless Sedation	OTHER RELEVANT INFORMATION:
ATTITUDES/EXPECTATIONS OF TREATMENT:	MOBILITY: No Assistance Some Assistance Total Assistance Remarks:	

PATIENT'S DESCRIPTION
Height
Weight
Scars
Deformities
Colour of Eyes
Colour of Hair
Distinguishing Features
Complexion
Habits

Temperature		Urinalysis	Specific Gravity	
Pulse		Glucose	pH	
Respiration		Ketones	Bilirubin	
Blood Pressure		Protein	Blood	

Source: Adapted from Clifton Hospital, York.

Figure 4.2: Nursing Care Plan

	First Names	Surname	Consultant
Address	Date of Birth Marital Status Occupation Religion Legal Status	Details of Occupation Details of Dependants	General Practitioner and address

Relative or person to be contacted Address Telephone no. Day Night	Date of admission Accompanied by Referred from	Social Worker Community Psychiatric Nurse Special dietary requirements
Recent history and reason for admission Sleep pattern	Reason given by patient Usual weekly routine	Hobbies/interests

Anxieties related to admission	Care of dependants/work anxieties
Previous history Number of admissions Details cf last admission	Present admission. Information and medical directives
Observation of physical and mental condition on admission	
Observation after 24 hours	

Source: Adapted from Northern General Hospital, Sheffield.

Figure 4.3: A Human Hierarchy of Needs

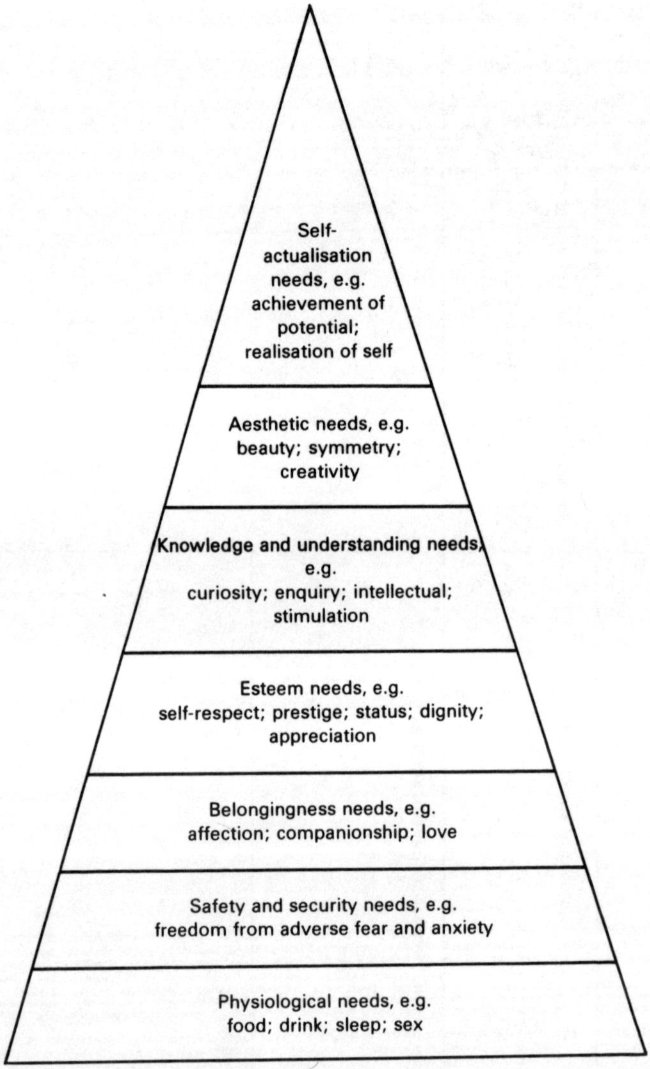

Source: A.H. Maslow (1970).

Table 4.4: Potential Problems

	Assessment Form	Care Plan
	Information (or observed behaviour)	*Nursing problem*
(a)	Mrs Little is expressing thoughts of unworthiness — stating she is —not worth the attention', and that 'she would be better dead'. She appears unconcerned about her appearance and personal hygience. This according to relatives has become increasingly worse.	Actual problems — poor self-esteem, lack of personal hygiene care. Potential problem — suicide or attempt.
(b)	Mr Brown, aged 72, is in a debilitated state, he has not been drinking and eating for the past three weeks, and has a chest infection. Requires nursing in bed.	Actual problem — refusing to take solids, reluctantly drinking some fluids. Potential problem — bed sores; breathing difficulties.

well as the obvious problems presented, as when a patient refuses to to drink, there is also the question of potential problems — in this example it could be dehydration. This becomes clear in Table 4.4.

It can be seen from the examples given, both preventive and curative action will be required in the planning of nursing care.

Planning

Once sufficient information has been gathered to enable specific problems to be identified, steps can be taken towards developing a unique care plan for the patient. It may be that circumstances require nursing actions to be implemented before any formalised plans can be drawn up (refer back to Mr Miles' admission). This is, of course, what happens in practice, and it is only after a period of days, and sometimes weeks, that a functional plan can be fully implemented. In nursing practice, however, there is no question of delay for the sake of the process, for 'the Nursing Process assessment cannot be carried out by a nurse alone ... Assessment must be a part of the nursing intervention' (Altschul, 1977). This emphasises that the assessment can facilitate the therapeutic relationship, if done skilfully, and that assessment requires a team approach as opposed to an individual taking sole responsibility. So, in fact, the planning of nursing care is ongoing from the first introduction to the patient and priorities are established very early on within the relationship. However, there is a need to systematise these plans in order to ensure continuity and measure progress. This involves setting short-term and long-term objectives of nursing care. In order to avoid confusion over terminology, it is necessary to clarify the terms that we intend to use.

A 'goal' (or long-term objective) is a statement of intent related to the long term:

Problem	*Goal*
Patient denies the death of her husband.	To facilitate the patient's acceptance of her husband's death.

An 'objective of care' (or sub-goal) is also a statement of intent, but more specific and related to the short term.

To achieve a single goal may require many objectives. One objective of nursing care for the above goal may be:

Goal	*Objective*
To facilitate the patient's acceptance of her husband's death.	To encourage gradual acceptance of her situation and feelings in relation to her husband, in order for her to be able to talk about his death within the next two weeks.

or

Problem	*Goal*	*Objective*
Fear of crowds, shops, public transport and lifts.	To help the patient overcome his fear to the extent of leading a life that is normal for him.	To help the patient overcome his fear of small groups of people before attempting to tolerate a crowd of people.

Note that in each objective there is a time factor which enables progress to be monitored, and facilitates evaluation. The long-term 'goal' will communicate to everyone concerned the direction of care and what it is hoped will be achieved. The short-term objective relates to what is being focused upon now and will encourage the patient towards improvement. The long-term objectives are often beyond the capacity of the patient to accept, due to the nature of his illness. However, the short-term objectives are more tangible and will often act as a reinforcer if achieved.

Before embarking upon writing specific objectives of care, several important factors must be considered. The objectives of care must be realistic and achievable, and the resources required available. The resources required are, almost invariably, the staff and their expertise. The objectives should be realistic from the nurse's point of view, but also from the patient's perspective. As far as is possible and appropriate, the patient should be involved in the planning of care, together with his family, which is often an integral part of a care programme and which, in many cases, is progressively involved as discharge of the patient approaches. This principle of negotiation is particularly important, for many of the problems presented are so complex that no one individual could realistically be expected to cater for them. So each care plan is drawn up by the care team, where necessary involving staff of other disciplines as well as the ward nursing team.

The specific, realistic and achievable objectives set allow the appropriate nursing action to be decided upon.

For the process to work effectively, the nursing action needs to be communicated extremely clearly and precisely, to ensure that anyone reading it will be under no illusions about what is required for that individual. To illustrate this, which of two nursing actions do you think will most likely help towards achieving the objective set for John:

Nursing Action 1
Observe John when he appears to be troubled by hallucinations, and prevent aggressive outbursts.

Nursing Action 2
When John appears to be troubled by hallucinations, sit by him and firmly distract him by reinforcing some aspect of reality. He seems to respond well to the subject of current sporting events.

The first 'nursing action' leaves much to the discretion of the nurse, whereas the second is clear and specific and more likely to result in consisent nursing practice.

When deciding on the nursing action to take, the consequences involved in its implementation must be considered. A final check is often useful before implementation:

— Is the nursing action based upon a careful assessment of the patient's problems and needs?
— Have all the appropriate and available resources been considered?
— Are the care team, patient and, if appropriate, the family, aware of the possible consequences of the implementation of the planned nursing care?

When the nursing team has achieved this state of readiness, implementation of the care plan can go ahead.

Implementation

This stage requires the nurse to carry out the agreed nursing action and proceed to initiate the action by the method chosen on the care plan. The skills required to do this are those of the psychiatric nurse, which this book attempts to identify. However, there are several general principles to be considered when implementing nursing care. These are:

(1) *Concentrate on the needs of the individual.* Is it possible to solve a nursing problem without considering the patient's needs? For example, a patient who becomes noisy and distressed and starts screaming at night is removed to a side ward and given sedation. The problem has been solved in the short term. By ensuring that the needs of the individual are identified and satisfied, the likelihood of the problem being solved in the long term increases. In the example given, if the nurse took time to sit with the patient, listen, talk, touch and reassure, it is possible that the needs of safety, security, warmth and love will be satisfied and the patient might sleep without sedation. The information gained in this incident, if appropriately communicated and followed up, could have a positive effect on the overall nursing approach.

(2) *Be sensitive to your feelings and behaviour when delivering nursing care.* When the nurse is aware of her own feelings, she increases the likelihood of understanding her own behaviour, thus preventing a 'blind' approach to the patient. It makes all the difference when a nurse approaches a patient whom she knows and appreciates exactly what she is doing. The patient certainly senses this difference and reacts positively. The nurse, being 'cued' in to her own state, is able to make a more effective evaluation: as well as looking at external factors when things go wrong, internal ones are also explored.

(3) *Make full use of the expertise around you: use a team approach.* Appreciating the resources available within any given nursing team will allow certain problems to be handled more efficiently. That is to say, if there is a nurse who relates well with a particular patient, then it may be appropriate that she undertakes the key role in his care. This can only happen if communication is accurate and consistent within the team. This is only one example; there are many others where the team approach is of more value than an individual one, e.g. dealing with aggressive incidents or other crisis situations, collection of 'data' concerning the patients, assessment of social, physical and psychological states, or the organisation of large group activities such as ward socials or outings. By the team taking a collective responsibility for the patient's care plan, the possibility of engendering trust and confidence in the patient will increase, thus forming a sound foundation for a therapeutic relationship to be established.

(4) *Never lose sight of the original goal.* To ensure that the direction of nursing care is appropriate to the needs of the patient, the nurse must not forget the original goal set. By frequently reviewing goals and sub-goals and ensuring that the methods chosen are appropriate, the nurse continually evaluates everything she does, which ensures effective use of time, resources and skills.

(5) *Be sensitive to the patient's changing environment.* An individual's behaviour changes, often dramatically, depending upon where and with whom he is. The nurse must be sensitive to this, and be aware that the approach in the care plan may have been based on a 'one to one' interaction. This approach may be quite inappropriate in different circumstances. The patient who talks freely about himself at an initial interview may be virtually mute in the company of other patients.

(6) *Ensure a safe environment at all times.* The nurse must be

alert to the environment and the feelings and behaviour of all the patients and staff within that environment when implementing nursing care. By doing this she will be able to intervene appropriately to minimise any risks or dangers the patient may take or be exposed to, e.g. being sensitive to changing moods, behaviours, disappointments, effects of emotional crises and using skills to diffuse a potentially dangerous environment or removing a patient from the same.

Evaluation

It can be seen from reading the previous stages that evaluation is far from a separate entity. The skills required for evaluation are virtually the same as those required for assessment, planning and implementation. Evaluation of nursing care starts from the first interaction with the patient to well after discharge and into continuing care within the framework of community services. It is an ongoing process, necessary to measure the effectiveness of the care given.

How is effectiveness measured? It could be said that effectiveness is proportional to the degree of goal achievement. If the goal was 'the patient will walk around the hospital without support' and the patient is able to do this within the time set, the nursing care has been totally effective and successful. Evaluation is not only an ongoing process, but a process during which individual nursing action is considered in the perspective of the total care given, for if the result of the above goal was 'the patient can now walk around the hospital without support, but resents the nursing staff for pushing him into this and refuses to participate further in his programme', the nursing approach in this case may have been inappropriate.

One of the ways to look at evaluation is by examining pertinent issues relevant to questioning what has been done so far:

— Was the goal originally set realistic and appropriate?
— Was sufficient time allowed for it to be achieved?
— Was the patient sufficiently motivated?
— Did the patient agree?
— Were all the resources available used effectively?
— Was the plan flexible enough to allow for patient progress or

deterioration?
- Were the methods chosen the right ones?
- When assessing the patient, were all relevant factors taken into consideration?

When exploring these issues, the evaluation of nursing care revolves around the evaluation of the nurse's 'performance'. Looking at the above questions from this perspective, the questions could read:

- Did I expect too much from the patient and myself?
- Was my explanation to the patient adequate?
- Did I consider sufficient alternatives?
- Was I too rigid in my thinking and approach?
- Was I insensitive to change within the patient?
- Did I make the right choice in my approach?
- Was my original assessment of the patient inaccurate?

A major step toward meaningful evaluation is acceptance of responsibility by the nurse and acknowledgement of her position as a major controlling factor of circumstances. Once this has been achieved, serious steps can be taken towards improving her performance and ultimately the care that is given. One step is to question and search for reasons for your behaviour in order to have greater awareness if a similar set of circumstances arises again, which will enhance the chances of coping more effectively. This search and reasoning can be achieved by attempting to look at yourself objectively and accepting feedback from other sources relevant to the situation, e.g.

Since David's admission two weeks ago, all efforts to relate to him have been rejected. He has become increasingly aggressive and now refuses to say very much to nursing staff except to hurl abuse, claiming that they are deceitful, dishonest, liars and want to keep him there for good.

It was only after an honest appraisal by the whole team that it came to light that one of the major contributing factors to David's condition was the conflicting information that nursing staff had given to him on different occasions. On admission one nurse said, 'You're an informal patient, here of your own free will.' Later another nurse said, 'You cannot leave, you are compulsorily detained.' The conflicting statements continued from different sources, e.g. 'You should be able to go home for the weekend,' 'The doctor says you're not to go home,' 'There's a trip to the baths tomorrow, you can come if you wish,' 'The trip is cancelled, I'm sorry, only a few can go on their own.'

It can be seen from the above series of comments to David that it could be interpreted as purposeful deceit, especially in David's case, as he was already in a very insecure and vulnerable state. It was only after this team's disclosure to each other about the various conflicting facts that had been given to him that a plan based on consistent, clear and honest communication was made. This went a long way towards helping David's acceptance of his situation. In this case, self-appraisal and acceptance of feedback led a team towards looking objectively at what had gone on so far, to analyse behaviours, feelings and circumstances in order to improve the care given to David.

Key Concepts

Assessment

(1) It is the skill of observation combined with effective listening and questioning that allows the nurse to build a profile by proceeding beyond the obvious needs of the patient, thus ensuring *all* needs are identified and catered for.
(2) Assessment is a continual process of gathering information in order to establish the needs of the patient.
(3) When recording, it is important to distinguish between observations made and conclusions drawn from them. Only actual behaviours should be recorded without the presumptive explanation of them.
(4) The reasons for assessment are:
   — to ensure specific problems are identified.
   — to help establish what is normal for the patient.
   — to provide a basis for evaluating the patient's progress and the effectiveness of nursing care.
   — to facilitate understanding, thus enhancing the nurse/patient relationship.

Planning

(5) The activities of living and hierarchy of needs are two major

concepts that should be considered when assessing and planning nursing care.

(6) Rather than choosing which needs should be catered for first, it is usually a question of emphasis, i.e. which need should be concentrated on, at the same time not neglecting the 'higher' needs, which of course become progressively more important as the lower needs are satisfied.

(7) The setting of short- and long-term objectives of nursing care ensures continuity and allows progress to be measured.

(8) The short-term nursing objectives relate to what is current. This will often encourage the patient towards improvement, for the long term is often unreal to the patient due to the nature of his illness. The short-term gains are more tangible and will often act as a reinforcer if achieved.

(9) Objectives of care must be realistic and achievable.

Implementation

(10) The nursing action should be communicated clearly and precisely to ensure that anyone reading it will be under no illusions as to what is required for the patient.

(11) The following should be considered when implementing nursing care:
- — concentrate on the *needs* of the individual.
- — be sensitive to your own feelings and behaviour.
- — make full use of the expertise around.
- — never lose sight of the original goal.
- — be sensitive to the patient's changing environment.
- — ensure a safe environment at all times.

Evaluation

(12) The effectiveness of evaluation is proportional to the degree of self-awareness and willingness to accept your own limitations as well as your own strengths.

(13) It will be useful for you to familiarise yourself with the language associated with the nursing process, as it has now become an established part of communication used in caring organisations. There is a tendency to dismiss this problem solving approach because of its language and technicality. To minimise the likelihood of doing this, we suggest that you focus upon the principles of evaluation and ask yourself the following:

— Is what I am doing for the patient what he really needs?
— How have I come to that decision?
— What am I trying to do for the patient?
— What are the implications of what I am doing likely to be?

If at the end of the day you can honestly say that what has been achieved has been for the benefit of that particular patient, then it is likely that the organisation and delivery of an individual care programme have gone some way towards being successful. The stages of assessment, planning, implementation and evaluation are all steps towards this aim, the outcome of which is dependent upon your relationship with the patient, and your ability to understand his needs at any given time during the process. This can be usefully demonstrated by a model adapted from Egan (1984), where E stands for evaluation and empathy, i.e. understanding throughout is imperative to the effectiveness of the nursing process.

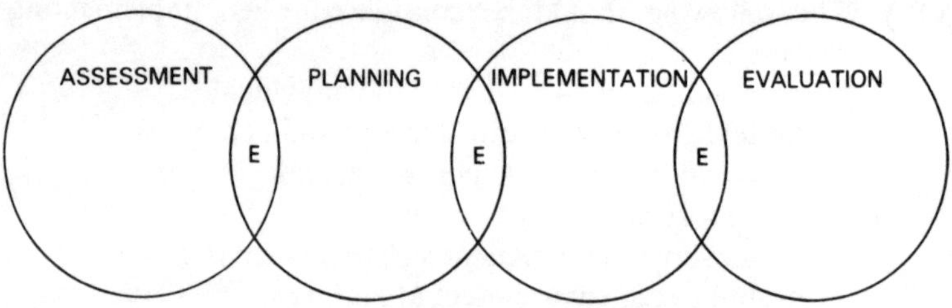

Suggested Further Reading

Crow, Jean and Kratz, Charlotte *The Nursing Process* (A *Nursing Times* Publication, Macmillan Journals, London, 1977)

Daray, P.T. *Mental Health Nursing Sourcebook* (Baillière Tindall, Eastbourne, 1985)

Heath, J., Law, G. and Cross, I. *Nursing Process — What Is It?* (NHS Learning Resources Unit, Sheffield, 1982)

Jones, M.P. 'The Nursing Process in Psychiatry', *Nursing Times*, 17 July 1980, pp. 1273-5

Keane, P. 'The Nursing Process in a Psychiatric Context', *Nursing Times*, 8 July 1981, pp. 1223-5

Kratz, Charlotte *The Nursing Process* (Baillière Tindall, London, 1979)
La Monica, Elaine *The Nursing Process: A Humanistic Approach* (Addison-Wesley, Reading, Massachusetts, 1979)
McFarlane of Llandaff, Baroness and Castledine, G. *The Practice of Nursing: Using the Nursing Process* (Mosby, St Louis, 1982)
Royal College of Nursing *Implementing the Nursing Process* (London, 1979)
Schrock, R.A. 'Planning Nursing Care for the Mentally Ill', *Nursing Times*, 17 April 1980, pp. 704-7
Ward, M. *The Nursing Process in Psychiatry* (Churchill Livingstone, Edinburgh, 1984)
Whyte, Lawrence and Youhill, Graeme 'The Nursing Process in the Care of the Mentally Ill', *Nursing Times*, 1 February 1984, pp. 49-51

PART II:

APPLICATION OF SKILLS

5 THE DEPRESSED PATIENT

Peter sat, staring at his plate of food. His head was bowed and his arms were hanging loosely by his side.

'Come on, Mr Birch, you must eat.'

Peter did not respond. It was as if he was oblivious to all around him, his greying hair seemed to stand in defiance of the nurse's attempt to straighten his appearance, his partly shaven face, motionless, and his reddened eyes seemed to appeal to all to leave him alone.

'Is there anything here that you don't like, Mr Birch?'

The nurse then lowered herself to attempt eye contact, and touched Peter's shoulder.

'Mr Birch, can you try and eat something?'

Peter's eyes feebly moved towards the nurse as if to acknowledge her presence. Slowly he lifted his right hand and with effort pushed the plate of now cold food away from him, leaving his arm on the table as if that movement drained what little energy he had.

The picture illustrated above is one of a man with severe depression. He has little or no motivation to move or talk, or when he does, attempts it with great effort and at a very slow pace (psychomotor retardation). During the three months before admission, Peter Birch had experienced a range of moods, varying from dejection and sadness, through despair and hopelessness, to total futility and emptiness. This continuum of depression (see Figure 5.1), however, is not necessarily experienced by all. Individuals may never proceed to the depths of hopelessness described, others may not experience sadness, but find themselves suddenly in the grips of despair.

There are many theories relating to the causation of depression (Mitchell, 1974), varying from the psychoanalytical theory of loss of a love object (Freud, 1917) to the neurophysiological theory of relating the alterations of feeling states to chemical disturbances. It is our opinion that it is unlikely that a single theory could adequately cover the aetiology of depression; it is probably a combination of factors that play a part in each individual. However, when dealing with someone with depression, the cause becomes academic, for each individual is unique, as is their experience.

Figure 5.1: A Continuum of Depression

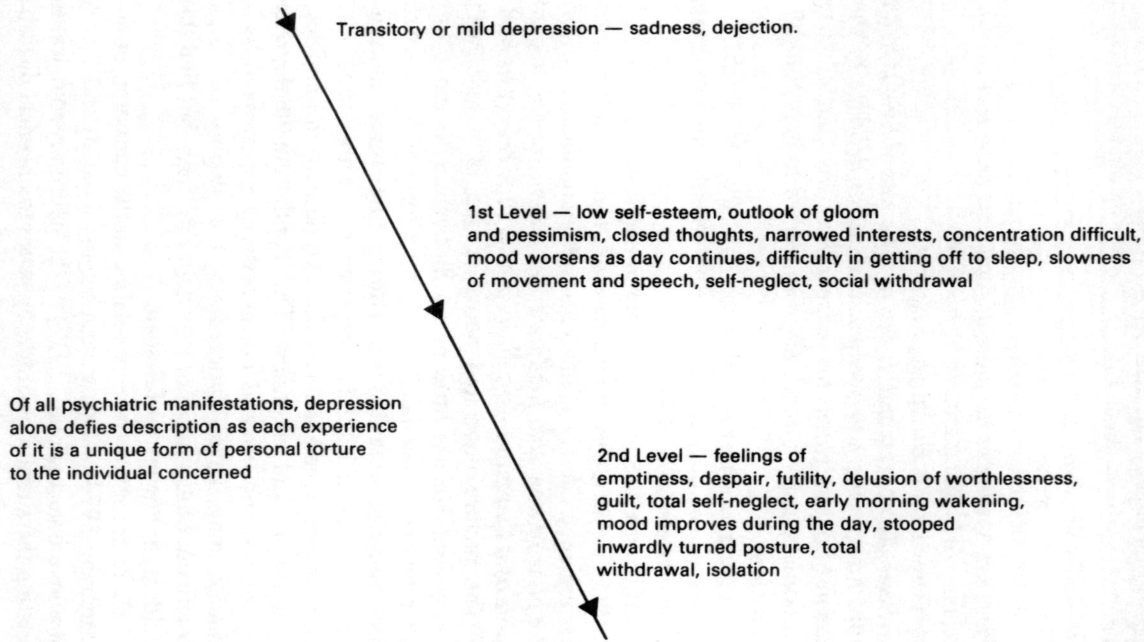

Consequently any attempt to generalise and find a common denominator between individuals who are depressed should have little effect, if any, on the nurse's attitude and skills in her interactions with people who are depressed.

The individual manifestations of depression are varied and many, and an outline of the most common features associated with feelings, thoughts, behaviours, communication and sleep will help to clarify this point (Figures 5.2-5.5).

Depressive reactions can occur at any age and in either sex. Individuals may communicate their feelings differently. People tend to be at risk from depression at times of crisis or during some developmental period of their life, e.g.

Loss of a loved one or separation anxiety	Bereavement
Having a baby	Puerperal depression
Entering the change of life	Menopausal or climacteric depression
Retirement	Depression of old age

Of course it is not just the process of change that gives rise to the depression, as many physical, psychological and social components will play their part, resulting in what can be referred to as a 'complexity of painful despair'. The following is a transcript written by someone recalling this aspect of depression.

I think I'll just sit here — but I've got so much I should do, it doesn't matter. If I do start something I'll only do it wrong. Oh God, why should there be so much pressure? I can feel them all wanting so much, almost like a physical pressure on me dragging me down. So I'll sit here — just sit. I refuse, no one can make me do anything — but they'll try. I'll fail again. They all expect so much, and I'm just not able. I try so hard, but I'm just not up to it. If only they could see, but they just keep smiling and saying it's all right. But I know it's not, just look at me, I'm a mess, if I ever feel better, how will I ever face them after they've seen me like this, I can't let them — but what can I do — why should I do anything? If I sit here I'll die eventually then I won't have to do anything ever again. I'll study that carpet until I die, it's better this way, I can never fail again. I don't even have to do anything, I couldn't even do what I've rehearsed so many times. I even bought a tow rope, tested the

Figure 5.2: Depressive Feelings

1st Level	2nd Level
Achievement of pleasure and satisfaction negligible. Feels helpless. Generally pessimistic. May show clear evidence of crying. Experiences feelings of heaviness and emptiness. Anxiety may be present mildly or intensely.	Often 'expressionless', as if without feeling. Experiences feelings of 'nothingness', 'bottomless', despair and futility, worthlessness and hopelessness.

Figure 5.3: Depressive Thoughts

1st Level	2nd Level
Thought process slow. Concentration becomes difficult. Interests increasingly diminish. Becomes unsure and indecisive. Ruminative thoughts interfere with problem solving, dwelling upon the lack of future prospects and a meaningless existence.	Orientation to reality becomes increasingly difficult. Delusional thinking may be present, often confirming negative feelings. Delusional content may be associated with guilt, poverty, 'nothingness' (nihilistic) and bodily functions.

Figure 5.4: Depressive Behaviour

1st Level	2nd Level
General slowness of movement. Every task takes a great effort. Very little effort to invest in self-care. Weakness and fatigue. May overeat or more often become anorexic and lose weight. Marked decrease in sexual interest. Agitation may result in persistent movement. Tendency to withdraw from others leading to isolation.	Becomes almost motionless or indulges in agitated purposeless movement. No evidence of self-care. Posture often slumped, head and eyes down and generally curled inwards. If left, would never move out of bed. Every task becomes a major ordeal.

Figure 5.5: Communication Observed in Depression

1st Level	2nd Level
Slow speech, often with long gaps between sentences, often delivered in a monotonous manner. May forget the original train of thought due to poor concentration span. Posture and facial expressions are often reliable aspects of non-verbal communication.	Often mute, or monosyllabic. Little acknowledgement of others present. Very subtle changes in non-verbal communication.

garage beams — but I couldn't even do that. I thought about the kids at the last moment — if I'd done it, then it'd be over now, the kids would cry, but at least they'd respect me for doing something right. Now all they see is this sorrowful pitiful mess they call their father. If I am their father, I wonder if I even did that right. Who would blame her for taking a lover, married to a mess like me? If only I could get it together just enough to get it over with, but it's just too much effort. I'll just stay here and look at this carpet till I die — please God if you'll just help me to do this. I even need help just to sit here and die. God — that's a laugh, he should worry about me. My God, what a mess I am just sitting here feeling sorry for me, I don't deserve to live when I can't even feel sorry for the people I've hurt. Please please someone help me die.

This transcript illustrates that suicide is consistently contemplated and is often thought of as the only way out of what is perceived as a desperate situation. It must be made clear that **any depressed individual may attempt to end his life by suicide**. It has been said that those individuals who have very little energy, drive or lack clarity of thought due to severe depression, as in Mr Birch's case, are unlikely to succeed in killing themselves, but the nurse cannot ignore the possibility of Mr Birch finding sufficient resources to fall through a window, walk in front of a car or wander off towards the river. When nursing patients who are depressed, it is safer to consider them *all* as potentially suicidal. Patients are most 'at risk' when their physical and psychological state has outwardly improved, but the feelings of desperation still remain. At this time the patient may resolve never to experience the same depths again, and, to ensure that does not happen, decides to 'end it all'.

Two weeks after admission it was clear that Mr Birch's state of 'retardation' was lifting. He now prepared himself before breakfast without prompting, he was no longer refusing nourishment, he responded to the usual social exchanges among the rest of the patient group and was even seen reading a newspaper for a short time. The day staff that evening in their report to the night staff stated that: 'Mr Birch appears to be making an effort to socialise, showing more interest in his environment and now seeing to his basic needs without prompting.'

The night staff's report the following morning read: 'During a routine ward round, Mr Birch was discovered to have a red plastic clinical disposable bag over his head, tied down around his neck by a shoe lace. The time of discovery was 3 a.m., last seen alive 2 a.m.'

The treatment given to Mr Birch was sufficient to lift his depression and enable him to think of an effective way to kill himself. He had sufficient drive to take and conceal a plastic bag, stocks of which are usually locked away in a clinical area, and also to take note of the timing of the night nurse's observation rounds. Between two and three in the morning, when his realisation of despair was probably at its highest, he succeeded in ridding himself of what was for him the continuous torment of life. Other risk periods related to depression are summarised in Figure 5.6.

It is not only people who suffer from depression who attempt suicide. Others are also at risk, e.g. those who are continually tormented by disordered perceptions and wish to rid themselves of the torment or as a direct response to hallucinations or delusions. Some people may not intend to kill themselves, but use an attempt at suicide as a 'cry for help' with problems which overwhelm them. *All* attempts at suicide are serious and raise many issues that require exploration by the nurse.

Implications for the Nurse

Imagine yourself walking across a bridge and in the distance you see a figure sitting precariously on the edge of the bridge, looking down on the busy road beneath. To fall would mean almost certain death. As you approach you recognise that she is an ex-patient who was discharged a few weeks ago. She had been treated for depression, but was considered fit to leave by all concerned. As you walk, you recall the conversations you have had with her, particularly the one that related to her wanting to commit suicide, arguing that it was her right to do so and giving what appeared to be quite logical reasons for this act. When you are almost at arm's length from her she turns and recognises you. She shouts, 'Leave me alone, this is something I must do.'

By putting out your arm and grabbing her, it is likely that you could stop her at no risk to yourself.

Attempt to answer the following questions:

— What would you do?
— Would you stop her?
— Would you let her jump?

Figure 5.6: Mood Variation Curve Showing the 'High Risk' Times for Potential Suicides

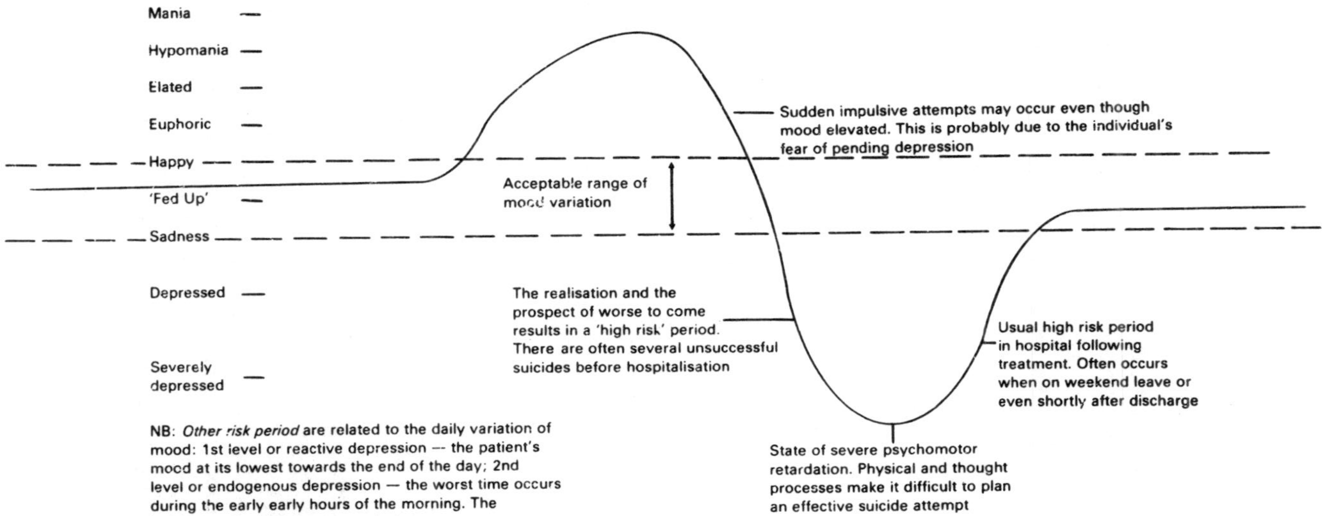

NB: *Other risk period* are related to the daily variation of mood: 1st level or reactive depression — the patient's mood at its lowest towards the end of the day; 2nd level or endogenous depression — the worst time occurs during the early early hours of the morning. The incidence of suicide increases during springtime and personal anniversaries are often significant.

— How would you feel if she jumped without your attempting to stop her?
— Have you the right to interfere with someone else's decision about their own life?
— Why is she about to kill herself in a place where she may be discovered and prevented from doing so?
— How can you be sure her thinking is logical and without distortion?
— How can you be sure she won't blame you for the rest of her life for saving her?
— How can you be sure she won't thank you for saving her when her depression lifts?

In our opinion, it is not for the nurse to collaborate with the intention of people who wish to kill themselves. As psychiatric nurses we feel we should preserve life and prevent this destructive act occurring if the chance arises. By holding this attitude we are being safe in that on one hand we can accept an individual having certain reasons for killing himself but on the other we must question the situation: 'How is it that I find myself in a position to stop this person killing themselves?' Who is going to make the judgement that the individual did not intend anyone to discover him? Can you imagine someone falling to his death shouting up at you, 'Why didn't you stop me?'

It is important for the nurse to explore these issues and questions in order to prepare for the situation occurring, thus increasing the likelihood of effective intervention taking place during a crisis. When the nurse is clear in her mind what she thinks, the issues are prevented from being distractions during the 'crisis intervention'.

Another potential distractor that could interfere with the therapeutic process is the expressed depression from the patient affecting the feelings of the nurse. It is possible to find yourself sad, low, irritable and often helpless during an interaction with someone who is depressed. It is necessary for the nurse to realise this possibility, as it could result in her avoiding the depressed patient, which may reinforce the patient's feelings of rejection. By being aware of this potential distractor, and sensitive to the way it is communicated, i.e. mainly by non-verbal cues, the nurse should be able to avoid interference from it and use the added awareness to 'tune into' the patient's problems and needs.

The Problems and Needs of the Depressed Patient

The problems and needs of the depressed patient are varied and many. We intend to outline these only in general terms in order for the student to perceive the total picture of complexity, thus appreciating the scale of the problem. As with any intention to embark upon caring for an individual, a thorough assessment must be made and priorities of care set. The priorities for a depressed individual will vary, depending upon the severity of the depression. Invariably there is some degree of self-neglect, which can vary from slight deterioration in usual standards of dress to a total neglect which can become life threatening. These aspects are summarised in Figure 5.7. It can be seen that if the potential problems were taken to their extreme state, death is a possibility. The needs and principles of care are therefore aimed at closely monitoring progress and preventing deterioration.

Some patients may actively refuse nutrition as a form of suicide, claiming that there is no point in living, so there is no point in eating. Actively suicidal patients pose an acute nursing problem. A suicide attempt can have a significant effect, not only on the nurse/patient relationship, but also the patient's family, friends and, if attempted within the hospital environment, the other patients on the ward. It can be seen (Figure 5.8) that the principles of care are related to the prevention of suicide attempts. The needs, however, are specific and should be considered an important factor within the nurse/patient relationship.

The nurse should be able to fulfil the needs of the patient and at the same time adhere to the principles of care. For example, if effective continuous observation is to take place, the nurse should be ideally be with the patient all the time. This is done most acceptably to the patient by joining in an activity with him and, if appropriate, conveying honestly to the patient the caring role: 'I'm "with" you because I fear you may take your own life. I don't want you to take your own life because I care for and value you as a human and believe that your intentions will change.' In this way the principles of care and the needs of the patient are considered together in a positive way without detriment to the relationship.

The psychological problems of someone who is depressed are uniquely entwined around their personality, environment, circumstances and relationships. There are, however, some clear common problem areas that can be experienced in varying degrees and

Figure 5.7: The Physical Problems and Needs of the Depressed Patient

Physical State

Neglect of

- **Hygiene**
  - Potential problems
    - Social rejection
    - Reinforcement of low self esteem
    - Body odour/soreness/infection
    - Infestation
    - Dental caries
- **Diet**
  - Potential problems
    - Loss of weight/anorexia
    - Dehydration
    - Constipation
    - General weakness

Needs (and principles of care)

- Assessment of usual self-care standards (if necessary obtain information from the family)
- Allow sufficient time to complete tasks of self-care
- Prompt and encourage efforts made towards improving appearance
- Give positive feedback — may increase self-esteem
- Encourage relaxing baths — may be a good time for the patient to talk

- Monitor intake (chart if necessary)
- Assess likes and dislikes and usual diet
- Complement diet with nourishing fluids
- Encourage roughage/fluids/exercise to prevent constipation
- Provide attractive, well presented meals — do not discourage with large amounts
- Allow sufficient time to eat — provide reheating facilities if necessary

Figure 5.8: Suicide Prevention

- Prevention of Suicide (principles of care)
  - Continuous observation
  - Removal of harmful objects/situation
  - Awareness of high risk periods
  - Help occupy patient, thus avoiding isolation
  - Other nursing considerations relate to acknowledging the feelings of:
    - family and friends
    - other nurses
    - other patients, especially when suicide is attempted or has occurred
- The Needs of the Suicidal Patient
  - Honesty from the nurse concerning her caring role
  - To be told of his worth as a human
  - Freedom to talk through his self-destruction without being judged
  - An accepting 'hand' to hold on to when he feels the sense of 'drowning'
  - A hand that conveys friendship and confidence in being able to help and support him

combinations. Not all depressed people experience them all, but most experience some of the problems outlined in Figure 5.9. This simplified diagram of some psychological problems shows how each one overlaps and often reinforces the feelings expressed. The needs related to these problems are concerned with allowing the patient to talk through and express his feelings to someone skilful enough to facilitate this.

Principles and Skills Required to Help the Depressed Patient

Sensitivity and Awareness Skills

A person who is severely depressed has limited resources to use in

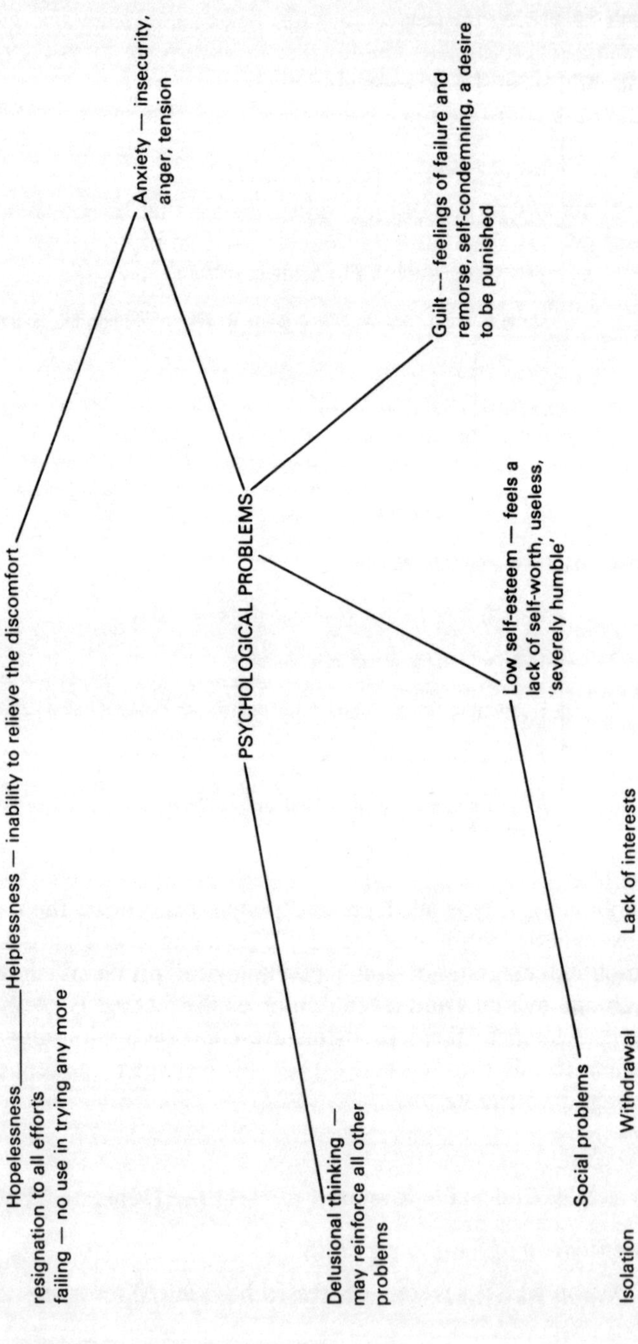

Figure 5.9: The Psychological Problems of the Depressed Patient

self-care. He may neglect his most basic needs to such a degree that many, if left alone, would just sit, oblivious to their own physical discomfort and environment. When this state exists to any degree, the nurse must be sensitive and anticipate the needs of the patient, e.g.

— he may sit in a draught and not state that he is cold;
— he may sit in his own urine and not admit to being sore;
— he may be severely dehydrated and not ask for drink;
— he may be crying out for love and acceptance yet deny himself tears.

Accepting that the patient may be unable or unwilling to communicate his own needs, the nurse must rely on her observational skills (see p. 113), in order to perceive accurately what is going on for that particular patient. The observations made should give sufficient information for the nurse to be able to approach the patient with appropriate sensitivity. It is important for the nurse to be aware of her own feelings and mood state, for it is common enough mistake to believe that superficiality and overcheerfulness may somehow help the patient who is depressed to change his mood. This does not occur and this insensitive approach can quite often have the reverse effect, making the patient withdraw even further. So by being aware and sensitive to the fact that people on the ward may not share the same degree of mood elevation as others, the nurse can and should adjust her approach appropriately when helping patients who are depressed. This process of mood influences can work both ways, for the patient's depressed mood may affect the nurse's mood as mentioned in the section on 'Implications for the Nurse'. This is why, particularly with patients who do not readily respond or comply, the nurse must always be prepared to look inwards and self-evaluate in order to ensure that the approach and care that she gives are tailored towards the patient's needs and not the needs of the nurse. The following are examples of some questions that would help the nurse to explore for herself a less than satisfactory nurse/patient interaction.

— Did I have a preconceived idea of what the outcome of the interaction would be?
— Did I enter the relationship with some negative feelings that may have been communicated non-verbally?

— Am I more concerned with the way I am feeling at the moment and this is distracting me from understanding the patient's feelings?
— Are my expectations of the patient and/or myself too high?
— Am I bringing my own frustrations into the interaction?
— Am I displacing my frustrations on to the patient?
— Is there something about the patient that reminds me of someone else with whom I did not have a good relationship?
— Do I see something negative in the patient that I see in myself?
— Am I being honest with myself and am I really interested in this patient?

This series of questions demands a degree of self-challenge, which is an aspect of self-awareness, and should be part of a continuous process of self-evaluation, to guard against rising barriers which prevent the formation of relationships based on honesty, trust, genuineness and understanding.

Non-verbal Skills

During the description of the interactions between a nurse and Mr Birch, the patient responded only when 'contact' had been made. It was through eye contact, touch and tone of voice, all of which were essential in order to break through Mr Birch's 'wall' of depression. When the aim in this sort of interaction is to gain a response, this approach is necessary for those who have withdrawn to prevent total isolation. Efforts to make contact with patients who are severely depressed should be aimed at gaining a response that will minimise the tendency to withdraw, reinforce reality such as the time and the nature of the environment, and increase the chance of further communication.

Sometimes just 'being with' someone experiencing depression may be enough to show the patient that you care and also to make contact. Sitting with the patient, acknowledging his presence and being aware of subtle changes in his breathing, eye movements and posture may give the patient a sense of belonging and acceptance, which they often lack. This awareness of the patient's posture may consciously or unconsciously aid the nurse to 'mirror' (see p. 42) by making subtle adjustments to her own breathing, leg positions, head and body movements and arm position. This mirroring is very powerful and is a physical way of communicating, 'I'm interested in you, I want to invest some time with you, and I'm prepared to accept you and your present state by understanding your life as much as I can.' So by using your own body language and being sensitive to the patient's it is possible to communicate, thus going towards helping him satisfy his need to be accepted and valued.

Verbal Skills

The principles underlying the use of verbal skills when talking with individuals who are depressed are that they must be allowed to verbalise and explore their feelings, without reinforcing their negative thinking (Beck, 1980). We believe that the state of 'depression' is in many respects similar to the state of 'bereavement' (see p. 277), and is particularly relevant when the importance of helping the patient work through his feelings is considered. It is generally accepted that unless someone who is bereaved works through most of the stages of bereavement, prolonged grieving and depression may occur. It is our experience that the longer someone who is depressed is left to dwell upon the 'complexities of his despair', the longer he will take to recover. The skills that seem particularly pertinent here are the listening skills of paraphrasing and reflecting, conveying to the patient basic understanding and allowing him to hear his own words and rationale, so that he can explore further his own world in an atmosphere of genuineness, warmth and empathy (see p. 26). This relationship between the nurse and the patient must be one where the patient can feel safe enough to explore many emotive issues that he may not have expressed to anyone before. His innermost conflicts may be verbalised, as he places trust and confidence in the nurse who is listening. She must respond to this trust by conveying acceptance and understanding, thus facilitating further exploration. The nurse must be prepared to accept verbalisation of some very strong emotions, particularly anger, which is directed inwards to the patient, to his significant others or even to members of the nursing staff. Anger is quite a common component of depression and one emotion that tends to be controlled, causing much inner frustration and preventing further exploration of other thoughts and feelings.

By using observation and sensitivity skills, tension, agitation and frustration can be detected. Emotional release can be encouraged by highlighting and communicating these observations to the patient, at the same time giving him permission to be angry. For example, while listening to Geoff, the nurse noticed his voice becoming less relaxed; he started fidgeting and his face began to look tense.

Nurse. Geoff, I've noticed when you started to talk about your mother you seemed to become tense, I'm wondering if there is a connection?

Geoff continues to talk about his mother in an angry frame, but still holds back on releasing any particular emotion.

Nurse. You seem to be holding back your feelings, as if you're saying to yourself, 'I shouldn't be talking about my mother like this.'

The theme of anger and guilt continued until Geoff found himself freely expressing anger without guilt, which helped him explore further his relationship with his mother.

Actively listening to someone who is depressed, encouraging him to ventilate his feelings in an atmosphere of trust, will help him to work through his despair as an important part of the overall care and attention he needs.

When responding to patients who are depressed, the nurse must consider their poor concentration span, which will have an effect on their ability to think and communicate. Therefore the response from the nurse must be appropriate to the degree of concentration from the patient, for the nurse may inadvertently reinforce complex issues and futility by summarising. Therefore, responses in the same language and level of patient awareness are essential.

Finally, when listening to depressed patients, the content is extremely important on two major accounts, the delusional content and the suicidal content. For the delusional content the same principles apply as for any delusional patient (see p. 236), but perhaps it is sufficient to say here that for many depressed individuals, the delusional content has some personal significant meaning. Suicidal themes, however, are often not so obvious, and if the nurse detects this theme, she should encourage the patient to verbalise and talk openly about his suicidal thoughts. Some common phrases may be:

— 'It doesn't seem worth going on much longer.'

— 'There's no point anyway.'
— 'It'll be over soon anyway.'
— 'Why should I struggle on like this?'
— 'No one can help me.'

By paraphrasing and reflecting back these responses, a clearer indication of the patient's intentions can be achieved.

Conclusion

Depression is potentially a life threatening state of 'being'. You must never underestimate the personal pain an individual may be going through. You will need all your personal resources to withstand the barriers of silence, monosyllabic utterances and futility expressed by the severely depressed. By your sensitivity, warmth and understanding, it will be possible to enter into the patient's world. In doing so you must be strong enough to withstand the enveloping nature of the patient's mood and stand back to respond with empathy. This will help you lead the patient out to look forward to some future where he can value his life.

Key Concepts

(1) The manifestations of depression vary in severity from sadness and dejection to despair and futility.
(2) The main areas of depressive symptoms focus around:
  — depressive feelings;
  — depressive thoughts;
  — depressive behaviour;
  — communication.
(3) People are particularly at risk from depression during developmental stages of life or by experiencing some personal crisis such as the loss of a loved one.
(4) Any depressed person may attempt to end his life by suicide.
(5) It is essential for the nurse to be aware of the 'high risk' factors in the potentially suicidal.
(6) The implications for the nurse involve exploring personal ethics and being self-aware during interactions with depressed patients.
(7) The problems and needs of the depressed patients revolve around:

— physical needs;
— prevention of suicide;
— psychological and social needs.

(8) The skills required are aimed at encouraging the patient to explore his own feelings and work through his despair without reinforcing his negative thinking. They include:
— sensitivity and awareness;
— non-verbal skills;
— verbal skills of listening, i.e. paraphrasing; reflecting; questioning; clarifying;
— avoiding overuse of summarising.

Suggested Further Reading

Beck, A.T. *Diagnosis and Management of Depression* (University of Pennsylvania, Philadelphia, 1973)

_____ *The Prediction of Suicide* (Charles Publishing, Bowie, Maryland, 1974)

_____ *The Cognitive Therapy of Depression* (John Wiley, Chichester, 1980)

Blyth, Marguerite M. and Pearlmutter, Deanna R. 'The Suicide Watch: A Re-examination of Maximum Observation', *Perspectives in Psychiatric Care*, vol. 2, no. 3 (July/September 1983), pp. 90-3

Freden, Lars *Psychosocial Aspects of Depression: No Way Out* (John Wiley, Chichester, 1982)

Hauck, Paul *Depression* (Sheldon Press, London, 1983)

Mitchell, A.R.K. *The Nature of Depression* (NAMHO, Penguin Books, Harmondsworth, 1974)

Morgan, Howard Gethin *Death Wishes? The Understanding of Deliberate Self Harm* (John Wiley, London, 1979)

Office of Health Economics *Suicide and Deliberate Self Harm* (Office of Health Economics, London, 1981)

Rowe, D. *Depression: The Way Out of Your Prison* (Routledge and Kegan Paul, London and Boston, 1983)

_____ 'Helping the Depressed Patient', *Nursing Times*, 26 October 1983, pp. 62-3

Stengel, E. *Suicide and Attempted Suicide* (Penguin Books, Harmondsworth, 1964)

6 THE OVERACTIVE PATIENT

'The tables are set and met with friends to lend money to honey who is my best girl sexlet, a flat that can't be changed because tyres are so expensive, I'll have a dozen please Mr Michelin X certificate for that sordid little film which should only be seen by.'

'Mr Miles, here's a cup of tea for you.'

'Don't interrupt, I'm composing the garden rubbish, I'll pour it in later.'

'Do you take sugar?'

'Sugar is sweet, so are you, give me a kiss for a generation of Miles, two please, shaken not stirred carefully into.'

'It'll taste nicer warm than cold.'

'Trivia, trivia, don't bother me now, so much to do and so little time lords to do it.'

Mr Miles proceeded through the ward having quickly taken his bath and wearing only an untied dressing gown. He had been admitted earlier that day accompanied by two police officers, his clothes in a dishevelled state, his jacket adorned with milk bottle tops representing 'the battles of marriage'. On him were sufficient details to contact his family in order to piece together his mysterious appearance. The priority now was somehow to slow him down sufficiently to enable him to take nutrition and rest.

Two nurses had followed him into the lounge, where he had started introducing himself to all around. It was a busy morning and a variety of people were there, including some visitors and the hospital chaplain. Mr Miles was bowing, nodding and insisting upon shaking the hand of everyone present. Unfortunately his dressing gown was wide open, his wiry but lively frame on view to all. Turning to the chaplain, he said, 'Ah my God Father, shake my hand but not my . . .'

The nurses intervened, distracting Mr Miles sufficiently to take him somewhere slightly less stimulating.

This situation warranted quick thinking and reaction from the nursing staff. Their skills would be tested for some time yet, probably until Mr Miles' mood had settled to a somewhat less demanding level.

The symptoms portrayed here — pressure of speech, flight of

ideas, overactivity — are indicative of someone experiencing hypomania bordering on mania, the latter being a rarer and more serious situation, sometimes culminating in a delirious episode. Hypomania is an 'affective disorder' with an insidious onset. It begins with mild elation or euphoria, a general feeling of well-being to general overactivity and grandiosity. It can occur in isolation but is more commonly associated with severe mood swings indicative of 'manic-depressive' psychoses. A complete picture of someone experiencing a hypomanic state would include:

— a feeling of well-being, denies that he may be ill;
— easily provoked, may be impulsively aggressive;
— mood can quickly change from laughing to crying (lability);
— pressure of speech and flight of ideas, comprising a continuous and rapid change of topics, often includes rhyming and punning as in Mr Miles' case;
— grandiose delusions may be present; if so, a history of gross overspending is usually common;
— neglect of or inappropriate self-care. Dress and personal hygiene may be generally neglected, or dress may be over-expressive and not in the patient's usual style. Aspects of clothing or additions may have special meaning, as the 'milk tops' did for Mr Miles;
— general increase in physical activity, always on the move, doing three or four things at once, continuously interfering in other people's business;
— disturbed sleep pattern, will often fight rest until close to exhaustion;
— sexually disinhibited, may describe indiscreetly and in expressive detail personal sexual exploits or engage in sexual acts foreign to his usual judgement;
— extremely distractable, focusing upon anything novel for short periods, often misidentifying and misinterpreting certain stimuli.

From the above description it is clear that this particular individual's situation has potential for many serious problems. It is essential that the nurse is aware of the needs required, for it is likely that the patient is not.

The Problems and Needs of the Overactive Patient

Assessing someone experiencing hypomania will require a quick establishment of priorities. These are usually related to the patient's *physical problems and needs*, e.g.

Problem: The patient will fight sleep, deny the need to rest, and may be at risk from physical exhaustion.
Needs: The nurse must be aware of the patient's general physical state in order to appreciate his limitations. General encouragement from the nurse is required to allow the patient to rest. Include the patient in activities that involve him sitting down, and do not discourage times when he is resting, even during the day.
Problem: The patient will neglect his diet, will claim he has no time to eat.
Need: His intake should be monitored and, if necessary, recorded. Rather than insist on him sitting down for meals, provide nutritious snacks and complemented fluids to enable him to include them in his demanding schedule.
Problem: May neglect his self-care, i.e. hygiene and appropriate clothing.
Need: Provision of opportunity to concentrate on himself with the skills of the nurse to encourage, suggest and persuade.

The psychological problems are more likely to be varied, depending upon the individual, but, generally speaking, they may be related to underlying conflicts and anxieties that are often neglected by others because of the front of 'well-being' and elation. A psychological problem arising from the patient's actual behaviour may be one of social neglect, i.e. other individuals avoiding or shunning the patient because of his demanding behaviour. The patient is vulnerable to feeling frustrated, insecure and not being accepted. Therefore the needs of security, belongingness and self-esteem should be considered in any nursing care plan.

The social problems and needs concern themselves with the patient's occupation and interactions with others. Social problems arise out of the patient's inappropriate behaviour and faulty judgement giving rise to potentially embarrassing situations. The patient will have to interact in the same environment as he improves, with the same people, which will involve him gaining insight into his previous behaviour. It is therefore essential that the nurse attempts to protect the patient from unnecessary embarrassment. This fact must be considered when assessing the patient's interests and abilities in order to plan suitable activities. When planning activities for someone who is overactive, the following considerations are useful:

— his interests, hobbies, occupation;
— concentration span and level of distractability;
— his physical limitations;
— his need to express his energy in some physical way.

Music and painting are often useful activities, involving large motor movement and sufficiently expressive to enable the patient to release emotions and frustrations in a positive way.

Implications for the Nurse

Nursing an overactive patient could make exhausting demands on the nurse. She will be expected to be patient and tolerant in her interactions with the patient, which becomes extremely difficult if she is tired. It is therefore necessary for her to be able to evaluate her own capabilities and limitations. All members of the nursing team must be sensitive to this and must allow for realistic expectations from all concerned. In practice this means finding a balance between the nurse 'specialling' the patient, getting to know him very well and possibly becoming exhausted, to several nurses working in rotation for a realistic time span, thus enabling them to use their skills effectively. Even so, patience and tolerance will be tested. It is important not to rise to the personal insults and argumentative tones of the patient for this would result in further stimulation, which may end in the nurse being assaulted. The principle of reducing environmental stimuli for the overactive patient has implications for nursing management. Realistically, very little can be done to control everything in the patient's environment, but at certain times, especially on admission and early on in the illness where distractability is at its highest, it would be beneficial to all concerned if the patient could be kept away from the busy and intensive areas of any caring unit. Therefore planned admission is preferred, unlike the case of Mr Miles (see p.

111), who was brought straight into the busiest area of the ward quite unexpectedly. It was only the skill of the charge nurse that prevented the police having to restrain Mr Miles again.

Principles and Skills Required to Help the Overactive Patient

In order to implement the principles already mentioned, certain skills must be specifically applied, one of these being a sensitivity to non-verbal communication. This is necessary in order to reflect observable emotions through the distraction of the verbal content. Is it possible to make sense of the opening paragraph illustrating Mr Miles' flight of ideas (see p. 159)? Looking at the content, very little sense can be made, but listening to how he said it and observing his non-verbal communication may give clues to how in fact he is feeling behind the barrage of the verbal communication. As he was talking, Mr Miles frowned, clenched his fist and tensed his shoulders.

Nurse. I'm not sure what you're saying, Mr Miles, but I detect that you may be feeling tense or angry about something.

Here the nurse uses her sensitivity to the non-verbal communication and the skill of reflection in order to gain some understanding of the patient. She also attempts to convey this understanding, which is important to establish rapport. We are not saying that the nurse should ignore the content, just its fine detail, for the overall theme of the content may also be helpful in detecting how the patient is feeling or what need he is trying to communicate. What possible feelings or direction of content may be useful to explore with this patient's communication, which is said rather sternly?

> 'If she thinks as I thinks and stinks I would knock twice before entering the pathway of punishment, no way is she cash and grabbing my little bird's nest before going in and doing hell.'

There seem to be two, maybe three, consistent elements to this content. They are:

— directed to someone — 'she';

— entering or going into somewhere;
— and possible fear about being harmed by that person on entering.

Now if we were to say that this patient stated this whilst pacing outside the interviewing room, waiting to see the doctor, then it may be appropriate to reflect:

> 'Am I right in thinking you're anxious about seeing the doctor this morning?'

Suggestion and Persuasion

Often a tactful approach is more successful than an authoritarian one in facilitating the patient in certain directions. This is illustrated again in Mr Miles' case. When he was first brought on to the ward, the staff nurse used suggestion rather than authority to coax Mr Miles into having a bath: 'How would you like me to run you a nice warm bath while they sort out all the boring administrative details?'

Suggestion and persuasion are often useful tactics to *distract* the patient from potentially damaging situations. This was required again when Mr Miles was busy introducing himself to the chaplain. The nurses who distracted him approached him in a friendly manner, saying 'There is someone extremely interested in meeting you now, Mr Miles, he's waiting for you in the office.'

This form of distraction is acceptable as long as it is not deceitful. If there was no one in the office waiting for Mr Miles, this would be dishonest and wrong. Distraction makes the best possible use of current situations based on the nurse's knowledge of and relationship with the patient.

Conclusion

When caring for someone who has very little time to share with you, then the contact you do make becomes very valuable. The patient will think he is always one step ahead and make out that he is coping extremely well. You must appreciate that under this perception of energy someone is fighting for survival, and indeed may be experiencing conflicts that only he is vaguely aware of. During this time of extreme activity, his basic needs must be met. As his mood drops, you need to be sensitive to the implications this may have for the patient. These may involve the patient experiencing embarrassment, guilt, remorse, insecurity and, in the extreme, he may swing very quickly to depression.

So you will have to be prepared for all eventualities, and rather than the patient being one step ahead of you, it becomes the reverse.

Key Concepts

(1) The patient may be overactive, disinhibited, distractable and easily provoked. He may express flights of ideas and grandiosity. Self-neglect and exhaustion are real dangers.
(2) The overactive patient needs sleep, nutrition, hygiene, security and to feel needed.
(3) Other important areas of assessment include interests, hobbies, concentration span, physical limitations and the need to express energy.
(4) The implications for the nurse involve having insight into her own limitations and realistic expectations, also using a team effort rather than a singular one.
(5) The skills required are:
   - being sensitive to non-verbal communication, particularly tone of voice and gestures;
   - reflecting any theme that may be present in the content;
   - using suggestion and persuasion rather than an authoritarian approach;
   - managing the environment, i.e. protection and reducing stimuli.

Suggested Further Reading

Buckwalter, K.C. and Kerfoot, K.M. 'Emergency Department Nursing Care of the Manic Patient', *Journal of Emergency Nursing*, Vol. 8, no. 5 (September/October 1982), pp. 239-42

Corker, E. 'Nursing Care Study. Manic Depression', *Nursing Mirror*, vol. 157 (July 1983), pp. 43-5

7 THE AGGRESSIVE PATIENT

Katherine has been in hospital for twelve years. She has become obese with prolonged use of major tranquillisers and hospital food. It is unusual to see her without a cigarette in her mouth or walking jauntily around eating a sandwich or sweets. It is possible that Katherine would not be noticed in a long-stay ward, except for the fact that whenever there is an incident, she can usually be found in the midst of it. She has almost achieved notoriety within the hospital. Staff are warned how unpredictable she is; if the fire alarm sounds, someone will remark, 'Oh, it's probably only Katherine'; when a pane of glass breaks, people expect Katherine to be the cause; if a patient or member of staff has been attacked, inevitably Katherine has been 'at it again'.

Katherine is 32 years old, has been married and divorced, has a child, and both elderly parents are still alive, but she has not seen any of these people for some years now. Trained nurses, doctors and other professionals are wary of her, so it is not surprising that her family became disenchanted many years ago. Yet when time is taken to get to know her, she becomes more than just a manifestation of an undesirable behaviour pattern: she is a warm, caring and sensitive individual. She does not consciously intend to hurt anyone, but simply finds great difficulty in controlling her emotions. She can sometimes be seen in great distress, crying bitterly into a hospital tissue, and, if she is listened to, she will tell how frustrated and depressed she is about her life. She will say how helpless she feels with despair in the knowledge that she will probably spend the rest of her life in hospital.

Katherine is not perhaps typical of the aggressive patient, but neither is she untypical. She represents and exposes a powerful phenomenon that can be observed in many institutions amongst residents considered to be aggressive: people tend to behave according to other people's expectations of them. We have to emphasise, however, that this is not the case in every story. People become aggressive for almost as many different reasons as there are aggressive people, and consequently it is important to investigate the causes, as they hold the key to dealing effectively with aggression. It is always more difficult to find the cause when the patient is distant from the nurse, if the nurse is afraid, hesitant or withdraws from the relationship. The patient's problems and needs can never be fully understood and dealt with if a poor rapport exists.

Aggression can take many forms. It is sometimes seen as a physical and violent attack upon a person or object, but more commonly it is a verbal explosion of emotion directed at someone or something. Even in more 'normal' adult interactions raising of voices indicates an aggressive intent and heightened emotion. Even more subtle is when self-mutilation, depression and sulky behaviour manifest as symptoms of aggression turned inward.

The Problems and Needs of the Aggressive Patient

The patient expressing aggressive behaviour patterns desperately needs help. It is probable that violence occurs because there is no other route to express the seething emotions that exist for the individual. It is despair due to an inability to find alternative more desirable strategies to vent feelings that results in violent behaviour.

The patient may feel misunderstood, isolated, lonely, frustrated and, in the absence of a constructive means of communicating this, he acts out his feelings in aggression.

Implications for the Nurse

The nurse has many responsibilities in dealing with aggressive and violent behaviour, and it is useful if she can pre-organise these mentally before an incident occurs, rather than after. If she can do this it may well assist her effectiveness in any aggressive interaction.

Responsibility for the Patient

The nurse needs to help the patient to resolve his problems, and protect him from himself, or others. This will include an honest appraisal of knowing what limits she will set on behaviour before she considers restraint. Does she have the courage, resources and williness to risk taking direct action which may jeopardise her relationship with the patient? If conflicts exist on the issue of restraint, she may need to challenge her belief, attitudes and thinking in this area until she is very clear on her limits. Restraint unfortunately is sometimes necessary, and is a reality we have to face. But what may be equally important is that when it is used its use is critically evaluated:

— Why was it necessary?
— What motivated its use?
  Staff anxiety for the patient?
  Other patients?
  Themselves?
— What other strategies were available?
  Were they inappropriate?
  Why were they inappropriate?
— What exactly happened?
  Cause?
  Effect?
— How did we all feel?
  Staff, patients with person restrained?
— How do we all feel now?
— How could it have been prevented?
— How can we prevent its recurrence?
— What action should be taken now?

This is only a sample of the type of questions teams should ask following incidents and restraint; it is up to the team to devise their own according to their unique situation.

Principles and Skills Required to Help the Aggressive Patient

(1) It is important that the cause of the aggression is sought in every incident. This may best be done by the use of reflecting (see p. 47) the patient's feelings as seen through non-verbal behaviour presented, and by facilitating discussion through an open question, e.g.

'I can see you are very frustrated and angry about something, Katherine, I wonder if you feel able to talk to me about it?'

'I would like to understand how you feel.'

'Tell me what's really bothering you.'

(2) It is also important that a relationship of trust remains

throughout every incident — facilitated through honesty.

Here the nurse needs to be totally honest about what she has in mind. If, for instance, she intends to get help to restrain the patient and give an intramuscular injection, she must not mislead the patient into believing she just wants to talk, e.g.

'Katherine, I can see you're very upset and I think you need some medication. You refuse to talk calmly to me about what's troubling you, and frankly you are frightening me and I fear for people's safety.'

'I've sent for some help to give you an injection, but I hope you will agree to have it without force.'

'I hope you will believe me when I say I'm only trying to help you.'

This interaction may be unrealistic if the patient is likely to react to it violently, but it needs to be said even if it is during actual restraint. The nurse needs to be frank and explain her actions to ensure some rapport remains.

(3) Even during physical restraint, the nurse may facilitate a caring relationship. Conversation should not cease with the patient even during restraint. If the nurse is able to continue talking in a calm soothing voice, explaining what is happening and why it is, much of the rapport between patient and nurse may be saved, e.g.

'Katherine, I'm sorry it has come to this. When this happens it means we've failed. If you feel you can't talk to us, and allow us to help without incidents like this, then something must be wrong.'

'I hope when you are feeling calmer we can talk and you may be able to explain how you felt and explore more productive ways of dealing with your feelings than aggression.'

'I'm going to give this injection now, I know it's difficult but if you can try to relax a little it won't hurt so much. It will help you to feel more relaxed and we'll stay with you till you *are able* to feel calmer.'

(4) In situations of verbal aggression a skilful approach may divert any actual violence. The principles and skills here are as follows:

Absorption: The nurse should be able to absorb any hostility or abuse directed at her without reacting. Obscene language may cause offence to the nurse, but it will not cause physical harm — however, retaliating or showing offence may well precipitate an actual physical attack. We suggest the nurse raise her awareness of exactly what may make her unable to absorb verbal abuse and deal with it in safe role play type situations.

Distraction: Nurses may be able to distract patients who are verbally aggressive by switching conversation completely by putting on some music, or the use of humour if the patient is known to be susceptible to this.

Approach: The nurse's approach may be all important. She should be non-threatening, and to facilitate this the following suggestions may be useful:

— a low posture — preferably sit near to the patient;
— hands in pockets — or similar;
— helpless posture may help;
— an open frontal approach wherever possible is recommended;
— a congruous smile may help alleviate the patient's fear that the nurse's approach heralds physical force;
— maintain eye contact to establish a willingness to listen, without constant staring which may be interpreted as confrontation.

Reassurance: Positive verbal reassurance may be very helpful, e.g.

— 'I'm trying to understand.'
— 'I'd like to listen to what you have to say.'
— 'Please don't feel threatened, I'm not going to hurt you.'
— 'I really do care — I want to help you.'

Disclosure: Somehow, probably as a legacy from the custodial days of psychiatric care, a belief that the nurse should be fearless has built up. We are not at all sure or impressed with this macho image of psychiatric nurses. In many ways it detracts from empathic, genuine and caring attitudes which need to be demonstrated. Far better perhaps to say to a patient, 'I'm trying to understand how you feel — but at the moment I'm frightened that you may hit me,' rather than the cool 'hard' image approach that often can be interpreted as challenging, taunting and an invitation to physical confrontation.

We suggest that the nurse disclose what she feels to the patient, whether it be fear, dismay or disappointment, providing it is honest and not derisive, at the same time communicating sufficient confidence to get over the fact that the nurse is able to take control if the patient desires this. We believe that this will close the gap between the two people, form a bridge and strengthen an existing, but perhaps fragile, rapport.

(5) General principles which may help prevent a violent incident:

(a) Observation of patient's behaviour may forearm the nurse to a potentially violent incident. There may be many tell-tale signs of imminent violence, such as scowling, pacing, shouting, clenched fists and so on. Knowing the patient well is the nurse's most effective weapon.
(b) The team of nurses must be working as a team, and there should be good communication so that there is consistency of care. There is nothing more frustrating for any individual than to have conflicting instructions or advice. If this situation exists, frustration will eventually build up and a violent reaction can be anticipated.
(c) Safety valves: in any well run ward there must be some established method of being able to express frustration, fears or general moans. Patients' meetings or group discussions are some such strategies that may be useful to help situations defuse before they become violent issues.
(d) If it begins to look as if a violent incident may be imminent, the person closest, with the best rapport with the patient, should normally be the nurse directed to deal with the situation. Any known antagonistic agents, i.e. particular people, should be removed.

Attention Seeking Behaviour which Takes an Aggressive Form

Suffice it is to say under this section that the nurse requires to know the cause of behaviour in order to facilitate its change.

When aggression results from a patient seeking attention, many factors will determine the response:

(1) Is the aggression likely to harm the patient or another person?
(2) Is an extinction programme established (see p. 82)?
(3) What other course of action is available other than reinforcing the undesired behaviour by attention?
(4) Can attention realistically be withheld long enough to wait for

some positive behaviour to emerge, so that this can be linked with attention?

In all cases of aggressive behaviour, the nurse will be called upon to use her knowledge, discretion and judgement, and the aforementioned suggestions are intended only as a guide. In reality the nurse must find her own appropriate strategies for the unique individual in her care.

Key Concepts

(1) It has been shown that aggression may take many forms. Physical violence, verbal abuse, hostility, self-mutilation, depression or sulkiness may all be manifestations of aggressiveness.
(2) Primarily the patient's problems centre around an inability to communicate effectively emotional, physical or interpersonal problems. If the patient is unable to use appropriate strategies to deal with emotions such as insecurity, loneliness, despair, frustration and uncertainty, they may very well be seen as frank aggression.
(3) It has been suggested that the patient requires understanding and someone to listen to him; he may subsequently be able to understand himself more clearly. It is only when he is able to do this for himself that he will be able to formulate new strategies to cope with his feelings.
(4) The nurse's responsibilities are to herself, her colleagues and the patient. It is possible that these responsibilities can only be discharged successfully on some occasions by the use of restraint. When these situations arise, the nurse should be able to restrain effectively with the minimum force, and subsequently investigate by critical evaluation the necessity for such action.
(5) The skilled nurse will be able to maintain the patient's trust by remaining honest, avoid violence by absorbing abuse, distracting the patient, and using appropriate positive reassurance. We would conclude by adding that this altruistic approach is only possible in an established climate when the nurse truly cares for the patient; has tried to form an empathic bond; and is

open enough to share with the patient her feelings and hopes for more positive ways of dealing with the causes of the aggression.

Suggested Further Reading

COHSE *The Management of Violent or Potentially Violent Patients: Report of A Special Working Party Offering Information, Advice and Guidance to COHSE Members* (COHSE, Banstead, Surrey, 1977)
Lorenz, Konrad *On Aggression* (Methuen, London, 1970)
Ownes, R.G. and Ashcroft, J.B. *Violence: A Guide for the Caring Professions* (Croom Helm, London, 1985)
Storr, Anthony *Human Aggression* (Penguin Books, Harmondsworth, 1979)

8 THE ANXIOUS PATIENT

Matthew sat wringing his hands and rocking backwards and forwards with a strained facial expression.

'Hello, Matthew, is there anything I can do to help you at the moment?'

'I'm scared sick, I don't know what it is, but I just can't seem to think straight, everything is so difficult. My head aches, my heart is pounding, it's as if I've got some dreadful disease.'

Matthew has been complaining of a variety of bodily symptoms for some time, but underlying all these are his persistent feelings of fear resulting in a severe 'anxiety state'. This fear incapacitates Matthew to such an extent that he finds it difficult to do the simplest of tasks. The nature of his anxiety clouds his thinking to such an extent that he finds it difficult to pin-point any specific area that causes it. This is generally known as 'free-floating anxiety'. However, anxiety can present in a multitude of ways, and may occur as a symptom in any psychiatric disorder. Another form of anxiety is where a specific fear can be isolated, which results in a 'phobic state'. Phobias such as fear of open spaces (agoraphobia) can be totally incapacitating and require very specific nursing intervention (see p. 88).

Anxiety occurs in an individual when he is confronted with some form of stress. It is a state whereby the body prepares itself for a 'fight' or 'flight' reaction to the stressful situation. Its physiological origin (see Figure 8.1) gives rise to symptoms such as palpitations, increased respiration, diarrhoea, frequency of micturition, tension, headache, nausea and potentially many others. However, an appropriate level of anxiety can be very beneficial. For example, before a race, in exam preparation and other situations where the individual is put to the test, anxiety usually increases the motivation to do well. Once the anxiety goes beyond its useful level, disaster can occur, e.g. exam or test failure. Examples of situations where anxiety is a major component of the individual's feeling state include exams, interviews, important personal occasions, e.g. marriage, birth of a sibling, loss of a loved one and funerals, competitive events, life threatening or personal danger situations. The body's response is geared towards helping the individual cope with these situations. But there are times when the physiological response remains when the stimulus situation appears to have gone. Recall how you felt before your interview, increase that feeling tenfold, and imagine feeling like that days and sometimes weeks on end; you will then be going towards some understanding of how it must feel to be suffering from an 'acute anxiety reaction'.

Some people are more anxious than others, which could be due to many factors, some being personality, family environment and influence, personal financial and occupational circumstances, education and ability to relax. The ability to cope with anxiety stems from an awareness of what causes it and then a purposeful attempt to either avoid the cause or cope with the anxiety. Avoidance, however, could lead to further anxiety when eventual confrontation of the 'stressful event' takes place, or just the thought of the event could be sufficient to set off an anxious reaction.

People have different ways of coping with anxious moments. These are often unconscious processes aimed at protecting oneself from the anxiety provoking situation or thought. These processes are termed 'mental defence mechanisms' and were first described by Freud (1958). Using defence mechanisms initially serves a useful purpose in that it allows time for an individual to work through the anxiety situation, e.g. the student who fails the exam for the final time may say or think initially, 'Well, it's probably for the best anyway, I'm a more practical person and if I had passed I would have been stuck with the office responsibility which isn't really what I want.'

This 'rationalisation' gives the person time, if they so wish, to work through to the actual thinking and acceptance of 'I have not got the intellectual or technical ability to pass this exam.' This form of thinking initially would have been anxiety provoking, so the 'unconscious' use of the mechanism rationalisation occurs. There are many other mechanisms that are used, depending upon the individual and the situation (see Appendix 1). Overuse of these, however, is not conducive to 'healthy living' and many patients with anxiety states tend to rely rather heavily on them. It is therefore necessary for the nurse to understand these mechanisms and be aware of when they are used excessively in order to appreciate the stressful areas in the patient's life.

Figure 8.1: The Physiological Origin of Anxiety

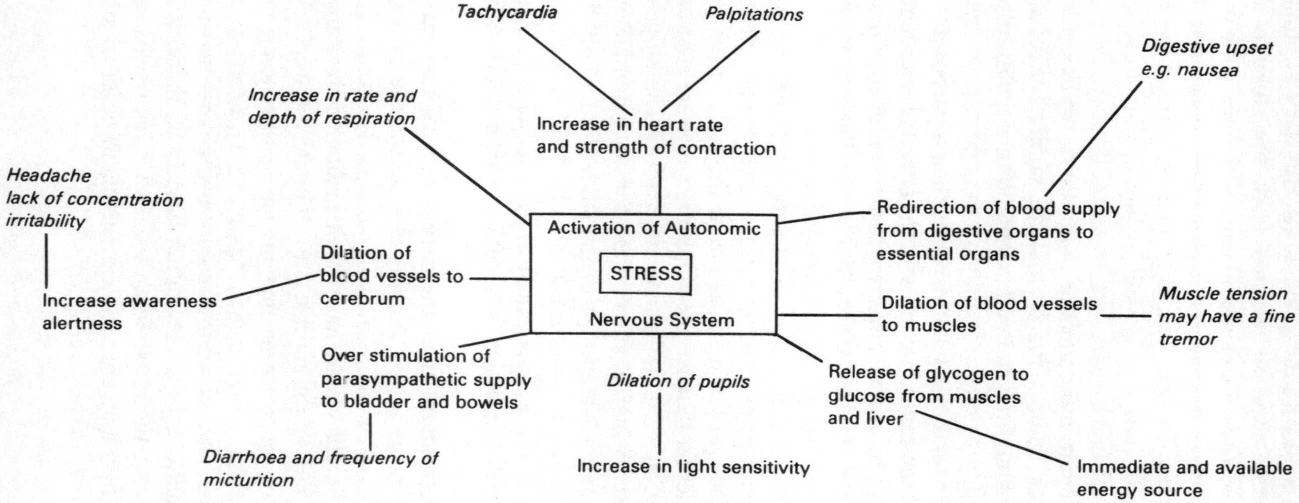

Other symptoms of anxiety are also due to alteration of sympathetic/parasympathetic action, adjusting blood supply and increasing function. These include: *increase in sweating, dry mouth, flushed face.*

Symptoms are shown in italic.

The Problems and Needs of the Anxious Patient

The problems and subsequent needs of the anxious patient are mainly twofold: those presented as a direct result of the physiological response, and those related to the psychological effects of fear (see Figures 8.2 and 8.3). On assessment it is often necessary for the nurse to take reasonable control of the situation, conveying a calm air of confidence in order to avoid the patient experiencing further anxieties related to 'Do they know what they are doing?' Clear explanations of 'what will happen next' are necessary in order to minimise the effects of the patient's anxieties concerning the outcome of his admission. A steady tour of the environment and an early introduction to the patient's personal space should help minimise his feelings of insecurity, at all times making clear the safety line of 'nurse availability'. It may be useful to concentrate on a one to one basis initially, until the patient's confidence grows.

Priorities of care need to be quickly assessed and acted upon. In severe anxiety states, it is likely that the nursing intervention will work in conjunction with the medical treatment. Prescription of anxiolytic medication, psychological testing, group therapy and relaxation techniques may all play a part in the care of the anxious patient.

Implications for the Nurse

The nurse when caring for the anxious patient must remain calm and confident, acting in a sense as a model for the patient. However, this is by no means an easy task, because the anxiety that is generated from the patient is often severe enough to cause anxiety in the nurse.

A situation can occur whereby, while the nurse is listening, the patient's expectations of the nurse to do something increase, the nurse's feelings of responsibility to do something for the patient increase, and at the same time the nurse realises how powerless she is to help, thus creating a 'mutual anxiety provoking' relationship. The danger then is that the nurse's anxiety reflects further on to the patient, and, instead of having a calming effect, the patient's anxiety increases. An extension of this could be when a patient detects his anxiety being reciprocated and becomes increasingly

Figure 8.2: The Psychological Problems and Needs of the Anxious Patient

Problem	Potential Problem	Need
Continual feelings of fear and dread	Panic attack	Calm, accepting presence of nurse. Clear safety limits explained
Insecurity	Uncertainty Loss of confidence	Highlight and reward any signs of progress. Give clear indications of any changes in treatment or care
Agitation	Exhaustion Social isolation	Encourage rest. Provide opportunity for privacy. Guide appropriateness of behaviour, i.e. protect from other patients' reactions to ceaseless agitation
Lack of concentration	Inability to complete simplest of tasks	Occupation given at appropriate level of patient's concentration. Regularly assessed and suitably changed to encourage distraction from personal worries
Frustration	Irritability, anger	Opportunity to vent and explore feelings, to be listened to and understood

Figure 8.3: The Physiological Problems and Needs of the Anxious Patient

Problems	Potential Problems	Needs
Digestive upset, e.g. nausea	Anorexia, loss of weight	Monitoring of dietary intake and weight. Small, regular, non-irritating nutritional meals. Appropriate medication for indigestion
Frequency of micturition and diarrhoea	Incontinence, accidental soiling, dehydration	Easily accessible toilet facilities. Clothes that launder well and are practical. Extra fluids to compensate loss. Appropriate medication for severe diarrhoea
Excessive sweating	Body odour, discomfort, soreness	Frequent opportunity for bathing. Encouragement of self-care
Increased respiration and palpitations	Exacerbation of anxiety fears of physical cause/disease	Clear and simple explanation of symptoms. Avoid dwelling upon patient's physical complaints. Focus upon feelings underlying the symptoms
Continual agitation, movement, restlessness	Irritability, frustration, aggression, exhaustion	Encourage rest and relaxation techniques at any opportune time

frustrated to the extent of directed aggression towards the nurse. The tendency for the nurse to withdraw with feelings of rejection is considerable, and may influence the nurse to the extent that she may avoid the patient in the future. It therefore becomes clear that whilst interacting with anxious individuals, it is important for the nurse to be aware of her own anxiety levels and to understand the possible causes within any interactions. The causes are often concerned with the nurse's self-doubt or lack of confidence (see Figure 8.4), the effects of which are minimised if she is prepared for this happening and given some idea of the strategies that she could use when anxiety levels increase in a nurse/patient interaction. These strategies are concerned with relying on genuineness, i.e. being honest to yourself about self-doubt and personal limitations. This will help to perceive intended interactions with realistic expectations, thus reducing what often becomes 'personal pressure' of having to do something well and in concrete terms. During interactions the strategy used is the practical application of skills, and the more effective these are, the less likelihood there is of 'personal distractors' causing anxiety in the nurse.

Principles and Skills Required to Help the Anxious Patient

The skills required to help anxious patients are mainly those associated with encouraging them to explore their feelings in order to identify in more concrete terms the areas in their lives that contribute to the anxious state. Referring back to Matthew's statement when he was asked by the nurse is there was anything she could do to help:

'I'm scared sick, I don't know what it is, but I just can't seem to think straight, everything is so difficult. My head aches, my heart is pounding, it's as if I've got some dreadful disease.'

Figure 8.4: Some Causes of 'Nurse Anxiety' during Interactions with Patients

Personal	Environmental	Patient
Am I helping? What am I doing? Will I be able to help? Am I saying the right things? What shall I say next?	Have I got time? Should I be doing something else? What about the other patients? I must go soon. How do I end this?	He is becoming more frustrated. He is becoming very emotional. What if he turns his frustration towards me? Can I cope with all this?

Nurse. You feel frightened because you are not sure what's happening, you have all these symptoms and you suspect there may be something physically wrong with you.

This response demonstrates the use of paraphrasing and reflecting in order to convey empathy to the patient, but also allowing him to hear again what he has just said, thus giving more time to focus on what he actually does feel. The tentativeness in the nurse's response at this stage is important in order to allow the patient to correct or focus in further on the nurse's response.

Matthew. Yes, it makes me wonder sometimes if there is something physically wrong, but at the same time, I know it's to do with my thinking, my feelings, the worry about home, relationships and work.
Nurse. So you realise that the way you are at the moment is to do with your thinking, feelings and worries about home, relationships and work. I'm wondering which of those is the crucial issue for you at the moment?

One of the skills when interacting with anxious patients is to distract them from dwelling too long on their bodily symptoms, as this is likely to increase their fears, yet at the same time the nurse must acknowledge and show understanding of the patient's feelings. The response above is a 'clarifying' skill, in that it is an extension of a paraphrase asking the patient to sort out priorities, which may mean the patient responding to something that is the most crucial issue, or something that the patient feels comfortable to talk about at this stage. Either way, it is helping him to explore his situation with the aim of identifying feelings and problems.

Matthew. Well, I suppose a lot of it is to do with home and my wife. She's changed so much over the last few years, she has so many new interests it's as if she's a different person.
Nurse. How does this change in your wife make you feel?

The open question is used here for two main reasons: one is to gain more information, and the other is to help the patient focus upon his own feelings in the present rather than his wife's behaviour in the past. This is important, for it enables the patient to continue talking about himself, whereas the details about the past and others, although relevant and possibly serving a purpose in some cases, may cloud the issue of the 'patient's feelings now' in this type of situation.

Matthew. I just know that I'm becoming less important to her, that one day she's going to go off with someone who's on her level that she can share more interests with. I just can't keep up with her.

It is often the case that because of the high level of anxiety within the patient, even when asked directly how he feels, he may still come back with more detail concerning his feelings but not identifying them. When this occurs, it is important that the nurse uses an empathic response to ensure that understanding has taken place and that the patient has a chance to pin-point his feelings:

Nurse. Are you saying you're feeling inferior in some way to your wife and this makes you feel insecure within the relationship?

The stronger the feeling words used, the more tentatively the nurse should say them, as they can sometimes be received with some surprise, and, if said dogmatically, the patient may become defensive and refuse to explore the possibility of owning the feelings put to him.

The skills described so far are the listening skills from the counselling model (see p. 34). To expect to use advanced skills in a severely anxious patient is unrealistic as much working through of the patient's feelings is required before problem solving should be considered. This 'working through' is facilitated by the nurse if the skills above are used in conjunction with observational skills. Sensitivity to the patient's non-verbal behaviour will help the nurse appreciate the general state of the patient through observing behaviour such as restlessness, pacing, rocking, wringing of hands, nail biting and many others that are indicative of anxiety. Also, being acutely aware of more subtle changes during interactions, e.g. looking away, resorting to closed posture, change in tone of voice, will help identify possible areas of particular difficulty in the patient's life. This does not necessarily mean that it would be right for the nurse to focus on these areas, as this would depend upon many factors, e.g. how secure the patient feels within the nurse/patient relationship and the ability of the nurse to cope with the possible consequences. At the very least, any appreciation of the patient's anxiety situations will enhance the empathy that the nurse achieves.

Another area of skills that is very useful for the care of the anxious patient is that related to facilitating relaxation and teaching methods of self-relaxation. There are many different methods of relaxation, but one technique that is commonly used involves the physical relaxation of the body by systematically tensing and relaxing groups of muscles. This involves following instructions either from someone or a tape. The skills needed to perform this are: appreciation of the appropriate environment, i.e. a quiet, comfortable, dimly lit room, the use of a tone of voice that is soft, clear and free from obvious distractions such as stutters, lisps or strong accents, and a sensitivity to timing, ensuring that while the nurse is taking the person through the experience, she allows sufficient time to carry out the individual exercises. This is one advantage over the tape recorder; another is that the nurse can be sensitive to a particular area of the body that is visibly more tense than anywhere else, and subsequently spend a little more time helping the patient to relax that part. Once the patient has learned the principles of physical relaxation, the nurse can help him to apply those principles to himself at times of stress, in order to minimise the effects of anxiety.

Summary

Anxiety is a part of all of us and can be useful in increasing our motivation to do certain things. However, when anxiety becomes the predominant emotion in our lives, its usefulness turns to destruction, fear and helplessness. Its physiological and psychological nature requires the nurse to have a clear understanding of its origin and effect, and the subsequent problems and needs. When caring for the anxious patient, the nurse must be in touch with her own feelings and be aware of her own anxiety levels, so as not to compromise the attention she gives to the patient. The skills required to help the patient explore his anxious world are the listening skills of paraphrasing, reflecting, questioning and clarifying. These are used to help gain empathy with the patient, at the same time supporting him through confused and sometimes painful emotions.

Key Concepts

(1) Anxiety can present in a multitude of ways and may occur as a symptom in any psychiatric disorder.
(2) It is a state whereby the body prepares itself for a 'fight' or 'flight' reaction.
(3) Its physiological origin is due to the overactivity of the sympathetic and part of the parasympathetic nervous system.
(4) Mental defence mechanisms are unconscious processes aimed at protecting the 'self' from anxiety.
(5) The problems and needs of the anxious patient are those presented as a direct result of the physiological response and those related to the psychological effects of fear.
(6) The nurse, when caring for the anxious patient, must remain calm and confident.
(7) The nursing skills required are those of effective listening to gain empathy and help exploration of the patient's emotions.
(8) Other skills are related to observation, sensitivity and the use of non-verbal communication and the facilitation and teaching of relaxation.

Suggested Further Reading

Girdano, Daniel and Everly, George *Controlling Stress and Tension* (Prentice-Hall, Hemel Hempstead, 1979)
Goodwin, Donald *Phobia: The Facts* (Oxford University Press, Oxford, 1983)
Hambly, Kenneth *Overcoming Tension* (Sheldon Press, London, 1983)
Madders, J. *Stress and Relaxation* (Martin Dunitz, London, 1980)
Melville, Joy *First Aid in Mental Health* (Allen and Unwin, London, 1980)
Monten, Edgar, A. *Anxiety and Phobias: Their Cause, Symptoms and Treatment* (Roseneath Scientific Publications, Worcester Park, Surrey, 1974)
Priest, Robert *Anxiety and Depression* (Martin Dunitz, London, 1980)
Rycroft, C. *Anxiety and Neurosis* (Penguin Books, Harmondsworth, 1971)
Spielberger, C. *Understanding Stress and Anxiety*, A Life Cycle Book (Harper and Row, New York, 1979)

9 THE OBSESSIVE COMPULSIVE PATIENT

'I must always wash my hands before putting the clothes into the spin dryer. If I can't remember whether I have done so or not, I think to myself, "It doesn't matter, I'll hang them out to dry anyway," but it will go on and on in my mind until the clothes are dry and I have to wash them again, this time ensuring I wash my hands first.' Mrs Armstrong evidently washes all her clothes three times, each time after drying.

'I must clean something before I touch it, then after I've touched it I must wash my hands. Sometimes I don't realise I'm doing it, but then I know if I didn't do it, I would never rest. I spend most of my day cleaning clothes and the house. My husband has been very tolerant up to now, he used to try and help by cleaning parts of the house for me, but that was no good, I had to do it, I had to make sure it was right.'

The above account illustrates obsessive compulsive behaviour from a woman whose life is now totally dominated by her rituals. An *obsession* is a repetitive thought which the individual is unable to control, which often leads to a *compulsion*, an urge to act in a way that the mind knows to be irrational but which can only be resisted with the greatest difficulty. In Mrs Armstrong's case, the obsession is the persisent thought of having to ensure something is clean, in an attempt to prevent contamination, and the compulsion was the actual act of cleaning and washing, in a precise order. If that order was disturbed, the ritual would have to be started all over again.

The obsessional person lives in a world in which every eventuality is taken account of and every counter-move calculated, so that in a sense he cannot be surprised. This eventually involves the significant people in his world, causing tension, anxiety and eventually distress. It is quite usual for someone with obsessive compulsive behaviour to be admitted with accompanying depression. This may be a reaction to being involved in and responsible for domestic chaos, and at the same time having the feeling of helplessness, yet also having insight into the irrationality of it all. This frustrating picture usually results in a cry for help from the whole family, in which case all should be involved in the care of the individuals concerned. The family in this case is likely to ask questions such as:

— 'What causes it?'
— 'Why should it happen?'
— 'Is it to do with us?'

It is often the case that the nurse will have to use her skills to explain to the family the nature of the behaviour and the possible reasons for its development. One theory is that obsessive compulsive states are a result of unresolved conflicts and anxieties unconsciously pushed back and taken over by various defence mechanisms (see 'Regression', Appendix I). It is also likely that the underlying conflicts are concerned with the 'significant others'. The obsessional character develops out of the need to obtain approval by being excessively tidy and controlled. A child will react to standards set by the parents and sometimes these standards may conflict with normal developmental tasks. This may lead to the child being very frustrated, which could contribute to the incidence of obsessive compulsive behaviour later in adult life. Whatever the reason for its occurrence, the family is usually very much involved, therefore the continuation of the principal aims of care should continue from the hospital environment to the home.

The Problems and Needs of the Obsessive Compulsive Patient

One of the initial and sometimes major problems for the obsessional patient occurs as a direct result of admission to hospital. It is often the case that the patient's ritualistic behaviour can only be carried out to a satisfactory degree at home because he has that element of control over his environment. However, in hospital, the potential to contaminate or disrupt has increased tremendously. This often becomes apparent to the patient on or shortly after admission, thus increasing the likelihood of someone presenting not only with the obsessive compulsive behaviour, and likely underlying depression, but also with acute anxiety symptoms (see p. 179). So the need of the patient in this situation, for the first 48 hours or so, is to allow him to find some form of security in his own personal routine in order for the anxiety to drop to tolerable levels. Therefore the constraints and demands that are usually placed on newly admitted patients should in this case be minimal. Once this principle has been taken into consideration, the problems and needs become evident, based on an individual nursing assessment. However, there are some problems that are common to many obsessional patients. Many patients with severe states are at risk from self-neglect, mainly in the areas of sleep and nutrition. Because of the time consuming compulsive behaviour these areas are given low priority by the patient. Their needs in this case are obvious, but it is through the skills of the nurse that these are met; by her providing opportunities to sleep and ensuring adequate nutrition, the patient can continue without the added complications of exhaustion. A physical complication that is common to those compulsive behaviours that include hand-washing is one of sore and abrased hands. Any measures that the patient finds acceptable to treat or minimise the risk of this occurring should be encouraged. This may vary from the use of creams to wearing gloves in order to limit the risk of contamination, thus cutting down on the need to wash the hands. We have observed in some individuals, where hand-washing is an important part of their ritual, red, sore and cut hands that are painful to the touch, yet these same people, because of the compulsive nature of their behaviour, will scrub these sore and injured hands with a nail brush. The physical pain experienced by them is minimal compared to the psychological pain of doubt, uncertainty and torment they would have experienced if prevented from doing so.

It may be that a nurse, in an endeavour to protect the patient from further damage, will inadvertently, by trying to stop the patient, cause more harm than good, for if the patient's ritual is thwarted he will feel compelled to start over again. The patient's needs in relation to this are to be able to conduct his rituals in an atmosphere of acceptance. At the same time the nurse encourages any limits the patient may place on himself and any behaviour other than that of an obsessional nature. The only time when this principle is not adhered to is when the patient is receiving response prevention therapy — which is when the patient is encouraged to face the fear, gradually increasing time with the anxieties until the tendency to carry out a particular ritual diminishes.

The patient's continual high level of anxiety and the potential risks of severe panic attacks if the rituals are thwarted make it necessary for the patient to know how to relax. Teaching and helping in the use of relaxation methods will be a useful tool when dealing with the patient's unresponsiveness due to anxiety. Activities and occupation must take into consideration that anxiety levels are likely to impair the ability to concentrate. When planning the care programme the nurse must allow for the fact that it is likely that the obsessional patient will find it difficult to follow any new instructions or tasks that would interfere with his routine. It is therefore essential that any changes in therapeutic occupation are carefully explained and planned in advance. How responsive and accepting the patient will be to any programme, especially if it involves group activities, will depend largely upon how the obsessional behaviour is perceived. The patient is open to ridicule by other patients and it may be that as well as modelling an accepting approach, the nurse may have to explain tactfully to other patients the need for acceptance throughout the ward. If the patient is subject to embarrassment and hilarity, the outcome is likely to be one of increased ritualistic behaviour.

Implications for the Nurse

Modelling an accepting approach can be very difficult with patients who seem not to respond to their own logic and insight. This can seem very frustrating not only for the patient, but also for the nurse. It may develop at times into a feeling of helplessness on the nurse's part, from which frustration can grow into anger. It is important that the nurse is aware of the possibility of this occurring in order to prevent these emotions compromising the delivery of care. Being patient, understanding and helping the patient set small achievable goals will help both parties to achieve realistic expectations. Part of acceptance involves being able to respect the obsessional patient's rituals and allowing time for their completion (depending upon the regime of care). The nurse may be in conflict at times, as the patient's demands may be interfering with the care and attention given to other patients. It will be up to individual judgement at the time, aimed at achieving some compromise between balancing out the needs of the obsessional patient and the needs of the other patients.

Finally, there are times when we see things in others that we see in ourselves. Obsessive elements in anyone's personality can be helpful, especially in certain occupations where precision, accuracy and detail are essential. The organised and conscientious mind is a useful asset to any team leader. It is when the organisation and responsibility become dominated by torment, doubt and uncertainty that they cease to be useful.

Principles and Skills Required to Help the Obsessive Compulsive Patient

Initially the skills required for the obsessional patient will be those most appropriate to dealing with severely anxious individuals. Objective assessment for future planning should be postponed until the patient is reasonably settled. It may be appropriate during this time for one particular nurse to be given responsibility to help the patient in this settling down period. By listening and reassuring the patient about the accepting attitude of those around him, she will increase the likelihood of a trusting relationship being established which is vital for the future of the care programme.

Once the nurse is confident that the patient's anxiety level will not inhibit assessment, then she can, by using her skills of listening, non-verbal sensitivity and questioning, gather information from the patient which will be significant for the planning of future care. At the same time, by understanding and giving empathic responses, she is bringing the bond of nurse/patient relationship closer.

It is important to establish baseline assessment early in order to assess progress or deterioration during the patient's care. This involves establishing the nature of the obsession and rituals and the extent to which they are impairing the patient's life. From further exploration specific details of Mrs Armstrong's (see p. 185) constraints were:

Her obsessional thoughts related to:

— sexual matters;
— contamination;
— disease.

The only way she could lessen the dominance of these thoughts would be to proceed and complete a comprehensive self-cleansing ritual which would sometimes involve being in the bathroom for up to three hours.

Her obsessional washing was mainly:

— of herself following her obsessive thoughts;
— around the house, particularly the bathroom and toilet;
— her own clothes.

For Mrs Armstrong, the combination of these factors (which is often the case) resulted in a further problem area, i.e. *avoidance.*

— of large gatherings, particularly social ones such as parties;
— public toilets;
— talking about any topic that was remotely to do with sex.

This, alongside the information gathered from the whole family, will give a comprehensive picture of the nature and extent of disruption the patient and family have been experiencing.

In addition to using the skills of listening, the nurse could also use questionnaires designed particularly for rating an individual's anxiety levels, extent of obsessions or even the patient's mood. It must be remembered that it is not uncommon for a patient tormented by obsessions and rituals to be severely depressed to the extent that suicide could be an option 'out' for them. The anxiety rating scale could be in the shape of a 'fear inventory', whereby a hierarchy of anxiety provoking situations is established ranging from the least provoking, e.g. being prevented from washing her clothes the third time, to the most provoking — being prevented from bathing following a particularly 'disgusting' obsessional thought. This hierarchy will become useful in setting realistic goals depending on the therapeutic regime used.

Up to the present, many of the principles of care involve allowing patients to express their behaviour in an atmosphere of acceptance, thus helping them to lower their anxiety sufficiently to facilitate the exploration of underlying conflicts and encouraging patient 'self-limit setting'. However, there are certain behavioural methods that have proved to be very effective and are mainly based upon helping the patient come to terms with his behaviour and consequently his anxiety more directly. This regime is ideally conducted in a specialised therapeutic environment where all staff are trained in behavioural techniques (see Chapter 3) and the patients on the unit are undergoing similar experiences.

One or a combination of the following techniques can be used.

Response Prevention

The patient is encouraged to face a particular fear, e.g. using the toilet without washing her hands and the toilet immediately afterwards. The length of time between using the toilet and washing increases as the anxiety diminishes.

Modelling

Involves the nurse showing the patient the appropriate behaviour and reinforces the fact that no harm has occurred.

Graded Exposure in vivo

A hierarchy of anxiety producing situations is constructed. The patient agrees to confront these situations, beginning with the least anxiety producing and working towards the greatest.

Flooding

The patient agrees to confront the feared situation until the overwhelming anxiety begins to reduce naturally.

Contract Therapy

A mutual agreement between the parties concerned is made so that it is very clear and explicit. It establishes a bond or an obligation in such a way that the actions of one party demand the conduct of the other according to the terms of the contract.

These 'behavioural' therapies are all dependent upon the agreement and commitment of the patient. The appropriate skills here are those related to being able to explain and educate the patient about the nature and benefit of the therapies involved. Before embarking upon these, however, the patient must be equipped with the ability and experience of relaxation techniques (see p. 183). The ability to relax physically may mean the differences between success and failure, especially with techniques that involve gradually increasing anxiety levels. A patient's reluctance to commit himself to these regimes is understandable, and it may be appropriate to challenge the patient skilfully here, e.g.

'You say you want to stop these rituals, and that you can see the benefit of these techniques, yet you still don't feel able to commit yourself to them. I'm wondering if there is anything else getting in the way?'

This response points out some discrepancies between what the patient says and does and gives him a chance to explore further his feelings and behaviour. Another challenge to someone who has already verbally committed themselves to a particular therapy could be:

'You've said that you see the value in these sessions and that you agree to participate, yet you consistently cancel appointments, make excuses or just don't turn up. How do you think that is perceived?'

If the patient replies honestly, then a description of the perception and reasons for behaviour will follow, but if the patient continues to follow the line of 'apology', 'I will try' or 'I keep forgetting,' then it is likely that further exploration of his anxieties and identification of needs is required.

The dangers of challenging (see p. 54) must be considered carefully, especially with people who have insight and are frustrated by the helplessness of not being able to act out their own logic. There is no therapeutic benefit from challenging the discrepancy between 'I know it's wrong, silly or irrational' and the continuation of their behaviour with obsessive compulsive patients, as this is the consequence of their conflicts and not its origin.

It is likely that when caring for individuals with these kinds of problems contact with the family is usually considerable and beneficial. Keeping them informed, especially the spouse, of the principles of care and progress will enhance the likelihood of some continuation of care from the hospital environment to the home. The community psychiatric nurse may be involved in helping plan a specific programme of care to continue in the home, and may be instrumental in encouraging 'family talk', if necessary conducting family therapy alongside individual counselling sessions. All of which will be in support of the patient fighting the battle against his own 'constraints'.

Summary

The individual whose life is governed by routine and who then becomes uncertain whether that routine is enough is expressing internal anxieties and conflict in his own way. The nurse in caring for this individual must aid him in conquering his personal loss of control, and at the same time must help him express his anxieties. A major obstacle to this is that one enhances the other, i.e.

attempting to control or limit his compulsion increases his anxiety, yet expressing his anxieties and exploring areas of conflict are likely to increase the occurrence of his compulsion. It is therefore essential to devise a balanced programme based upon individual needs and problems and the resources available to cater for them.

The overall skills required, however, are: those needed initially to facilitate exploration to a level essential for accurate assessment, i.e. exploratory counselling skills, and, later, to help the patient express personal conflict areas; teaching skills to aid the patient through his therapies; behavioural skills (see p. 70), depending upon the regime set; challenging skills for the reluctant patient; and, finally, 'family skills', i.e. those skills required to enable a family to work together, communicate and support each other throughout this crisis.

Key Concepts

(1) An obsession is a repetitive thought that the individual is unable to control, often leading to a compulsion, which is an urge to act in a way that the mind knows to be irrational, but which can only be resisted with the greatest difficulty.

(2) As a direct consequence of admission, someone with obsessive compulsive behaviour is also likely to present with acute anxiety symptoms.

(3) Because of the time consuming nature of many rituals, patients are often at risk from personal self-neglect of physical needs, e.g. nutrition and rest.

(4) It is important for the nurse to be aware of her own feelings of helplessness less this turns to frustration and anger, possibly compromising the care that she gives.

(5) It is not uncommon for a patient tormented by obsessions and rituals to be severely depressed to the extent that suicide could be an option 'out' for him.

(6) Many of the principles of care involve allowing the patient to express his behaviour in an atmosphere of acceptance, thus helping him to lower his anxieties sufficiently to facilitate exploration of underlying conflicts and encouragement of 'self-limiting' behaviour.

(7) Certain behavioural methods have been found to be very useful and effective, mainly: response prevention; modelling;

graded exposure *in vivo*; flooding and contract therapy.

(8) Keeping the family informed of the principles of care and progress made may enhance the likelihood of some continuation of care from the 'hospital' or 'unit' to the home.

Suggested Further Reading

Melville, Joy *Phobias and Obsessions: Their Understanding and Treatment* (Allen and Unwin, London, 1977)

Monten, Edgar A. *Obsessional Neurosis: Its Causes, Symptoms and Treatment* (Roseneath Scientific Publications, Surrey, 1974)

10 THE HYSTERICAL PATIENT

Sheila is a 25-year-old married woman with two young children. Prior to admission she had a history of fainting, giddiness and amnesia for certain events. This made the domestic situation at home rather difficult, as she had very little support from friends, neighbours and other family members. Also, her husband had recently taken up a position which involved him working away for most of the week. Her admission came about following a referral from her doctor via the police. She had told the police that her children, aged five and seven, had been missing for two hours, and it was only after a comprehensive search of the neighbourhood that they were found at a friend's house a few streets away. This, according to her friend, was organised and agreed upon the day before, and in fact that morning Sheila had dropped the children off herself.

Shortly after admission, Sheila began to develop a loss of sensation and movement in her right arm. In response to a nurse's encouragement to use her right arm in order to maintain the muscular strength remaining, Sheila's response was 'It's all right, I can always use my left'. Sheila had undergone a variety of physical diagnostic tests prior to admission, and all were negative. The GP suggested to her that she might be under a lot of stress and admission to a psychiatric unit might give her time to rest. Her attitude to this was positive with the proviso that no one should consider her 'mentally ill'.

The above case demonstrates several patterns of behaviour and responses common to many forms of hysteria. Although hysteria can take several forms, they all have a common factor: an emotional reaction to stress which is characterised by some form of physical disability or mental disturbance. The physical symptoms are ways in which individuals protect themselves from conflict and anxiety that they find unbearable or unsolvable. By unconsciously converting the anxiety into something physical, which can be as serious as 'blindness' or 'total paralysis', the individual gains attention from others and becomes preoccupied with the 'self', to the extent that the original areas of distress is repressed (see Appendix I, 'Repression' and 'Conversion'). Consequently the anxiety reduces and what often occurs is that the patient achieves 'secondary gain' — when an individual is rewarded for whatever symptoms are portrayed. In Sheila's case, the secondary gain is the attention she achieves, primarily from her husband.

After carefully listening to and assessing Sheila and her husband, it became apparent that the relationship between them and his change of job were major areas of concern. So, by unconsciously converting this area of anxiety, she gained the proximity and concern of her husband, which were previously lacking. Other 'secondary gains' may inadvertently come from the nurses caring for her. By reinforcing the 'sick role' and offering sympathy as opposed to empathy, it is possible to develop an acute hysterical reaction into a chronic one, where muscle wasting and weakness can occur in a paralysed limb through lack of use.

Another common factor to hysterical behaviour is that of the patient's attitude towards the physical symptoms. A comparison of someone's response to paralysis with known cause to someone with hysterical paralysis will show the apparent lack of concern, e.g.

Questions and responses from organic paralysis

'Is it permanent?'
'How long will it last?'
'Will I gain any movement?'
'What chances have I of walking/running again?'
'What are the complications?'
'Why me?'
'What effect is this going to have on my family?'
'Can I/they cope with this?'

Questions and responses from hysterical paralysis

'It's one of those things.'
'I'll have to live with it.'
'I'll be all right.'
'I've got experts around me.'
'I'll have plenty of care.'
'Life goes on.'
As in Sheila's response (see p. 195): 'It's all right, I can always use my left.'

This attitude of inappropriate concern is generally known as 'la belle indifférence', and quite often the patient can describe the symptoms in great detail with the 'nonchalance' of describing everyday activities.

Hysterical symptoms, and in particular hysterical paralysis, can be quite easily distinguished from organic symptoms. The physical symptoms portrayed usually follow a pattern that is congruous to the patient's knowledge or insight to the affliction concerned. For example, Sheila's loss of sensation in the arm was complete from her elbow down to her wrist, but she could still feel below and above. This loss of sensation does not follow any known established nerve pathway, and therefore from a physiological basis cannot occur. It is known as 'stocking paralysis'. The response from the patient when confronted with this information is usually akin to:

'I don't know, I'm no doctor, all I know is that I can't feel anything and it's not helping matters when you're suggesting I can.'

At some time during interactions betweeen professionals and people presenting with hysterical symptoms there occurs an element of doubt: is this hysteria or organic? It is often the observations of the nurse which help to confirm this one way or the other. An example of some specific distinguishing observations are those related to hysterical convulsions. When the following characteristics are present, then convulsive hysteria is likely:

(1) No full loss of consciousness.
(2) The convulsion occurs only in the presence of others.
(3) No dangerous falls occur.
(4) Pupillary and deep reflexes are present.
(5) No biting of the tongue.
(6) No loss of bladder or bowel control.
(7) Facial flushing present, but no cyanosis or pallor.
(8) Attempts to open the eyes are resisted.

The problems and needs generated are very real for the patient, so the pain, discomfort and inconveniences are all important aspects of the patient's reality.

The Problems and Needs of the Hysterical Patient

The priority of care for the patient with suspected hysterical conversion will depend upon the severity of the symptoms. Symptoms like paraplegia or blindness will play a major role in determining the emphasis of care. The care must incorporate the physical consequences of the symptoms, e.g. for paralysed limbs the risk of soreness and muscle wasting exists, therefore hygiene, positioning and passive exercise are required. Any preventive measure to avoid complications must take place. However, it is important that the nurse, while carrying out these procedures, avoids sympathising and dwelling upon the effects of the symptoms. The nurse can, by suggesting the occurrence of independent movement and giving praise and encouragement, help the patient initiate slight and sometimes major movements, especially during passive exercises.

Some patients with hysterical symptoms have a low frustration threshold and are prone to extreme outbursts of temper, often at the most inopportune moments. What the patient wants is attention, but what he needs are alternative coping strategies. In between the 'want' and the 'need' is a nursing management problem. The action of the nursing team will depend upon the immediate environment in which the incident is occurring. If the patient's behaviour is totally inappropriate and is disruptive to those around, he may need to be removed to a place where he can act out his own behaviour without the attention he seeks. However, if there is no harm to himself or others, ignoring his behaviour in the environment where it occurs may be more beneficial. Any signs of acceptable behaviour can be rewarded by the attention he initially sought. Discussion on why the incident occurred in the first place needs to take place some time after the event, when the patient and the effects of the incident have hopefully calmed down. One of the negative effects of this sort of incident is the pervasion of tension and anxiety in the ward. This may have an adverse effect on interpatient relationships. The lack of understanding and potential rejection from the other patients may reinforce the already low self-esteem the hysterical patient may have. The patient's needs, in respect of this, are for him to be accepted for what he is. The chances of this occurring are enhanced greatly if he is surrounded by understanding and accepting individuals. The nurse can help the other patients by example and attitudes of approach generating acceptance throughout the unit. Including the patient in group activities and encouraging responsibilities within the ward environment will increase the patient being accepted as a group member by his fellow patients. Another form of behaviour that is often exhibited from a patient with hysterical symptoms is making extra demands upon an individual nurse. This may also interfere with the patient's chances of being accepted by the other patients, but also has specific implications.

Implications for the Nurse

Generally the demands on the psychiatric nurse are great, but they become particularly so when one patient seeks personal and additional attention over and above what can realistically be given. There is a tendency for patients with some element of hysteria to seek emotional attachment or demand special attention from the nurse. They may expect the nurse to give up her breaks, stay behind, or even contact outside working hours. It is at these times that the nurse must find a balance between appropriate amount of attention given to the patient and the time needed for herself.

She may need to communicate honestly the effects of the demands the patient is having upon her and the need for personal time. Stressing the professional role and the need for team work is particularly relevant at these times. All this should be communicated with an attitude of acceptance, but even this can be stretched with some patients, particularly those who emphasise the sick role. The nurse must be aware of the dangers of judging 'hysteria as false, and labelling them as lazy and immature malingerers'. Malingering is quite different. It is an intentional and often malicious effort to deceive and in some way gain. Hysteria is the result of totally unconscious processes, and no malice is intended by it.

Principles and Skills Required to Help the Hysterical Patient

It must be remembered while dealing with patients exhibiting hysteria that they have within their life history an area of serious conflict. This area would likely cause great psychological trauma if they were coldly confronted with that particular part of their life. So one of the aims when caring for them is gradually to help them identify these areas and to help them gain the confidence and strength to cope with them in reality.

The skills required to do this are the assessment skills, mainly observation and questioning, sensitivity to the patient's non-verbal communication, empathy and challenging. From first contact with the patient, the nurse must gather as much relevant information as possible, paying particular attention to possible areas within the patient's life that show signs of sensitivity, defensiveness, reluctance to disclose or discomfort. With the appropriate use of open questions and noting particularly the non-verbal response, useful information can be obtained for later rather than present counselling. For example, the nurse's notes on Sheila's admission read:

'When asked about how she felt about her husband working away from home, the patient replied in an angry tone of voice, "I've enough on my plate without bringing that up," at the same time folding her arms and looking away.'

Continual use of observational skills, focusing upon changes of behaviour and the circumstances in which they changed, may give further clues to areas of conflict.

The dangers of the nurse reinforcing the 'sick role', and consequently allowing the patient to achieve secondary gain, have already been mentioned. The skill of empathy is essential here, not only to avoid sympathising, but also to distract the patient into feelings that are in keeping with problems other than 'symptoms of conversion', e.g.

Sheila. This whole business is getting worse, I just can't cope, I'm losing control, even my arm is feeling foreign to me now.

Inappropriate response. You feel your arm is becoming less a part of you?

Useful response. You're not sure you can cope with things getting worse and you're feeling more out of control as the days go on?

These responses would bring very different replies from the patient. The first is likely to continue on the theme of Sheila's increasing paralysis, but the second is more likely to continue on the theme of her feelings and thoughts about her general progress. The former may reinforce the sick role; the latter is more likely to allow exploration towards identifying areas of personal conflict. Other skills the nurse may use in facilitating exploration are those that encourage the patient to express himself in the therapeutic environment of art and drama (see Chapter 22). These activities may help express painful areas in a safer and more personal way than in verbal expression. This level of exploration is all part of the process of gradual realisation and acceptance of the life difficulties that initially caused the patient's psychiatric predicament.

Once the nurse is confident enough that a fair degree of exploration and attempts to identify conflict have been made by the patient, and that the nurse/patient relationship is well based on trust and confidence, then challenging the patient's continual use of avoidance, denial and discrepancies at this stage may help the patient gradually to confront herself with her reality, e.g.

Nurse. On one hand you say you've accepted that your husband must work away from home, but on the other, every time we talk about it your tone of voice changes and you seem to become more uncomfortable.

If the patient is ready to explore this issue further, she will, but if not, she will continue to deny that there is anything wrong in that particular area. It may be appropriate to challenge further:

Nurse. I'm wondering why it is that whenever the topic of your relationship with your husband crops up, you quickly and quite inappropriately change the topic?

Challenging can sometimes be quite painful and the nurse must be prepared for an emotional response. It is unrealistic to expect to break through the defences without some pain, but it is realistic to expect the nurse to facilitiate the breakthrough gradually and to handle the consequences in a skilled way.

Once breakthrough has occurred, the nurse, with the help of the ward team, must offer support and create an appropriate environment for the patient to solve or accept the particular conflict realised. This may involve utilising specialised help and follow-up and community resources, in order to allow the patient to be aware of and use alternative coping strategies.

Summary

Certain individuals in an effort to defend themselves against the path of certain aspects of reality will unconsciously convert one area of pain into another. The converted pain offers a reprieve until someone can offer appropriate skills to help them face the initial reasons for escape. These skills are those related to creating an environment of acceptance, genuineness and trust, one that the patient can feel secure in, so that when pain is eventually experienced from a skilful challenge, it bonds the relationship rather than breaks it.

Key Concepts

(1) Hysteria involves an emotional reaction to stress which is characterised by some form of physical disability or mental disturbance.
(2) The converted symptoms are ways in which individuals protect themselves unconsciously from conflict and anxiety that they find unbearable or unsolvable.
(3) The priority of care for the patient with suspected hysterical conversion will depend upon the severity of the symptoms.
(4) There are times when the nurse may need to communicate honestly the effects of the demands the patient is making upon her.
(5) The patient who is 'defending' an area of serious conflict is vulnerable to serious psychological trauma if inappropriately and coldly confronted with the 'evidence'.
(6) The use of skills is aimed at gradually helping the patient to identify these areas and to help him gain the confidence and strength to cope with them in reality.
(7) The skills required to do this are assessment skills, mainly questioning and observation, sensitivity to non-verbal communication, empathy and challenging.
(8) It is unrealistic to expect to break through the defences without some pain, but it is realistic to expect the nurse to facilitate this gradually and handle the consequences skilfully.

Suggested Further Reading

Mershey, Harold *The Analysis of Hysteria* (Baillière Tindall, London, 1979)
Mitchell, A.R.K. 'Hysteria and Malingering', *Psychological Medicine in Family Practice* (Baillière, 1971)

11 THE INSTITUTIONALISED PATIENT

Some 15 years ago, David was admitted to hospital with a diagnosis of anxiety/depression, following an attempt to commit suicide. Although David remains in hospital, it is not due to his anxiety or depression, but because the institution is now the only place he feels safe and secure. Any attempt to converse with him about the subject of his discharge into the community is met with a blank stare, an anxiety attack, or an aggressive response.

David has become institutionalised to the extent that his original diagnosis is rather mild in comparison to the debilitating state in which he now finds himself. Other than on the issue of his discharge, David is obedient, and is complacent to an extraordinary degree. His mask-like features would persuade the observer that he was suffering from Parkinson's disease. This would be equally supported by the blank expressionless eyes and the shuffling gait. The give-away clues of his actual disability can be easily observed when for some reason his chair in the day room is taken by an unsuspecting stranger, or a new nurse changes his routine for some reason. It is then that this blank eyes become expressive, and David becomes animated, for his security and safety are threatened.

For the last 15 years, David's choices and decisions have been largely decided by other people. Having accepted that David's judgement was impaired due to his initial mental illness, it is still a sad reflection of the care he received that his decision making was excluded even to the simple decision of what time he should go to bed. From almost the first day, David's routine was set. What time he would arise, what he ate, where he slept, what occupied him, even how he should be entertained were influenced almost totally by what someone else felt was best for him. It can be noted by observation that, even within a short period of time in an active acute admission ward, patients will adopt predictable patterns of behaviour. If these behaviours are reinforced by the figures of authority, i.e. the staff, these behaviours tend to be repeated. The newly admitted patient, even if fully aware of his wishes, needs and his own assertiveness, may still be subject to anxiety and insecurity in a strange environment. The tremendous psychological pressures of the 'group' (other patients), 'authority' (the staff) and the established routine for him to comply and blend in will be extremely difficult to resist. Institutional behaviour is essentially behaving as the controllers of the institution expect and demand the patient to behave.

In his book *Institutional Neuroses* (1959), Russel Barton considers many causes and effects of the lack of choices within a patient's environment. We support Barton's ideas and add that it is the authorities' expectations of patients' behaviour that tends to stereotype, confine and constrict individuality. The following is a short list of just a few expectations staff may have. Any thoughtful nurse may easily double this list.

(1) Patients should comply to staff regulations (? regardless of whether explained, reasonable or difficult).
(2) Patients should not complain (they are here for treatment, and we're trying to help, aren't we?).
(3) Patients should adapt to the standards of the institution (whether this is improvement or decline).
(4) Patients should be grateful (we are helping them, aren't we?).
(5) Patients should be ... (substitute here almost any emotional description, and add) when ... (a time considered suitable in our values, e.g. patients should be 'happy' when told 'good' news. Patients should be 'tired' when it's bedtime).
(6) Patients should share our values about life, death, health and illness (at least).

The list can become endless. The intractable staff attitudes, whether 'good' or 'bad', will be *their* attitudes, and we suggest that the only therapeutic attitude to have concerning expectations of patients is: I expect patients to have different attitudes from mine and I respect their entitlement to have and keep them. To expect people to be the same, to fit in, to be 'normal' and to have similar standards and to accept this is in our opinion as likely a cause of institutionalisation as any suggested by Barton.

How long does it take to become institutionalised? This is a question often asked. There is no set or standard answer, as it will depend largely on the forces for and against such a situation. Some patients will be more resistant to complying with the institution, and some institutions will be less influential in making patients comply. To be fair to the latter, some progressive institutions are very aware of this problem and take active steps to avoid institutionalisation developing.

It is not in any case an 'all or nothing' concept: it is a process. It begins on the first contact with an institution, and ends only when contact is broken with that institution. The effects to the individual exposed to this process, as previously intimated, can vary tremendously. It is not entirely confined to patients: some staff may show signs of institutionalisation relatively quickly, and in some cases most severely. To look at the specific factors that affect the development of pathological states of institutionalisation in anyone exposed to the institution would require a longer discussion. We recommend that students interested in this area read both Barton's work and the work of Irving Goffman (see 'Suggested Further Reading').

The Problems and Needs of the Institutionalised Patient

Probably one of the most ironic problems that David has is that he has very few fundamental needs. His needs are almost entirely catered for by the institution. His primary needs of food, shelter, warmth and comfort are indefinitely available without anxiety of them ever being withdrawn. Even some of the higher order or complex needs, such as belongingness and companionship, may be supplied in the ward environment. It is only the very highest human needs of self-respect, self-esteem and prestige and what Maslow (1971) calls self-actualisation that the institution fails to supply.

It is in fact exactly this that the patient who has become institutionalised lacks: he has been bereft of self-esteem and self-respect, and he has been robbed of his humanity in his higher expectations. His dreams have become mundane or non-existent, and he has lost motivation to strive for the ultimate goals of personal satisfation that Maslow aptly described as self-actualisation. David's problem is not that his basic needs are not met — his problem is that his basic needs are met. It is because he no longer suffers any anxiety, because he experiences no challenge that he feels no sense of satisfaction. Having no prospects for the future, no plans and no expectations deprives an individual of his hopes and desires. Without incentive to fulfil basic human needs, the individual human spirit is deprived of motivation and dies, just as a flower dies without water. As if to substantiate the truth of this statement, the institutionalised patient is often described as 'dehumanised'. We take this to mean having lost the human spirit and leaving only the body shell.

The patient needs to be restored somehow, to have this human spirit rekindled, to have his dignity, his hopes and his dreams returned to him. What we must remember, however, is that if the process of robbing David of his humanity took 15 years, we must not expect to restore it in seven days. The process of 'rehabilitation' for David will not be a simple task. It may be painful for both parties to engage on a project that neither will enjoy, and the pay-offs are indefinite and distant.

Implications for the Nurse

The first crucial factor the nurse needs to sensitise herself to is that each approach she makes to each patient must be flexible. Having respect for a patient means much more than simply calling him 'Mr'. Respect denotes that you are aware of his rights as an individual, that you consider him to be a unique human being and that you will not cut across his values. To understand that what he holds to be valuable, no matter how silly it appears to you, must be respected.

This may mean that on some occasions the individual's wishes will clash with the customary routine and the nurse's expectations of patient behaviour. Rather than immediately dismissing this refusal or non-compliance as awkward, or unreasonable, allow a few minutes' contemplation of exactly how unreasonable it is and, more importantly, how unworkable it really is. Sometimes patients' suggestions are not at all silly and it has been known from time to time that listening to patients' views has brought about significant and desirable change. Adopting a flexible approach will probably do no more than offset some of the institutional processes in the more acute patients, and it will have much less effect on the longer-stay patients. Understanding this from the outset may help nurses become less frustrated, for if they are expecting startling results from simply altering their approach they will undoubtedly be disappointed.

Another factor nurses need to be aware of is the risk factor that a 'rehabilitation' approach requires. There are many risks nurses must take if they are intent on restoring a patient's dignity and the first is perhaps the damage to their own prestige. Nurses become nurses primarily, we believe, to help patients. Unfortunately, all too frequently the nurse's concept of 'helping' means making the patient dependent upon her. Stepping back from the patient and encouraging him to take more responsibility for himself, refusing to give advice and insisting on the patient making his own choices may initially result in damage to the nurse's self-image of her helping skills. It is only after several months of gradually observing the patient become more independent that the rewards received from such 'non-behaviour' can be appreciated. A further risk the nurse takes with this approach is the threat of reducing standards. It is often used as a convincing argument that when the nurse stops working on the patient, that the patient stops too. In other words, if the nurse does not insist that the patient has a bath, he probably won't have one at all. Fundamentally we disagree with this philosophy. We consider that although in practice this is largely what happens, it is used quite unfairly as an example. It fails to take account of the fact that the institution incapacitated the individual in the first place, that before the institutionalisation process took place the individual was quite capable of taking responsibility for his own bath. It would be ridiculous to 'remove an engine from a car and replace it with pedals and them exclaim, "See, I told you it wouldn't work on its own if we stopped pedalling."' It seems to us the exponents of the argument for nurses doing everything for the patients in order to stop standards falling are saying exactly this. Standards of dress, hygiene, table manners and ward tidiness may indeed decline, and obviously some degree of monitoring and subsequent persuasion may be necessary, but surely this is a very small price to pay for beginning the process of restoring the patient's motivation, self-respect and decision making.

Dispensing with the role of parent and entering into a more equal partnership with a patient can increase the risk of anxiety feelings within the nurse. This is perhaps because operating from a superior position had in the past engendered a feeling of security. When instructing or directing from a position of superiority it is not necessary to understand or explain the reasons for such prescriptions. Once you enter into an equal partnership with a patient, it is possible to be challenged. It may even be possible that you are wrong, and that, on introspection, no valid reasons can be found for some of the things you have been doing. Who knows, some of the traditions which have been respected perhaps need to be challenged?

Is it possible to imagine the ramifications of the following brief dialogue?

Nurse. Mr Brown, come along for a bath please, it's Thursday night again.
Patient. I'm sorry, nurse, although I would really like to please you, I'm not sure I care for a bath tonight, and definitely not just at the moment as I'm having a conversation with Mr Smith.

Nurse reports to charge nurse:

Nurse. Mr Brown refuses to have a bath.
Charge Nurse. Oh does he, I'll soon see about that.

Some nurses may recognise some of the dialogue, if not all of it. We appreciate that Mr Brown would be a very unusual patient to be so unreasonable, resistive and unco-operative, but we would be most happy to see many more Mr Browns none the less.

Principles and Skills Required to Help the Institutionalised Patient

We believe nurses need to be skilled in the following areas:

(1) Knowing and accepting the patient's values. This will entail the nurse listening to the patient, spending time with him, and trying to understand how he feels about himself and his life.
(2) Encouraging the patient to make choices. This requires some behavioural skills (see Chapter 3), especially using positive reinforcers and the shaping process to reward successive approximations towards independent choices. This process may begin by adding at least one choice to each daily activity, and gradually increasing the choices, i.e. increasing choice of bedtime from 8 p.m. to 9 p.m. and varying the times during the week; one choice of food at meal times increasing to several choices; proceeding eventually to choices of clothes, activities and recreation.

(3) Ensuring that the patient remains secure when faced with choices he is not used to. This will involve a special relationship which is trusting and open, but without being restricting, advising or over supportive. Establishing such a relationship can be extremely difficult, and can only be achieved by having a sensitivity to the patient's anxiety levels and an understanding of what he can cope with. It especially involves the use of non-verbal reassurance, especially gestures of encouragement and touching when appropriate without encouraging dependence.
(4) Being able to accept the negative feelings of hostility and aggression should the patient feel insecure. Not reacting to displays of temper caused through frustration, but by verbal skills helping the patient ventilate his feelings, and sharing your own.
(5) Being able to model and teach mature and intelligent decision making. This requires the nurse to behave appropriately in various situations, and relate to the patient why it was appropriate (see 'Social Skills Training', Chapter 3). Facilitating intelligent decision making can be demonstrated by sharing your own recent domestic decisions with the patient. This should illustrate how appropriate choices are made by choosing from a larger rather than smaller list of options, and linking the choices with possible outcomes or consequences.
(6) Being aware of the interactions responsible for reducing independence. To be able to reduce these, and deal with the adverse emotional reactions within yourself. Objective self-awareness is probably the surest way of preventing yourself making the patient more dependent. One system of achieving this self-awareness may be found by recording the day's events in a diary, and evaluating how often, and how necessary, each of your daily interactions is in relation to patient independence.
(7) Being sensitive to the patient's needs for higher values of self-respect, individuality and purpose. This is achieved by constantly updating your ideas about each patient. Try to forget how they behaved last year or last month, and concentrate on the undeveloped potential yet unrealised.
(8) Facilitating verbally and non-verbally increasing responsiveness between the patient and the real world outside the institution. This means the nurse encouraging patients to write letters, read newspapers, catch buses and generally proceed

away from rather than towards reliance on the institution. Smiles of surprise are usually far more reinforcing than apathetic shrugs of the shoulders.

(9) Being able to let go of your responsibilities for the patient once he is able to retake possession of his own destiny.

Conclusion

We hope we have helped you to see in this chapter that helping patients is not always doing everything for them. That institutions tend to rob the patient of his individuality, independence and uniqueness and that it is the nurse's job to try to return these to him. Developing empathy with the institutionalised patient is difficult because he is so far away from the nurse's own orientation. The nurse who is very independent and capable often has difficulty accepting that her patient may be able, given the opportunity and skilled help, to emulate her.

Successfully nursing the institutionalised patient can be extremely rewarding, but requires patience, positive attitudes and trust in the human being's limitless potential. We hope this brief chapter has stimulated some insight, challenged a few attitudes, and offered some useful guidelines to nurses engaged in this difficult and frustrating area of care.

Key Concepts

(1) It can be noted by observation that, even within a short period of time in an active acute admission ward, patients will adopt predictable patterns of behaviour. Institutional behaviour is essentially behaving as the controllers of the institution expect and demand the patient to behave.

(2) The authority's expectation of patient's behaviour tends to stereotype, confine and constrict individuality.

(3) Some patients will be more resistant to complying with the institution and some institutions will be less influential in making patients comply.

(4) Institutionalisation is not entirely confined to patients; some staff may show signs of institutionalisation relatively quickly and, in some cases, most severely.

(5) Having no prospects for the future, no plans and no expectations deprives an individual of his hopes and desires.
(6) Institutionalisation robbed David of his humanity over 15 years; we must not expect to restore it in seven days.
(7) Respect denotes that you are aware of his rights as an individual.
(8) Unfortunately, all too frequently 'helping' means making the patient dependent upon the nurse.
(9) Some of the traditions which have been respected perhaps need to be challenged.

Suggested Further Reading

Barton, R. *Institutional Neuroses* (John Wright, Bristol, 1959)
Goffman, Irving *Asylums* (Penguin Books, Harmondsworth, 1968, reprint 1978)
______ *Stigma* (Penguin Books, Harmondsworth, 1974)
Morgan, Roger and Cheadle, John *Psychiatric Rehabilitation* (National Schizophrenic Fellowship, Surbiton, Surrey, 1981)
Paine, Thomas *Rights of Man* (Penguin Books, Harmondsworth, reprint 1982)
Shepherd, Geoff *Institutional Care and Rehabilitation* (Longman, London, 1984)
Townsend, J.M. 'Self Concepts and the Institutionalistation of Mental Patients: An Overview and Critique', *Journal of Health and Social Behaviour* (1976), pp. 17, 263-71

12 THE MANIPULATIVE PATIENT

Jane has been in hospital for six months; it is her 25th admission. She will probably be discharged soon, but there is little hope she will remain in the community.

Jane comes into hospital usually following an overdose of aspirins, or having slashed at her wrists. This has become a regular occurrence and generally follows some unpleasant incident in her life. She has many boyfriends, but no close friends. Her parents say they cannot cope with her and no longer visit. She has a long list of offences, mostly minor, and is well known to the local police — she is only 22.

Jane's whole life appears to have been like a racetrack circuit — going from one dangerous bend to the next, the straights, like her relationships with people, being very short. The bends in Jane's circuit are perhaps only minor events for us, like keeping a job, friendship, resisting temptation to steal or to tell lies, even just getting up in the morning — for Jane they represent major hurdles almost impossible to negotiate. Even while in hospital, Jane seems unable to stop telling lies, going from one member of staff to another with requests until she receives a favourable answer. When she doesn't get her own way she causes terrible scenes, makes suicidal gestures, breaks windows and furniture. Attacking patients both verbally and physically is her way of responding to frustration or boredom.

Jane would probably be labelled personality disordered, sociopath, maladjusted, inadequate or just a plain psychopath. Whatever the diagnosis, the case history is probably a recognisable one. An awfully high percentage of people like Jane end up in psychiatric hospitals on acute admission wards, with nurses not quite sure what to do with them.

Jane's case is by no means unique, but is seen in various guises. Some drug addicts and alcholic patients have similar backgrounds and problems to Jane; their overt symptoms of dependence are simply their individual ways of portraying their unhappiness. Excessively aggressive people, child molesters, baby batterers, prostitutes and recidivists may have in their ranks people not dissimilar to Jane. Indeed all the people like Jane have one factor in common — they have great difficulty in forming meaningful relationships with other human beings. They have learned ways of behaving which are not endearing to others, and seem incapable of changing.

It is our belief that many of their problems are inherent in their absence of values, due perhaps to a failure in learning in their early psychological development. Some of the elements most noticeable in Jane's character are as follows:

(1) an inability to love or to recognise love, warmth and friendship when it is offered;
(2) an inability to make thoughtful decisions to be independent and free;
(3) an underlying insecurity which breeds mistrust and anxiety;
(4) feelings of inadequacy — being different and unable to change;
(5) an overwhelming frustration that life is not fair, that people do not care about her.

This being the case, perhaps rather than condemning the Janes we nurse, we should try to understand them and help them to fulfil their needs. It is our belief that Jane can be helped with skilled nursing. The psychopath, like any other person, has potential for growth. We believe skilled nursing may be the facilitator for that growth.

The deficits highlighted in Jane's character suggest the needs that nurses may help her fulfil. For instance, if Jane is shown a consistent warm and caring approach, does she not have a better chance of developing these qualities herself? If the nurse is able to listen and try to understand her, will she not be more eager to try to understand herself? If Jane is offered some trust, will she not subsequently be able to grow to trust others? If she is offered a stable and committed relationship, will she not be more stable and committed in return?

The answer to these questions is undoubtedly in the short term — NO.

Jane will take advantage of your trust, manipulate your weakness, for that is how she perceives it. She will laugh at you, pour scorn on your genuineness, continue to be deceitful and lie and cheat whenever the opportunity arises. Indeed why should we be so arrogant as to believe we can change a process that has taken 22 years in a few weeks? It does not seem likely. We do, however, suggest that it *will* work. Your warmth, genuineness and empathy, if used skilfully and consistently, will overcome even the most difficult of manipulators if it is continuous and is given time.

Implications for the Nurse

When nursing the manipulative patient the nurse must be prepared for a long campaign. It is not one that can be won in weeks, and may take years. During this time you will have to have the patience of a saint to put up with all the disappointments and frustrations you will encounter. Jane will consistently let you down when you have faith and trust in her; she will misrepresent you, betray you and tell lies about you. When she realises you still accept her, do not resent her and remain warm towards her — things will probably get worse. At this point she may abuse you, threaten you, even physically attack you. If, despite this, your approach is immovably consisent, then, and perhaps only then, she may eventually learn to trust you. It is important to remember that in her disordered perception she has always been let down, no one has ever been reliable, no one has ever accepted her totally before. It is almost as if her entire previous behaviour has been an elaborate and marathon test of your honesty.

During this process, it has to be said that unless the nurse is a paragon of virtue, many crises will have occurred. Conflicts of loyalty, strain on emotion and just plain physical tiredness may have interfered with this therapeutic process. When Jane has stolen or bullied other patients, or had tantrums to seek attention, you may have given up. We believe the reason these patients have such a poor prognosis is that they require such intensive and continuous nursing that few establishments or individuals can fund it financially or emotionally.

Principles and Skills Required to Help the Manipulative Patient

Communication

At all times accurate and consistent communication must be maintained between patient, nurse and other staff involved.

It is important that the nurse is totally honest at all times with the patient. If possible the ward should have planned policies of dealing with antisocial or undesirable behaviour, and these should be understood by both parties, e.g.

Jane. But why can't I have my weekend leave this weekend?

Nurse. We discussed this when you first came into hospital, and you knew if you were found stealing patients' cigarettes, you would not be allowed home for weekend leave. You stole Brian's cigarettes on Wednesday, so you can't go home this weekend.

Jane. It's not fair, I don't get enough money to buy cigarettes, and I feel so frustrated here at weekends, I'll probably end up smashing something. You don't really care about me.

Nurse. I understand you are very upset about not going home, but you're wrong about me not caring. I care very much. It would be easier to let you go, but it wouldn't do you any good in the long run. We have a deal and we have to stick to it. If you break something this weekend, I'll be upset and disappointed, but I hope you think about it seriously before you do, as I'm not sure it will help anything. Wouldn't it be better to discuss your frustration and deal with it more realistically?

It can be seen from this exchange that the nurse shows she is totally honest, she is firm in her decision and is not interested in the 'inferred blackmail'. She takes the opportunity to say how she feels — that she does care and also suggests a possible more appropriate behaviour.

It should be emphasised that there is no attempt to judge Jane's statements; the nurse simply listens, understands and responds in a calm, consistent and caring way.

Dealing with Undesirable Behaviour

Essentially the ground rules have to be set early in the relationship. Although it is difficult to generalise, these suggested guidelines may be helpful.

Aggression

See Chapter 7 on aggressive patients, but note that when this is attention seeking it is best to ignore it as much as possible, and then to discuss the behaviour subsequently, i.e. 'I noticed how aggressive you were this morning — when you act like that I will ignore you. I think you were just trying to get my attention, and I'm sure there are more positive ways of doing that than with aggression.'

Self-mutiliation/Suicidal Gestures

Suggest to the patient that this behaviour is unacceptable, but you will not intercede unless life threatening situations occur. Explain that you do not intend to take responsibility for his life, as that robs him of his independence. Explore more acceptable ways of dealing with problems.

Telling Lies/Stealing

Discuss the situation with the patient, being careful to listen and not to judge. Present the evidence as it appears and discuss this openly. When you have decided, say honestly how you feel, take any action you think is appropriate, or according to ward policy, and state that this is the way it will always be dealt with in the future. It is important that even though sanctions may be operated against her at this point, your accepting attitude does not change, e.g.

Jane. So you don't believe me, and now I can't go on the trip tomorrow.

Nurse. Look, Jane, I believe you did steal Harry's soap, and yes, that means you can't go on the trip, but I am trying to understand why you behave like this, and I really want to help.

It may be seen from this that although the nurse may have judged guilt of the act, she did not judge Jane as a person, and continued to offer help in a caring way.

Antisocial Behaviour

Swearing, spitting and vulgar sexual behaviour are not uncommon in these patients. Largely ignoring this appears to be the most effective way of dealing with it. Intervention may be necessary when other patients are distressed by it. Once a trusting and respecting relationship is attained, the nurse should be able to model appropriate behaviour for the patient to learn more skilled social interactions.

Disloyalty and Selfishness

These traits are commonly seen, and can only be dealt with by a total acceptance of them, and disclosure of the nurse's feelings when appropriate, e.g.:

Nurse. I think I understand that you needed to complain to Dr Jones about my behaviour, because it seemed to you I was being unfair and asking a lot of you — I don't feel resentful about it, but perhaps a little disappointed you think so little of me.

This becomes more difficult, however, later in the relationship when trust has been built and yet disloyalty still occurs. Nevertheless no profit is gained by hostility and confrontation.

Once a rapport is struck between the nurse and patient, the nurse becomes a teacher. Her effectiveness in her teaching will depend largely on the respect, trust and integrity she engenders.

In all interactions the nurse should attempt a positiveness so that she is perceived as honest, reliable, stable, warm and caring. We believe that if this is maintained for any length of time, more positive outcomes are possible, and probable.

Summary

We have tried to show in this chapter that the manipulative patient suffers from an emotional deficit which has been potentiated by learned maladaptive behaviour. In order to help the patient, the nurse has to be aware of his needs. These are concerned closely to the underlying condition that the patient suffers. To reverse the maladaptive behaviour and repair the emotional deficit, the patient needs to be accepted and to be shown honest regard. New learning has to begin, as the patient needs to learn acceptable behaviour patterns and to be more trusting, warm and honest.

It has been suggested that the patient may seek attention by suicidal gestures, aggression and antisocial behaviour. Indeed the nurse should expect dishonesty, disloyalty and selfishness on the part of the patient. Although this paints a rather gloomy picture, and the nurse may be frustrated, disappointed, irritated and at times feel completely defeated, if the patient is to be helped the nurse must battle onward. Her main allies are good communication with the patient and her colleagues, a consistent approach, and her underlying qualities of honesty and warmth. If these qualities can be taught, modelled and suggested to the patient, the task, although awesome, may be considered more realistic. Considerable patience is required to listen to and try to understand the patient, especially when the nurse feels like giving up.

Finally, it would be ridiculous of us to suggest that successful outcomes will always result from this approach, but we do commend it to you as a caring approach that will at least enhance your self-respect and professional standards, when perhaps it is tempting to submit.

13 THE DEPENDENT PATIENT

Frank is 43 years old, thin and emaciated. He looks much older than his years, as he is completely grey, rather stooped in posture, with wizened skin and decaying teeth. He started drinking alcohol in his early teens and, as most young people do, considered it to be socially acceptable and a rather adult thing to do. He went to university, where his drinking habit was sustained, and achieved a degree in engineering. In his early twenties he married a schoolteacher and had a happy domestic life. He had two children whom he loved very much, and life generally seemed to be progressing pleasantly.

As his career developed and the subsequent pressure of his ambitions developed, he began to drink rather more heavily. He would pop out at lunchtime and stop on his way home for a drink at a bar. The significance did not really occur to Frank at this time, and his habit simply evolved. It wasn't long before he began keeping a bottle in his desk drawer for 'after a hard day' and his visits to the pub at lunchtimes and evenings became longer. Having a drink before important meetings became the normal practice, only shortly before it became normal for Frank to have a drink after an important meeting.

It was probably around this time that his boss at work reprimanded him for the first time and his wife began to nag him to spend more time a home with her and the children. Frank responded to these criticisms by getting absolutely drunk. He came home, hit his wife and shouted at the children. He had never behaved like this before. The next day Frank was shocked when confronted with his own behaviour, and swore it wouldn't happen again.

Frank managed to stop drinking completely for nearly a month after this incident. However, the pattern began to repeat itself the next month when Frank told himself that it was the pressures at work and his wife's lack of understanding that precipitated the incident and it had very little to do with drink. In fact drink was the support he was getting. No one really understood how he felt; hardly anyone knew he had a problem. This cycle continued getting worse and worse.

Six months later Frank was drinking all the time, consuming a full bottle of whisky a day with very little effect. His work deteriorated, as did his relationship with his wife. Six months later he lost his job. His wife tried to help and remained with him for another three years. The final blow for his wife was the realisation that she was working only to support his drinking, and on discovering he had remortgaged the house to its maximum and had spent several thousand pounds of this money on his habit, she left.

After his wife left, Frank gradually sold the furniture to buy drink, and spent all his social security money designated for mortgage repayments similarly. When the building society foreclosed he was left penniless and homeless. His first appearance in court was for stealing money from a parking meter. His second was for assault in an attempt to steal from an elderly woman. His third appearance led to his first admission to hospital and now, five years later he is up to his thirtieth admission. The pattern of his admissions has been similar over these five years. Admitted in a dreadful state, he is given good nursing care and 'dried out'. Subsequently he remains sober for some weeks. He enters group therapy determined to shed his problem, becomes depressed with his insight and discharges himself. He usually then remains stable for several weeks, then gets hopelessly drunk for several days and is readmitted to hospital.

Frank has become dependent upon alcohol. Like many other drugs, alcohol is capable of causing both physical and psychological dependence. For our purpose in this book we make no distinction between the individual who is dependent upon diamorphine, cocaine, alcohol or, for that matter, tranquillisers. Although there may be significant differences in physiological disorders or abnormalities, there is, we believe, a common component of psychological dependency. For example, there is no difference in principle between the socially acceptable cigarette smoker who finds it impossible to give up his drug or the young adolescent who inhales toxic fumes from glue to effect a 'high'. They are, of course, completely different subjects, but there is some common ground in that both are in some way dissatisfied with their strategies of dealing with their lives. Both demonstrate a need for outside agents to influence their internal emotional state. These dependences, whether linked to physiological craving and bodily disorders or a more immediately destructive form of suicidal wish, would both benefit from skilled intervention in order to achieve a healthy state. In the case of the alcoholic or drug addict, averting a premature death is the more serious objective.

Effective treatment of the alcoholic or drug addict begins with an understanding of 'Frank' as a human being. Clearly his physical dependence was built up by years of excessive drinking, but what originally motivated him to begin and continue to consume alcohol? A most popular contemporary theory is that we model our behaviour on others. For example, observing our parents and our peers consume alcohol or drugs will inevitably reinforce the idea that it is permissible. But, conversely, rebellious adolescents may act in diametrically opposed directions to their parents, simply to show independence and control over their lives. No research we are aware of has conclusively shown that alcoholic parents create alcoholic offspring, or, for that matter, total abstainers, so clearly these influences must be only one factor in consumers and not the end of the story.

Another current theory is that dependent patients have peculiar personality traits. However, although Frank may be a typical 'personality type' seen today, there did not appear to be any significant features in his early years to single him out as at particular risk of becoming an alcoholic. Neither is there some particular IQ range which suggests he is more at risk. Any evidence collected so far suggests that becoming dependent on drugs or alcohol seems to be a cultural phenomenon having no respect for class, age, intelligence or personality type. Neither would it appear that physiological factors are significant in the development of dependency, in as much as women and men are just as much at risk: fat, thin, tall or short people are not in any way, as far as we are currently aware, particularly susceptible.

From this short résumé of what can only be described as 'non-facts' we may take some comfort in thinking that dependency is not predictable, but by the same logic, but less comfortably, neither is it inevitable for any individual. Many people still believe that it is their own weakness of character, that they have some qualities attributable to others in less quantity and perhaps that they do not deserve our help. They appears to be a section of the patient population almost universally unpopular, evoking very little optimism, or, for that matter, sympathy. Many people would maintain they do not even require our help. Our feelings are most adamant on this subject — we believe that if a certain set of circumstances is applied to a certain type of person at the optimum time, at the most critical pressure 'X' is the result. If X turns out to be an alcoholic, a sex maniac or a potentially suicidal patient, all are equally entitled to our help. To withhold our help and our skills detracts from our own value. To allow our prejudices and preferences to interfere with our care casts doubts on our professional integrity. Despite our previous experience and our jaundiced views concerning the 'success' rate of such patients, we must attempt to consider each 'readmission' as another start afresh – to reassess, replan and implement our care as if no previous admission has occurred. To take any other course tends to predetermine the result. If it is debilitating for us to view potential success pessimistically, think of the detrimental effect it will have on the patient. Unless we are able to inject hope into his perception of himself, he is bound to fail again. A thirty-first attempt to succeed is far more positive an outlook than his thirtieth failure.

The Problems and Needs of the Dependent Patient

Alcoholics Anonymous considers the fundamental breakthrough in the rehabilitation of an alcoholic the point when he finally admits he has a problem, when he finally admits he is an alcoholic, Following this logically through (and we have no reason to dispute this theory), it appears that the alcoholic is protecting himself with the mechanism of denial and that he is very able to project and rationalise his situation and misery (see Appendix I). Indeed this largely supports our own experience of the dependent patient. We would agree that in our experience the most remarkable rehabilitation has occurred when sudden insight has inspired the individual from a position which could only be described as the depths of degradation. The patient appears to have reached rock bottom, has no self-respect, and his emotions and thoughts are left naked and open for all to see. The choice appears to be life, and change, or to die in this sorry state. It is at this junction perhaps that, if help is not forthcoming, if someone is not able to show they care, or if we are not alert to this potential for change, the patient may be completely failed by the nurse.

The patient who is motivated to change will meet many obstacles, and he will almost certainly have to contend with the unbeliever. After all, who in their right mind would employ a self-confessed alcoholic? Who would offer him a home and trust him in their house? Who would believe on seeing a history such as Frank's that such a person could change, would not steal, lie and cheat to obtain a drink? Certainly not an individual who had known him.

The patient needs someone to trust him, to have faith in him, to care enough to encourage him. His uphill battle for sobriety will not be made easier by people doubting him. How can he be expected to have faith in himself when others do not? Every aspect of his environment, of people's experience and his own thoughts tell him he will not succeed — but he knows he must. Even his own physical condition casts doubt on his ability to survive. How could such a frail, run-down body hold down a job? His thinking, memory and problem solving ability have also been diminished by *his habit.* All the assets he had within himself have been taken from him by his drinking.

Frank's past life is of no consequence or credit to himself or others — he has proved to be unreliable, dishonest and aggressive and only time can extinguish this stigma. He needs more than ever before some attainable goals and some distant dreams. He will need strength to work tirelessly towards remaining sober until the end of the day and the next, and the next, and he will need perseverance ultimately to be able to hold up his head again in society and to see his children in a climate of mutual respect. Starting all over again with a clean slate is almost impossible, indeed undesirable, for he needs to remember how easily his resolve can be lost, and how awful his previous existence really was.

Implications for the Nurse

The fundamental belief the nurse must have to be able to nurse Frank skilfully is: should he want to change, he is capable of it. If the nurse has any doubt about this concept then it will inevitably reflect itself in the attitudes she conveys towards him. To believe that Frank doesn't want to change is human; to believe he can't is debilitating. The second most important prerequisite to effective treatment is for the nurse to believe she can help Frank should she find herself in the position of being asked for help. Casting aside all evidence and statistics that spell failure for dependent patients and with an objective knowledge that most attempts at rehabilitation will fail, she must undertake each successive attempt at rehabilitating Frank as if it were the first and consequently the most likely to succeed.

The skilled nurse will be able to appreciate that at times Frank will be ungrateful, so she must not seek gratitude. She must know that he will test her trust and support, so she must be trustworthy and supportive. She should know he requires honesty, so she should reward him with the truth in a way he will not feel is punishing.

We believe dependent patients can only be treated voluntarily, but many alcoholics and drug addicts who commit crimes may be compulsorily detained. We do not necessarily think this is a good policy, although it is probably better than custodial care in a penal institution. However, simply because they are compulsorily detained does not preclude their voluntary submission for help. Neither does it mean that we should not continue any therapy recommended. It simply means that it may not be as effective.

Nurses dealing exclusively with the dependent patient may well become disenchanted and cynical. This is of course a very human and natural course of events, but we recommend that nurses be aware of the possibility and of the consequences of such an attitude developing, recognising that, once it has developed, the nurse's usefulness to the patient is seriously limited. Positive strategies to prevent cynical attitudes developing need to be devised to offset this possibility. We suggest that nurses in this environment should develop strong skills of debrief and group support (see Chapter 20, 'Community Skills').

Principles and Skills Required to Help

No matter how little the patient shows motivation to change, the nurse must show the core conditions of empathy, warmth and genuineness. She must continue to listen accurately to both his verbal and non-verbal behaviour. To establish an empathic bond with the patient is the only secure way of knowing *when* he requires the encouragement and support he needs to change his life.

The nurse needs to be skilled at challenging the patient's discrepancies from a positive position, challenging the strength of his resources when he is feeling down and unable to fight back, e.g.

Patient. I don't think it's really worth it, I've lost everything, my wife, children, job, house, what's the point of going on?

Nurse. You're feeling a little down, reflecting on all your losses, but in a way doesn't it prove something that you survived all that and are still game for another try? All those things you say you've lost are still within your grasp if you succeed this time, aren't they? Or were you being dishonest earlier when you said that this is what you have been aiming for?

The nurse needs to raise the patient's esteem whenever possible by reinforcing his strengths, especially in view of his uphill struggle – noting his resolve, how well he is looking, his ability to go into town without going for a drink. Eventually, he may be able to go into a bar and order a soft drink. All these strengths require positive reinforcement in the form of genuine regard. Even if the patient regresses and has a drink, concentrate on how well he did for so long, rather than punishing him for his failure.

The most important skill is being able to communicate the trust and faith the nurse has for him, and that that trust cannot be shaken even by a setback or disappointment. One word of caution: the nurse must not fall into the trap of becoming the patient's drink substitute when adopting this approach. It would be easy for the nurse to begin to feel sorry for the patient; and by being overly 'sympathetic' rather than empathic, she may reinforce his 'dependence' on her. This dialogue shows how the nurse must continually put the responsibility back to the patient to prevent dependence.

Patient. I really don't know what I'd do without you, nurse, when you're here I feel so secure, I don't ever feel the need for a drink? I don't even think you would mind if I did have a drink, would you?

Nurse. I sense you're beginning to doubt yourself and are putting the responsibility on to me. I have enough trust in you to know you will succeed giving up drinking if you want to, and yes, I would mind if you had a drink, because I'd be disappointed that you had lost faith in your resolve. I trust you can give up drinking but I need to remind you that you're giving up for you not me.

This approach needs to be tactful, but firm otherwise the nurse may become a replacement crutch for the patient's emotional instability. The patient needs to walk on his own.

Role play techniques may occasionally be helpful to patients, where they can enact the emotional situations which precipitate a bout of drinking and through this enactment find alternative strategies for dealing with their emotions other than alcohol. The nurse's role in this would be of great value, due to her closeness to the patient. Any role play situation may be emotionally tense, and knowing a nurse well may help this technique to be less threatening.

It may be seen that the nurse must practise all her behavioural and counselling skills to be an efficient helper with the dependent patient. It is an exhaustive and frustrating task, but none the less the rewards for success with patients like Frank are incalculable and the satisfaction of helping the 'unhelpable' immense.

Summary

Many drugs, including alcohol and tobacco, are capable of causing both physical and psychological dependence. This dependence is not predictable in, nor inevitable for, any individual; dependence can be developed in almost anyone. It follows from this argument that the effective treatment of the drug addict or alcoholic should begin with an understanding of the patient as an individual. This understanding can easily be jeopardised by prejudiced views and attitudes held by nurses. It is not enough to want to help. Helping requires the nurse to believe that the patient can be helped, to have faith and trust in the patient, whether this is the first or fiftieth attempt to control his dependence.

We have suggested that it is the nurse's task to stimulate attainable goals for patients, and to encourage restoration of longer-term aims and even distant dreams in patients. This approach is necessary to rekindle the patient's belief in himself. Probably one of the most important implications for the nurse is to avoid cynical attitudes developing within herself. We are aware that this is not easy, but any cynical approach will undoubtedly sabotage the patient's self-esteem and undermine any possible successful outcomes. Skilled challenges aimed at the patient's discrepancies of thinking and behaviour are strong medicine, and should be respected as such. There is a significant difference between inviting the patient to see himself more clearly by skilful challenge and destructively telling him what you think in cold hard terms. Challenging skilfully can only be successfully achieved from a position of empathy and, similarly, this is achieved from listening to both verbal and non-verbal communication. The nurse needs to raise the patient's self-esteem wherever possible by reinforcing his strengths, not continually pointing out his weaknesses. If the nurse is able to do this effectively and communicate how much faith and trust she has in him, it will help him to be independent. This latter point is most important, for it may help to avoid the potential trap of the nurse becoming a substitute for the drug the patient has become dependent upon.

Finally, it is worth mentioning that we have concentrated on an abstinence programme, which we believe, remains the more common practice in dealing with dependent patients. Some clinicians are of the opinion that patients dependent on alcohol may be rehabilitated to some form of continued social drinking, in perhaps the same way a heavy smoker may cut down, and registered drug addicts are maintained on lower-dose opiate substitutes. Although we have no personal experience with this approach, we see no reason why it may not be possible with some individuals. We would, however, recommend that the same skilled approach be undertaken.

Suggested Further Reading

Dawtry, Frank *Social Problems of Drug Abuse* (Butterworths, London, 1968)

Edwards, Griffith *The Treatment of Drinking Problems: A Guide for the Helping Profession* (Blackwell Scientific Publications, Oxford, 1982)

—, and Grant, Marcus (eds.) *Alcoholism: New Knowledge and New Responses* (Croom Helm, London, 1977)

_____ Jaffe, J. and Arif, A. (eds.) *Drug Use and Misuse: Cultural Perspectives* (Croom Helm, London, 1983)

Heather, Nick and Robertson, Ian *Controlled Drinking* (Methuen, London, 1981)

Jaffe, Jerome, Peterson, Robert and Hodgson, Ray *Addictions: Issues and Answers* (Harper and Row, London, 1980)

Kessel, Neil and Walton, Henry *Alcoholism* (Penguin Books, Harmondsworth, 1979)

Kinney, Jean and Leaton, Gwen *Loosening the Grip: A Handbook of Alcohol Information*, 2nd edn (Mosby, St Louis, 1983)

Rix, Keith and Rix, Elizabeth Lumsden *Alcohol Problems: A Guide for Nurses and Other Health Professionals* (Wright, Bristol, 1983)

Smith, Richard *Alcohol Problems* (BMA, London, 1982)

Williamson, P. and Norris, H. (eds.) *Personal Skills Training for Problem Drinkers: A Counsellor's Guide* (Aquarius, Birmingham, 1984)

Willis, J. *Drug Dependence* (Faber and Faber, London, 1969; 2nd edn, 1974)

14 THE HALLUCINATED PATIENT

Thomas was sitting in the corner of the ward staring at the floor. Occasionally he would lift his head, look to the side and smile. The nurse approached and sat down beside him.

Nurse. 'Hello, Thomas.'

There was no response. It was as if the nurse did not exist.

Nurse. 'Hello, Thomas, how are you?'

Slowly Thomas turned and stared. It was as though he could see right through the nurse. He suddenly opened his mouth wide, took a deep breath and groaned as if expressing some agonising pain.

'This place I am in is warm and dark. I can see the depths of colour moving around my feet. The mist is all around, everyone seems to be moving slowly. Someone is laughing up there, it is very funny.'

'Stop looking up there, Thomas, listen to me.'

'Don't listen to him, Thomas, he's only out to hurt you.'

'Who's this coming to laugh at you?'

Nurse. 'Hello, Thomas.'

'Open your mouth and swallow his pain.'

'Let out the hatred from your bowels.'

Nurse. 'Hello, Thomas, how are you?'

The above sequence is a description of one event from two different perspectives. The first is how the nurse attempts to communicate to a patient who appears to be preoccupied about something. The second description attempts to convey the experience from a patient who is being distracted by hallucinations. It can be seen that two completely different worlds can exist and, in such a situation, a bridge must be formed between these two worlds to allow effective communication to take place. To do this, an appreciation of how a hallucinatory experience can affect an individual is needed.

'An hallucination occurs when an individual experiences a sensory stimulus without any apparent external cause for that stimulus.'

It must be clearly distinguished from an 'illusion', which is when a '*misinterpretation* of a sensory stimulus' occurs. The following examples should clarify this.

A person may experience *'illusions'* when delirious. For example, he may see shadows, or the shape of a curtain as an intruder, or misinterpret a nurse's identity.

In contrast to this, however, a patient could experience *hallucinations* without any external stimulus:

- he may hear voices or other sounds during silence (auditory);
- see lights, colours and/or faces while staring at the floor (visual);
- may smell rotting vegetation or burning rubber when no one else can (olfactory);
- may sense the taste of faeces in his mouth whilst eating what seems an ordinary meal (gustaciary);
- he may feel the sense of things crawling in his hair or under his skin (tactile).

Any one or a combination of the five senses can be experienced in an hallucinatory form. The auditory and visual are the most common forms of hallucinations.

The Problems and Needs of the Hallucinated Patient

When caring for someone who is experiencing hallucinations, it becomes apparent that the problems and subsequent needs all relate to the patient's conflict of two worlds — one which involves very real and personal sensations with a compelling nature, the other a rather vague and somewhat impersonal world of everything going on around him. The actual effect of this can vary, depending upon the intensity and nature of the hallucination: the problems and needs of a patient who is hearing continual auditory stimulation will differ from one who occasionally sees bright lights flashing in front of him. This emphasises the fact that every patient is an individual and every experience is unique to him. So, although we describe skills and principles, it is the application of these in the context of knowing the patient that makes them effective. The fact that caring for one hallucinated patient may differ greatly from caring for another is made clear in Figure 14.1. It can be seen then that the problems vary from lack of adequate diet and personal hygiene to self-injury, with different feeling states depending on the nature and reaction of the patient, e.g. anxiety, depression, confusion and frustration. The needs will be specific to each problem, but generally speaking we can summarise as shown in the figure.

Implications for the Nurse

The question arises whether you should approach a patient who is showing evidence of hallucinating, but seems quite happy in his own world and does not seem to be hurting himself or others. Here, knowledge of the patient is crucial. It may be that, for example, if Thomas were left on his own he would go further and further into his hallucinatory world and might eventually act upon it to the detriment of himself or others. So by attempting to communicate and distract Thomas from his world now may prevent future difficulties. Conversely, if it is unlikely that he will deteriorate as a result of the hallucination, it may be that with minimum persuasion or interference he can function effectively. This really emphasises the point that you do not need to direct your attention to all patients who are hallucinating, only to those who might deteriorate if left to their own devices or, as shown in Figure 14.2, where the needs become evident because of a particular experience.

Figure 14.1: Contrasting Hallucinatory Experiences and Effects

Patient Experience	Problem	Need
Continual loss of reality	Self-neglect	Nutrition Safety Hygiene Sufficient sense of reality to maintain or improve quality of life
Loss of reality — with distress	Self-harm Isolation Depression	Defined limits Acceptance Reassurance
Loss of reality — interfering, annoying, embarrassing	Confusion Frustration	Sensitivity, listening, reassurance
Loss of reality — directed outwards	Dangerous, disruptive behaviour Effect on self and others	Clear identifiable nursing action with explanation.

Figure 14.2: The Possible Effects of Hallucinatory Experience

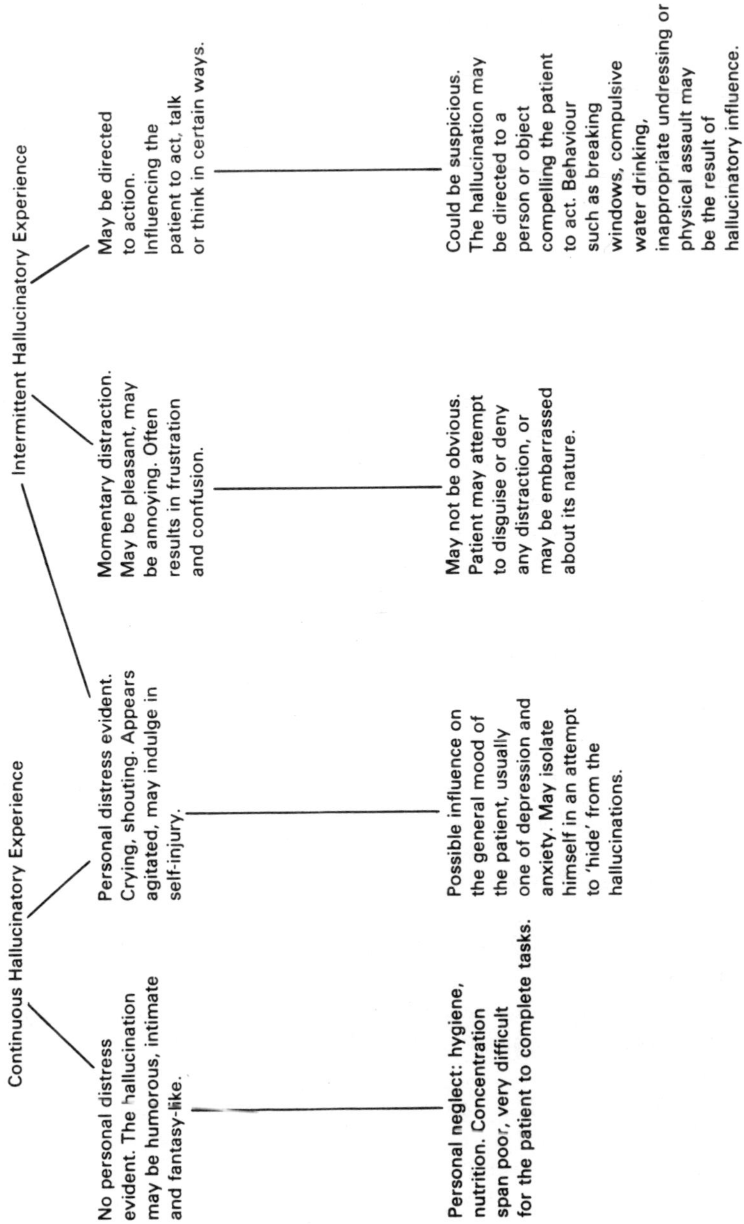

The signficiant issues for the nurse relate to the fact that she cannot validate what is happening to the patient. For example, she cannot see or hear what he does, which may be very frustrating for the nurse, so it is important that she is aware of her feelings and avoids arguing with or denying the reality of the patient's perceptions.

Principles and Skills Required to Help the Hallucinated Patient

Appropriate Use and Sensitivity of Non-verbal Communication

Sensitivity to non-verbal communication, an essential aspect of the skills required, is necessary in order to detect the more subtle signs that show a patient may be hallucinating. The patient may laugh, talk to himself, smile, grimace or distort his face inappropriately, he may turn his head to one side as if to listen, all probably out of the context of usual interactions. The patient's use of gestures, body movements and tone of voice may give the nurse vital information as to the nature or theme of the hallucination, thus increasing the chance of her responding appropriately. The verbal response is often enhanced by using *appropriate touch, posture, eye contact and tone of voice.* It often requires the effect of all these used at the right time in order to bridge the gap from the patient's world to that of the existing environment.

Thomas began shouting, then jumped out of his chair and started banging on the window.

'Leave me alone, leave me alone!' he screamed and started crying. The nurse approached Thomas, stood close, placed her arm firmly around his shoulders, turning Thomas towards her, and looked straight at him.

'Thomas, it's all right, I'm here and I won't let anything happen to you. You're safe with me, come away from the window and we'll have a chat.'

The nurse led Thomas away, still holding him and talking in a firm positive manner, communicating to him that she was in control.

The likelihood of the above situation turning out successfully will depend largely upon the degree of trust that exists between the nurse and the patient. If the nurse is to interfere or enter the world of a patient's hallucination, then the *development of trust* is vital in increasing the likelihood of positive outcomes when intervening with this type of patient.

This is an ongoing process whereby the attitudes and qualities of the nurse are communicated to the patient at all times, alongside the confident use of skills, showing that in the event of the patient losing control, there is someone capable of taking hold of the situation safely. This usually involves *reinforcing reality*. The patient's world is often frightening, but also compelling for that patient. It often occupies the whole person, sometimes to the extent that all reality is lost, as in Thomas' case, where the internal visions and voices were indiscernible from the external ones. It is the use of reality that can often bring back and maintain the patient away from the distractions of his hallucinations. The nurse, by acknowledging the patient's *feelings*, at the same time denying that she shares his perceptions, is reinforcing the reality of the feelings experienced, e.g.

Nurse. I do not hear the voices you hear, Thomas, but am I right in thinking that you feel confused and may be frustrated?

The same principle of reinforcing reality can be shown by:

- use of appropriate touch;
- questioning about the patient's current interests;
- asking about the patient's recent activities, how he feels about them;
- encouraging the patient to do something that requires connecting his thoughts directly with actions, e.g. going for a walk, joining in an activity, making something constructive;
- use of appropriate tones of voice, i.e. firm and calm when limit setting is required, but also loud enough to interrupt auditory hallucinations, especially when they are predominant.

So, by knowing the patient and his likely response the nurses can utilise the skills of questioning and reflecting to attempt to bring the patient out of a world foreign to us and often frightening to him.

Finally, never underestimate how real a hallucination can be to the patient, never argue with the patient about its validity, and always accept the individual without judgement or analysis. By doing so the person lost in a world of strange perceptions may be found.

Summary

The Patient

He may experience disordered perceptions concerning one or a combination of the five senses, resulting in auditory, visual, tactile, olfactory or gustaciary hallucinations. These may occur in varying degrees of intensity, giving rise to a multitude of *needs and problems.* Some of these may be related to the following: nutrition; hygiene; safety; self-esteem; isolation; depression; anxiety; confusion; frustration; suspicion and dangerous behaviour.

Implications for the Nurse

These are mainly to do with the discerning use of skills. The nurse should never underestimate the reality of the disordered perception to the patient, and should also be aware of her own feelings, especially when the patient requires control to be communicated to him in a crisis situation.

The Skills Required

- Sensitivity to non-verbal communication:
  - detection of hallucinatory experiences;
  - awareness of patient's feelings and theme of hallucinations;
  - appropriate use of non-verbal communication, mainly:
    - use of touch;
    - tone of voice;
    - posture;
    - eye contact;
    - reinforce reality;
    - development of trust.

Suggested Further Reading

Berkavitz, Ruth and Heinl, Peter 'The Management of Schizophrenic Patients: The Nurse's View', *Journal of Advanced Nursing*, vol. 9, no. 1 (January 1984), pp. 23-33

Falloon, Ian R. and Talbot, Ralph E. 'Persistent Auditory Hallucinations: Coping Mechanisms and Implications for Management', *Psychological Medicine*, vol. 11 (1981), pp. 329-39

Hiler, Penny 'Schizophrenia: An Inside Story', *New Society*, vol. 68 (14 June 1984), pp. 439-40

Slade, P.D. 'The External Control of Auditory Hallucinations: An Information Theory Analysis', *British Journal of Social and Clinical Psychology*, vol. 13 (1974), pp. 73-9

West, L.J. (ed.) 'A General Theory of Hallucinations and Dreams', in *Hallucinations* (Grune and Stratton, New York, 1962), pp. 275-91

World Health Organization *International Pilot Study of Schizophrenia* (WHO, Geneva, 1977)

15 THE DELUDED PATIENT

Mary was recently admitted believing herself to be perfectly well. She insists that she is a victim of a Soviet plot to destroy her. Her brain is receiving transmissions from Russia which are gradually interfering with her thinking. Her next door neighbours are spies. She knows this because it was they who informed the doctor that she was 'unwell'. At one time she trusted her GP, but that was probably her big mistake, for he is undoubtedly the head of the local spy ring, and by admitting her to hospital, he has prevented anyone believing her story.

Mary's belief is typical of the deluded patient receiving treatment in psychiatric hospitals all over the world. The great tragedy is that whatever is done for Mary, until such time as her ideas become more logical, she earnestly believes them. Any attempt to treat her may simply be incorporated into her delusional system as another plot and make her more resistive.

Delusions are said to be *false beliefs which cannot be shaken by reason or argument, and not in keeping with the person's cultural or religious background.*

They may take many shapes and forms, but we can list the more common.

Paranoid

Primary delusions, i.e. having an initial theme. Usually taking the form of suspicion of plots or malice towards them.

Systematised

From a primary delusion new ideas or experiences are incorporated and weave a complex linking network of delusional ideas.

Nihilistic

Usually these are found in depressive and withdrawn individuals believing themselves to be without organs or parts of their bodies, e.g. 'I have no stomach — I have swallowed my tongue.'

Unworthiness

Again associated with depressive illness — 'I'm not worth your time, I deserve to die.'

Grandiose

The delusions are often seen in organic dementia types — especially in neurosyphilis. Here the patient believes himself to be omnipotent or vastly wealthy. Some patients invent past lives for themselves, e.g. 'I was a Stuka pilot/tank commander/prime Minister/the Queen's hairdresser.' These become even more difficult to deal with when linked to hallucinations which support them, e.g. when the doctor arrives, he is perceived as Prince Philip, General Rommel, Margaret Thatcher, etc.

Ideas of Reference

Here the patients believe that words, gestures, television announcements or any innocent communications have a hidden and special significance to them, e.g. when the nurse sits opposite the patient and looks at her watch, he may say or think that this is a coded message directed at a hidden observer to signal some malicious act towards him.

The Problems and Needs of the Deluded Patient

The patient has difficulty discerning reality from fantasy, but no amount of persuasion seems to help. He may be very distressed that no one believes him and is at a loss to understand why. He may search desperately for an ally, for someone to place his trust in, but a great anxiety surrounds him as he has every reason to be suspicious. After all he is well, and perhaps being held against his will, and the people he feels he should trust, the doctors and nurses, seem to be totally in disbelief.

The deluded patient may have physical problems due to lack of nutrition. The grandiose patient could not eat such a basic diet — 'Bring me some caviar,' — the paranoid patient believes it to be poisoned and the nihilistic type cannot chew or swallow it, and, anyway, without a stomach what is the point? The taking of medication becomes equally difficult for similar reasons.

Implications for the Nurse

Using Mary from the original introduction, several principles and skills can be illustrated to show how nurses can best help the deluded patient.

Non-verbal Communication

This will be the first exchange of information between Mary and the nurse, and as such will largely influence the positiveness of the eventual outcome. It is important to approach Mary openly and directly, giving no hint of surreptitiousness, and certainly without any posture or facial expression that could be misinterpreted as threatening. Perhaps one approach may be to speak to several other patients in the same vicinity before speaking to her, using a consistent approach to each patient so that Mary does not suspect she may be a specific target. We have found that making very positive eye contact is very important with deluded patients, as this reinforces an honesty and a desire to be open. Tone of voice should be firm rather than hesitant, plus clear and loud enough so as to leave no room for misinterpretation. Adopt a posture that is non-threatening. We would suggest sitting next to Mary at the same height, or slightly lower, so that she may feel in control of the interaction. It is very likely that Mary's potential for misinterpretation is extremely high, so a minimum use of possibly ambiguous non-verbal signals should be used. For instance, touch can easily be interpreted as threatening, so although its powerfulness for reassurance may be useful, it should be avoided initially until a safe rapport is established.

Listening and Attending Skills

Here listening and showing Mary that you are listening (attending skills) are imperative. The skill of reflecting (see p. 47) is probably most important. Whether you are able to believe what is being said is largely irrelevant; to show her you care enough about her to listen is essential.

It is often argued that delusions should not be 'reinforced', i.e. agreed with, nor should they be argued against. Therefore by employing the skill of reflecting, the skilled nurse should be able to build up an empathic understanding and concentrate on Mary's *feelings* rather than the thoughts and ideas that form the delusion, e.g.

Patient (distressed). Nobody believes me when I tell them I'm being interfered with by these dreadful Russians. You believe me, don't you?

Nurse (carefully, thoughtfully and slowly). I can see that you feel very distressed by your beliefs and that's what I'm concerned about. I would like to be able to help you feel less anxious.

Patient. I would feel calmer if someone believed me, then I'd feel safe.

Nurse (ensuring maximum eye contact). I can see you feel very frustrated that no one believes you, and that makes you feel in danger. I hope you will believe me when I say I only want to help you and I'll do everything I can to make you feel safer.

We believe that this approach would be typical of a skilled response — note that the nurse is not dishonest, she does not agree with Mary, neither does she argue with her. She carefully concentrates on how the patient feels, without discussing, and thereby risking reinforcing, the delusions. This may help Mary to feel better understood; that the nurse is honest and deserving of trust. This approach may help Mary confront the feelings attached to her ideas and deal with them more effectively. When she is able to deal with her feelings of anxiety, her behaviour may change and her ideas may accordingly become less disturbing.

Once an atmosphere of trust is established with the patient, intervening in the patient's ideation is more likely to be effective. By listening to Mary, other interests, concerns and problems may well emerge. The nurse who is able to establish an empathic relationship with Mary will have more channels available to distract her into when her thoughts turn back to her delusional ideas. The skilled nurse will be aware that Mary has problems in her relationship with her mother, that she likes to play badminton, or that she is interested in music, cooking and art. These are the areas into which Mary's conversation is profitably directed. For instance, look at these two different interactions:

(1) *Mary.* I'm not really sure, but I think Dr Jones is working for the Russians.

Nurse. I can see you are starting to feel anxious again, Mary, perhaps it would be a good time to:

(a) write to your mother;
(b) see if we can get a game of badminton in the hall;
(c) go out to the shops and fetch something for your tea;

(d) listen to some soothing music.

(2) *Mary.* I'm not really sure, but I think Dr Jones is working for the Russians.
Nurse. Let's watch TV.

The difference is of course obvious in its depth, skill and appropriateness. Distraction is a useful skill, even in the second response, but it only becomes a powerful skill potentiating the patient's recovery when it is an integral part of the empathic relationship.

Similarly, the use of encouragement and persuasion is only skilful if the nurse uses them after a safe rapport is established. If they are used initially in order to *make* Mary do something, they will create resentment. They may even be responsible for the nurse being incorporated into the delusional system. This inappropriate use of encouragement and persuasion may be as damaging as arguing with the delusional ideas.

The skilled nurse will know when the rapport of trust has been established sufficiently to stand the use of encouragement and persuasion to eat meals and take medication. The nurse's judgement is critical in this area, and should be respected by other members of the caring team. In our experience, nothing is more damaging to a relationship of trust than a premature use of persuasion.

Devices such as eating with the patient and encouraging the patient to prepare her own meals may be useful but should be used carefully with thought. After having tasted her food for her, consider what she will think when you refuse to taste her medicine also.

Nurse. Mary, here's your medicine.
Mary. I'm not ill, why do I have it — it may be poisoned — will you taste it like you did my dinner?
Nurse. I know you believe you're not ill, but I think you are very anxious, I can see that now in your face. This medicine will help you feel calmer. If I was anxious like you, I would need some, but as I'm not, it would only make me sleep.
Mary. I'm only anxious because you're making me drink poison.
Nurse. I can see you are very anxious, I won't make you drink it, but it isn't poison and I think it would help you feel calmer. I'll ask you again later.

The nurse here may or may not get through to the patient, but the relationship remains intact, with more possibility of success next time.

Many experienced nurses reading this may feel that this is rather idealistic and that it may be expedient to give intramuscular medication in this case – the hope being that the medication, when effective, will succeed where the relationship failed. We do not rule out compulsion as an expedient; as we have said, these patients are extremely difficult. We do, however, suggest that the slower route is safer and more lasting if it is possible to implement, and should be given every opportunity first.

Summary

There are many forms of delusional thinking, and we have offered but a few of the most prevalent within this chapter: grandiose, nihilistic, ideas of reference and feelings of unworthiness, systematised and paranoid delusions. All these, but particularly the latter two, may lead to severe difficulties in forming and maintaining a rapport. This is especially true if the nurse becomes incorporated into the system as a suspect. This lack of trust in the patient will almost certainly produce management problems when attempting to implement care, which is often manifested as problems arising in the administration of medication, diet, hygiene and the patient's sleep disturbance.

We have suggested that it is possible that the frustration this creates within the nurse may result in nurse interaction difficulties. The nurse may become reluctant to approach or spend time with the patient. This occurs most often after she has been subjected to hostility by the patient.

In order to be of some help to these unfortunate patients, it may follow that some very practical skills and principles are needed and employed. We suggest the following:

(1) Do not argue or agree with delusions.
(2) Maximise the potential empathic relationship by using:
   (a) clear non-verbal communication;
   (b) an open honest approach;
   (c) skilled listening;

(d) reflecting the feelings of the patient, and sharing your understanding of his emotions.

(3) Use distraction to limit delusional thinking.
(4) Use encouragement, praise or any other rewarding responses to reinforce 'normal or non-delusional' behaviour.
(5) If possible, without jeopardising rapport, use persuasion to increase his occupation or activity into productive areas — i.e. resocialisation, work, projects, recreation.

Conclusion

Initial interactions are extremely important when dealing with people suffering delusions. It is vital to gain their trust, and to understand them by establishing an empathic relationship. In this way the nurse uses herself as a therapeutic agent to help the patient recover. Restoring these patients to health may largely depend on good physical care and appropriate medication, which will not be accepted until some valuable and trusting relationship is established. The nurse is therefore the central focus of effective treatment and her skilled interaction is imperative.

Suggested Further Reading

Berkavitz, Ruth and Heinl, Peter 'The Management of Schizophrenic Patients: The Nurse's View', *Journal of Advanced Nursing*, vol. 9, no. 1 (January 1984), pp. 23-33

Buckley, M. 'Nursing Care Study. Tormented by Delusions (Treatment and Care of Chronic Schizophrenic Patients)', *Nursing Mirror*, vol. 157 (November 1983), pp. 43-6

Frost, Monica *Nursing Care of the Schizophrenic Patient* (Kimpton, London, 1974)

Hill, Lewis B. *Psychotherapeutic Intervention in Schizophrenia* (Chicago University Press, Chicago, 1973)

16 THE CHILD

To appreciate the complexity of a child's world and its influences, an understanding of the normal milestones of development is required. It is not our intention to explore in any depth the psychological, physical or social background of any particular child problem, but rather to give some guidance as to how general principles of care must be applied in a special way to children because of the nature of the child's state of development.

When a child is admitted or attends a psychiatric unit, it is often viewed as a symptom of failed care approaches in the system. It is often a last resort to admit a child and in our opinion should remain so, for prolonged absence from a normal family unit can produce more maladjustment than it is designed to relieve. However, there are times when it becomes clear that the child and the family, no matter what intervention takes place, are in such turmoil with each other that some space placed between them is necessary. For example:

David's behaviour had become increasingly demanding. He would change from a state of withdrawal to a state of hyperactivity, with frequent temper tantrums. He suffered from encopresis and had a fear of men. The decision to bring him into the unit was due to the fact that his presence at home was causing a strain on his mother, who directed her frustration at her boyfriend, who in turn regularly beat David in the face, on one occasion causing severe bruising and bleeding. David's father, who has since left the household, also had a history of violence, mainly directed towards David's mother. Admission was brought about shortly after David had caused severe bruising to his two-year-old stepsister. David was six years old.

In this case, it seems that David and his family's safety was in jeopardy, and the space provided by admitting him gave a chance for the multidisciplinary team to assess the situation without the fear of further risk to David or his sister. During the first 48 hours, David was totally withdrawn, refusing to speak and cowering or moving away from any approach made towards him by any male member of staff. It took a long time before he could appreciate and enjoy the security of a loving and trusting relationship.

The following is a list of the more common behaviours a child may present with on admission to a children's psychiatric unit:

anorexia;	school phobia/refusal;
behavioural disorder	autism;
elective mutism;	encopresis;
enuresis;	hysterical behaviour;
psychosomatic states;	obesity;
language and learning difficulties;	depression/suicidal;
	states of deprivation/failure to thrive.

The Problems and Needs of a Child

The nurse must appreciate that when a child enters the 'caring unit' away from home, he or she is probably experiencing yet another traumatic event in a long history of confusion, conflict and rejection. The child could view the admission as another way of telling him/her that they are trouble, a burden, worthless and should be rejected. It is therefore necessary for the nurse to make herself accessible to the needs of this child, in order that she may provide the warmth and acceptance that has been so lacking up to then in the child's life. Figure 16.1 illustrates some common problem areas with children in care away from their own family and the needs required to counteract these.

The following is a list of questions or statements that a child of seven or eight may ask him or herself when they find themselves in care:

Why am I here, I don't understand	Confusion
What is going to happen next?	Anxiety
What is going to happen to me?	Fear
Why can't I stay with my mum/dad?	Rejection
What should I say or do?	Conflict
It doesn't matter, anyway, no one can hear/ understand me	Frustration

Figure 16.1: The Problems and Needs of a Child in Care

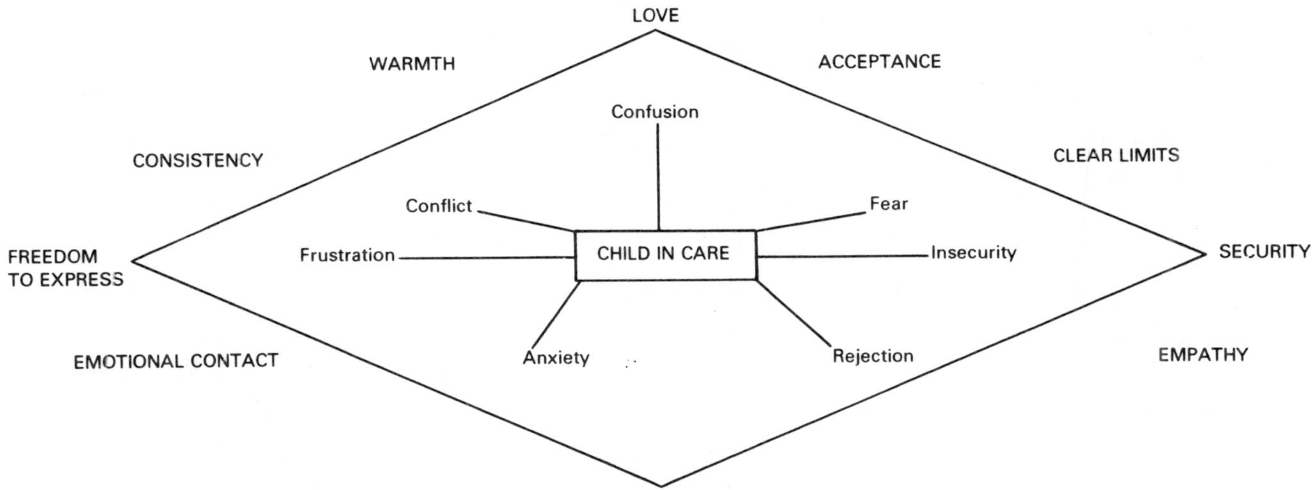

The Skills

The skills required are developed from an awareness of the needs of children in distress. They involve understanding what the child is trying to say and being able to communicate in his or her own language. The child, when communicating, does not always take into account the needs of the listener. For example, a seven-year-old may talk about an event but not the background or build up to the event, thus making full grasp of the story difficult. The listener therefore needs to be able to ask appropriate questions in order to clarify the full meaning. Another important aspect when 'listening' to a child is to take note of the non-verbal communication offered, as this is particularly strong, accurate and expressive. For example, observing a child playing with dolls may convey more about concerns, conflicts and anxieties than questioning would.

When communicating with children the nurse 'must have an awareness of the developmental stage in relation to the child's ability to understand and think at certain degrees of complexity'. Young children are very concrete in their thinking and often believe they have caused certain events — hence the common feeling of guilt often expressed by children from broken marriages. It is for this reason that it is vital for the adult to check understanding and ask the child what he or she understands from what has just happened or been said.

The key to handling 'disturbed' children is the appropriate use of communication skills and a sensitivity to the appropriateness of their use. We have identified seven skills areas used in conjunction with the principles of caring for children (Norbeck, 1980). They are:

(1) *C*rises skills.
(2) *T*eaching skills.
(3) *B*oundary setting.
(4) *R*easoning skills.
(5) *E*xploratory skills.
(6) *C*reative communication.
(7) *C*onveying Acceptance.

The seven areas can be remembered by using the mnemonic: Children's Traumas Become Repressed Causing Endless Agony.

1 Crises Skills

There are times when the child loses control and vents all feelings through some destructive act. As with dealing with any aggressive incident, factors such as harm to someone or self must be prevented. The skill in this situation is aimed at gaining control in the quickest and safest way possible. This may involve physical restraint; if so, it should be used with the minimum of force and ample opportunity should be given for the initial physical contact made by the nurse to restrain the child to be transferred to that of warm embrace, enabling the child to relax in a secure environment. It may be necessary to remove the child to a place where there would be less stimulation and less attention. This should be done for a minimal time only. In all incidents, a thorough exploration of the causes and consequences is essential with the ward team and the child, in order to establish alternative ways of behaving. One specific skill in the area of crisis intervention is that of distraction. This is used to gain immediate co-operation or obedience by the child. It involves telling the child what to do rather than what not to do, and intervening sufficiently loudly enough to gain the initial attention, in order to input the command. This 'resetting mechanism' clears the channel for the child to focus attention momentarily away from the destructive set. For example:

After hearing a commotion in the TV lounge, the nurse on entering saw Peter about to throw a cup at another boy. Her response, 'Peter, put that cup down now' was sufficiently loud enough to startle Peter into hesitating, allowing the nurse to stand in front of him and take the cup away.

It is important during an incident like this to allow the child to express his frustrations in another way, ideally verbally expressing his anger or acting it out in some form of activity room where a child can vent pent up feelings safely.

2 Teaching Skills

These involve enhancing the child's environment in order to maximise his or her awareness of the things around. It is necessary for the nurse to be enthusiastic about activities and choices, giving the child every opportunity to use his or her powers of judgement in order to make decisions. Giving the child a choice will increase the sense of autonomy and may reduce the opportunity or need to defy. For example, by asking what the child wants to wear it may be possible to avoid the issue of whether or not to get dressed. Conversely, unnecessary choices should be avoided as these may lead to additional conflict. For example, rather than say, 'Do you want to go for dinner now?' say, 'It is time for dinner now.' Maintaining the child's interest and pointing out the value of activities may give the child a sense of purpose and increased self-esteem. All too often, children are given toys, a room and told to play. This is satisfactory only to the extent to which the materials given and the supervision offered are sufficient to generate and enhance the child's imagination.

3 Boundary Setting

This is the consistent practice in the application of clearly defined and totally understood behavioural boundaries, sometimes referred to as 'limit setting'. If boundaries are left for the child to discover, this may lead to the child feeling guilty over the behaviour and unsure about further loss of control, fearing potential retaliation and/or punishment and rejection. However, if the boundaries are clearly set, this offers a sense of security to the child, allowing confidence for self-expression and exploring other directions. Some boundaries are based on avoiding injury to other children, nurse or child. Others could be reality issues such as time limits and property limits.

H.G. Ginott (1964) proposes four steps to successful limit setting:

(1) Recognise the child's feelings or wishes and help him to express them as they are. ('You feel angry, and you'd like to hit me.')
(2) State clearly the limit on the specific act. ('Hitting is one thing I won't allow you to do' or 'I won't let you hit me.')
(3) Point out other channels through which the feelings can be expressed. ('You can hit or kick the pillow.')
(4) Allow the child to express resentment or anger for having his behaviour restricted or redirected.

The four steps can be applied to any area where boundaries must be applied and should always be negotiated and clearly communicated on an individual basis to ensure that the meaning is fully understood.

4 Reasoning Skills

This relates to the nurse's ability to explain, enabling full understanding on behalf of the child. In order to do this, the nurse must consider the child's developmental level and anxiety levels. There is a need to be sensitive to what the child is anxious about and to appreciate what the likely outcome of an explanation will be. Consider the effects of these two explanations on a seven-year-old child about the same event:

'Tom, I want you to come and sit with your mum and dad and have a chat with Bill the doctor, Shirley the lady doctor, me and Dave the other nurse, is that OK?'

'Tom, I want you to sit in on a session of family therapy so we can all express what's going on and see if we can make things better.'

The latter's use of ambiguity and 'foreign language' is much more likely to cause fear and resistance than the former explanation where the intention is clear.

5 Exploratory Skills

These skills are aimed at helping the child to explore his own feelings and thoughts and express them. This is a two-way process and particularly important with children as they need to know what others are thinking and feeling also. The nurse can elicit the child's thoughts and feelings in many ways, often the more imaginative the better. Rather than direct questioning, generate interest in the topic first through wishes or fantasy or by allowing the child to correct the adult's incorrect information. The saying 'Actions speak louder than words' is particularly relevant to the communication of thoughts and feelings to and from the adult. Physical contact and hugging to convey acceptance are very powerful. If the child feels anxious about communicating feelings verbally, then alternative outlets could be using play or puppets; even just being with them can serve as a bridge for the message.

6 Creative Communication

Understanding the value of play, art, exercise, drama and other forms of creativity and their use in the therapeutic regimes of children in hospital is essential. These activities can have several functions at each developmental level:

— development and mastery of specific motor skills;
— expression of imaginative or symbolic content;
— repetition and working through of inner conflicts.

The nurse's role in relation to these activities can either be as a participant or as an observer. The nurse must ensure that she does not interfere with any 'working through' process by the child — just being there is usually sufficient to offer support during anxious moments or times of skill acquisition. These times offer a chance for the child to be him or herself, expressing thoughts, fears, conflicts or desires freely. The nurse could also express her own world through this media and by sharing with the child may enhance the bonding sufficiently to engender trust. From this the child's confidence may grow and readiness to disclose and share may increase.

7 *Conveying Acceptance*

Counteracting the child's feelings of rejection can be started by conveying acceptance to the child through the nurse/child relationship. The nurse must be open and honest with the child about the relationship and also consistent, especially in the form of communication. This can be shown through the use of the 'skill areas' mentioned above, but can be summarised (Norbeck, 1980):

(1) Providing a safe environment.
(2) Providing developmentally appropriate equipment and activity.
(3) Positioning oneself at the same level as the child.
(4) Engaging in appropriate activity as the child directs.
(5) Being with the child and attentive to him.
(6) Talking in language appropriate for the child.
(7) Respecting the child's need for social distance.
(8) Respecting the child's pace of activity.
(9) Demonstrating warmth and concern for the child.

If the nurse can accept the child as a valued member of society, someone who needs love, warmth and security, then she can begin to rebuild what is often perceived through the child's eyes, a shattered and fearful adult world.

Family Involvement

We feel it necessary to say that no child should be cared for in isolation from the family. That is to say, a child's problem is a family problem, and any therapeutic intervention should incorporate the needs of the parents and siblings. This may occur in several forms.

Mothering Groups and Fathering Groups

This is where the respective parents gather to talk about their roles and relationships, offering each other different perspectives on the mother/child or father/child relationship. The nurse may play the role of prompter and information giver in relation to helping the group work together.

Family Groups

Here the whole immediate family are invited together, either with a specific therapist and/or a nurse. The dynamics, relationships, issues and conflicts are aired openly in order to maximise the best possible opportunity for communication between the parties and reduction in barriers.

Other activities the nurse is likely to be involved in when working with children in a psychiatric unit are those supportive and therapeutic activities aimed at helping the whole family as well as the child, e.g. individual counselling of parent or parents; marriage guidance; helping the parent work or play with the child; teaching and modelling for the parents, and generally offering a consistent support system where the parents can feel confident and safe to communicate anything that may be of benefit to the child and family.

Implications for the Nurse

Working with children can be very emotionally and physically demanding. The nurse must be aware of the possible consequences of what often is a very close relationship with a child. The following is an outline of the most common mechanisms which, if the nurse is unaware of them, may interfere with the giving of care.

Over-dependency

This is where the child takes to the accepting nature of the environment to such an extent that the thought of anything outside it fills the child with dread, thus impeding eventual independence.

Emotional Involvement

When the nurse becomes particularly attached to a child to the extent that she finds it difficult to view the situation objectively, her judgement may be compromised and cause additional conflict within the ward team.

The continuous demands a group of children will make on a nurse will depend very much on how realistic the nurse is. If she provides uncensored attention, she will not survive. It is therefore imperative when caring for disturbed children to be aware of the emotional demands made and the limits to which you can give. Feelings of inadequacy, frustration, ambivalence and anger are all common emotions experienced by the nurse towards staff, self and the children. The need to accept these as normal processes and have the channel to explore them in a supportive staff environment is necessary in order to protect yourself, thus increasing the likelihood of consistent delivery of care to the child.

Conclusion

The child in care may look upon the carers as a substitute family. The nurse must find a balance between being mother or father, brother or sister and nurse. It may be that the nurse can amalgamate all roles into one, but this is acceptable only to the extent to which she can satisfy the demands a child may make on one particular role, within the constraints of her own professional judgement. The common factor to all these is the need for affection and love. To be able to give this, often in the situation of personal attack and what may seem like endless frustration, is a very valuable personal asset.

Finally, we have tried to identify specific skills the nurse may need to use when caring for children within a psychiatric setting. There is a wealth of material that revolves around the skills described; we hope our description is sufficient to stimulate you into further study.

Suggested Further Reading

Barker, Philip *The Residential Psychiatric Treatment of Children* (Crosby Lockwood Staples, London, 1974)
Bhoyrub, J.P. and Morton, H.G. *Psychiatric Problems in Childhood: A Guide for Nurses* (Pitman, London, 1983)
Bumbalo, J.A. and Siemon, M.K. 'Nursing Assessment and Diagnosis: Mental Health Problems of Children', *Topics in Clinical Nursing*, vol. 5, no. 1 (April 1983), pp. 41-54
Cromshaw, D. 'Careers. Child Psychiatric Therapy', *Nursing Mirror*, vol. 156 (July 1983), p. 56
Field, Michael and Bhoyrub, J.P. 'A Limit to Child's Aggression', *Nursing Mirror*, vol. 149 (December 1979), pp. 36-7)
Goodyear, I. 'The Recognition and Management of the Depressed Child', *Maternal and Child Health*, vol. 8, no. 9 (September 1983), pp. 381-3
Haber, J., Leach, A., Schudy, S. and Sideleua, B. 'Promotion of Mental Health in Families' in *Comprehensive Psychiatric Nursing* (McGraw-Hill, New York, 1978), ch. 32
Haldene, J.D., Lindsay, S.F. and Smith, J.D. 'Nursing in Child Adolescent and Family Psychiatry', *International Journal of Nursing Studies*, vol. 8 (1971), pp. 91-102
Hamilton, W.B. 'Role of the Nurse in Child Psychiatry', *Nursing Mirror*, vol. 144 (May 1977), pp. 21, 29-32
______ 'Children at Odds with the World', *Nursing Mirror*, vol. 147 (October 1978), pp. 16, 32-6
Kolvin, I. *The Nursing Therapist in Child Psychiatry. The Psychiatric Nurse as a Therapist* (*Nursing Times* Publication, London, 1973)
Quinn, D. 'The Conduct Disordered Child — A Psychiatric Nursing Approach', *Nuring Times*, 24 March 1977, pp. 426-7
Treacher, Andy and Carpenter, John *Using Family Therapy: A Guide for Practitioners in Different Professional Settings* (Blackwell, Oxford, 1984)
Wilkinson, Teresa R. *Child and Adolescent Psychiatric Nursing* (Blackwell Scientific Publications, London, 1983)
Wolff, S. *Children under Stress* (Penguin Books, Harmondsworth, 1973)
Wong, S.C. 'Child Psychiatric Care', *Nursing Times*, 16 June 1977, pp. 918-19

17 THE ELDERLY CONFUSED PATIENT

Mrs Garland's admission was due to a culmination of several month's gradual deterioration in her behaviour. Her family had coped quite well up to now, but recently Mrs Garland had been wandering about at night, turning the gas on without lighting it, or cooking things and leaving them to burn. What seemed to be the last straw for her daughter, who had been caring for her, was when her mother squatted in a corner of the kitchen and defaecated. This resulted in her daughter approaching the doctor with pleas for help. Mrs Garland had been on the waiting list to come into the elderly assessment unit, but this increase in deterioration had warranted immediate admission, as her daughter could no longer cope and Mrs Garland was a risk to herself and indeed to others.

On admission, Mrs Garland was accompanied by her daughter and son-in-law. They were taken to the reception lounge and offered a cup of tea. It was usual for the nurse in charge and another to introduce themselves and record essential information for records, and to give the relatives and the patient information they would need. Mrs Garland was sitting next to her daughter. She seemed nervous, and was continually fidgeting with her dress, pulling it up to her face.

'Do you take sugar, Mrs Garland?

She looked towards the nurse with a vacant gaze.

'Go away.'

She got up and walked towards the window.

'What is this place?'

'I've told you, Mum, it's a place where you can rest and get better.'

'There's nothing wrong with me, take me home.'

The nurse intervened, 'Come and sit down, Mrs Garland, and have a cup of tea and then we'll explain everything.'

'Where's my Billy?'

She started to cry. Billy was her husband, who had died four years ago. By this time her daughter was becoming distressed. In an effort to distract Mrs Garland, the nurse took her hand.

'Come on, Mrs Garland, I'll show you our garden, it's lovely out here.'

Her mood changed quickly and she seemed to go quite willingly with the nurse. The remaining nurse then spent a considerable time with the daughter, helping her explore a whole range of feelings, varying from frustration and anger to guilt and sadness, until she could accept the situation sufficiently in order to leave her mother in the unit with some sense of personal relief and reassurance.

This progressive loss of contact with reality, highlighted by intellectual, emotional and memory disturbances are manifestations of 'dementia'.

The following is a list of symptoms and examples of behaviour illustrating these.

Memory Disturbance

At first, Mrs Garland became absent-minded and forgot things like appointments, items of shopping and where she left things in the house. This, however, progressed to seeing someone one day and forgetting that she had seen them the next, or setting out to do the shopping and arriving back late at night, via the police, distressed, saying, 'I got lost.' Her memory for recent events had become extremely bad, but during this period she would recall past events of her childhood and early adult years very well. Recently she had started confusing dates, events and anniversaries: she could not recall whether her husband had died one year or four years ago, and occasionally she had stated that he was not dead. This severe memory disturbance results in a major manifestation of confusion.

Disorientation in Time, Place and Person

The disorientation in time illustrated by Mrs Garland's wandering at night is quite common, and an extension of this is the complete reversal of the sleep pattern, i.e. asleep most of the day and awake during the night. Disorientation in place is often highlighted by the constant questioning of 'What is this place?' or 'Where am I?' despite persistent answers and reassurance. This particular aspect is extremely frustrating, as you will appreciate when relating back to a time where unfamiliar surroundings dominated the environment; the insecurity, anxiety and fear will often result in anger and frustration. Probably the most disconcerting form of disorientation is that of 'person'. This becomes distressing, especially for relatives who visit the patient who turns and states, at best, 'I am not who you say I am and I certainly don't know you' or, at worst, gives no response or acknowledgement of their presence at all.

Emotional Disturbances

Mrs Garland's sudden change from crying to contentment at being shown around the garden demonstrates the 'emotional lability' that is often present. This is the inappropriate switching of extremes of emotion from sadness and crying to euphoria and laughter. Others, however, may exhibit a shallowness of emotion and lack of responsiveness. Associated with the confusion, especially early on in its development where moments of insight are apparent, are anxiety and depression, which can dominate the patient's mood.

Intellectual Impairment

The first signs of this occurring are usually seen when the patient finds it difficult to make decisions, or chooses inappropriately. The ability to make judgements diminishes rapidly and the ability to think in abstract forms becomes difficult.

It can be seen from the description of these behaviours that someone experiencing this devastating process can be transformed into someone hardly recognisable by those closest to him. These changes often exacerbate an already fragile body, resulting in an individual who is probably the most difficult person to nurse in terms of physical and psychological demands made upon the limited resources available. This brings a challenge to all those who undertake this particular caring role.

The Problems and Needs of the Elderly Confused Patient

The problems and needs of the elderly confused are often considerable, varying from the basic needs of nutrition and warmth, through those of love and belongingness, to esteem (see p. 126). It is therefore imperative that when assessing these patients, priorities are taken into consideration and the best use of resources made. There are a variety of assessment forms available (see p. 122), all of which are designed to establish the physical, psychological and social needs of the patient.

Physical Problems and Needs

A thorough medical assessment on admission is required in order to establish the extent of the patient's physical well-being and also to eliminate a variety of other causative agents which can cause confusion and would mean a different course of treatment and care. Two other causes of confusion in the elderly are toxic states and depression, which would warrant alternative regimes of care. Nursing observation in this area should be related to physical needs and ensuring that safety factors are considered. An elderly confused person who is very unsteady on his feet is agitated and restless. Because of the combination of these factors, the potential danger of falling is very real, so it becomes a priority to assess the degree and cause of immobility in order to rectify the problems if possible, and also to minimise the extent of restlessness. There is a need to pay particular attention to all the essential needs of the elderly confused because each one is at risk from self-neglect due to the incapacitating nature of the 'dementing' state. Assessment and planning of the individual's needs in the areas of nutrition, elimination, hygiene and sleep are vital in every case.

Psychological Problems and Needs

Consider yourself in a building where you wander round in a circuit, yet every room you come to is different, never returning to the first room you set off from. In each room there are people whom you have never met before, yet they seem to know you and tend to coax you from one area to another. When you try to speak to them the message comes out garbled and when they speak to you it seems like a foreign language. Some of these people pull at your clothes, enter into your bathroom and sometimes even your toilet area. Food and drink are thrust at you at any time during the day and if you don't eat it then someone will spoonfeed you. How would you react in this situation?

It is not surprising that many elderly confused patients are agitated and distressed, for it must be for them something like the scenario just described: a world of strange places and faces, not knowing the intention or purpose of being there, yet being helpless to do anything about it. This situation invariably leads to the psychological problem of:

Frustration
|
Anger/aggression ——— Confusion ——— Distress
|
Apathy/withdrawal/depression

Their needs in relation to these problems are those of reassurance, repetitive explanation, clarity of actions, all conducted in an atmosphere of acceptance, without condemnation and ridicule.

Social Problems and Needs

The nurse should never assume that because the patient is grossly disorientated, what could be perceived as more complex needs are not required. The needs for pride, dignity and independence are high in all of us, but possibly more so in the elderly. The fear of losing these must be very distressing, and it is therefore up to the nurse to be sensitive to this and provide every opportunity for the individual to maintain independence through which pride and dignity can be maintained. By careful choice of activities, the nurse can generate some course of usefulness in the patient, thus avoiding possible isolation. It is a common mistake to underestimate the insight and capabilities of some, especially when they are living with those whose orientation is limited to the vague acknowledgement of their surroundings. It must be stressed that each individual must be cared for on his own merits.

Implications for the Nurse

When caring for the elderly, the nurse is confronted with the reality of 'human decay'. The progressive deterioration of these patients is inevitable and no matter what the nurse's interventions are, she cannot change this course. This may cause feelings of helplessness and despondency in the nurse and may even progress to questioning the futility of maintaining this quality of life. There are serious ethical questions that the nurse must personally explore until a value can be found that is conducive to the maintenance of life and enhancing the quality that remains, by dedicated and skilful care. The dangers of working in this area without exploring and coming to terms with the reasons and personal demands may reflect the nurse's approach to her patients. She may, as a defence, withdraw emotionally and deal with her patients in a mechanical and impersonal way, without the 'giving' that is essential in any therapeutic relationship. It only takes one or two individuals with this sort of attitude to have a negative effect on the whole ward. It is particularly important that the morale on this type of ward is maintained as high as possible, so that an air of hopeful optimism can be reflected on to the patients.

No matter how well staffed these wards are, the physical and psychological demands made upon the nurse are considerable. The pressure of dealing with the essential needs of patients, and working in a team aiming to finish in time for another event to start, i.e. being constrained by the ward routine, increase the likelihood of nurses taking short cuts, sacrificing the quality of their care for the quantity of tasks completed. Ensuring adequate staffing levels and using an individualised nursing care approach will help minimise the risk of this occurring. However, in reality, we live in a society where care of the elderly will always lend itself to limited resources, partly because of the ever growing demand, but also because of the lack of importance and value we have for our ageing population. Despite what often seems a gloomy picture, nurses can and do gain tremendous satisfaction from caring for the elderly confused, as illustrated in this quote from a student nurse writing about her experience with the elderly.

> The last three months have instilled in me a new sense of tolerance, responsibility of care, and knowledge which I hope will continue to grow in me. I almost feel guilty because I have got so much out of this experience and if I have given a part of what I have taken, then I think I have justified my stay there. (Anne, 1982)

Principles and Skills Required in Nursing the Elderly Confused Patient

The major areas of skills necessary to care for the elderly confused effectively are non-verbal, verbal, psychomotor, group and management skills.

Non-verbal Skills

The nurse must utilise every personal asset she has to enhance communication to the patient. This involves effective use of non-verbal skills: talking in a tone of voice that is conducive to his hearing, which does not necessarily mean intensity, enhancing contact by appropriate use of touch, listening face to face with eye contact, being close with an open posture and leaning towards the patient all show non-verbally that the nurse cares and wants to be involved.

Verbal Skills

Verbal skills encourage the patient to communicate through his confusion. The nurse must allow the patient to express his fear and desires, no matter how confused they are, and at the same time she must be sensitive to his feelings and needs. The verbal skills are those related to specific questioning, clarifying and giving repetitive explanations. These must be exercises without patronising, for it is easy to fall into the mistake of playing the role of parent as opposed to helper.

Psychomotor Skills

If one were to analyse the physical tasks involved in caring for someone who was virtually helpless, they would vary from the large movements of lifting to the intricacies of applying a sterile dressing. Indeed the role of the psychiatric nurse can seem diverse, but the common factor when carrying out these psychomotor skills is the attitude of the nurse and the manner in which they are conducted. Whenever a physical task is performed, be it feeding the patient or assisting him to the toilet, there is always a need for the use of appropriate verbal and non-verbal skills in order to facilitate socialisation.

Group Skills

Group skills involve being aware of the needs and abilities of each individual within the group and coming up with a formula that will be sufficient to facilitate a common interest. With the elderly confused, the common denominator is often the past, mainly because that part of memory is often more intact than the recent and it leaves them with a sense of reality. Reminiscence therapy is a particular method conducted as a part of 'reality orientation'. Other group activities related to reality orientation serve this purpose of socialisation well, and at the same time it often stimulates and helps maintain the patient's usage of resources to its maximum.

Management Skills

Most relevant are management skills related to being in control of the environment. Besides the essential management of resources, i.e. manpower and facilities, there are specific skills involved in making the most of limited resources to the benefit of orientating the elderly confused. By utilising the skills of the care team, it is possible to create an environment which is bright, colourful, functional and clean. The sensible positioning of signs and the use of any aid to reinforce reality will help orientate its confused residents, e.g. calendar, clocks, menus, activities sheet, directional arrows and name-plates are all examples of materials that can be used as a continual reality orientation programme (see Appendix II).

Summary

As our hospitals become filled with our ageing population, the demands made upon the personal resources of the nurse increase. As the elderly progressively deteriorate, the skills to cope with this become stretched. It requires tremendous dedication and application to experience and care for those that require so much, yet appear to many to give so little. Yet they do give: they give with their eyes, their touch, their smile and their confused acknowledgements of gratitude. And, who knows, there may be more going on in that mind than we think. Therefore, let us assume the best possible state rather than the least; after all, we will be old one day.

Key Concepts

(1) The progressive loss of contact with reality highlighted by intellectual, emotional and memory disturbances are all manifestations of dementia.
(2) This severe memory disturbance results in a major manifestation of confusion, i.e. disorientation in time, place and person.
(3) It is imperative that when assessing these patients, priorities are taken into consideration and the best use of resources is made.
(4) There is a need to pay particular attention to all the essential needs of the elderly confused, because each one is at risk from self-neglect due to the incapacitating nature of the 'dementing' state.
(5) It is not surprising that many elderly confused patients are agitated and distressed, for they are living in a world of strange places and faces, not knowing the intention or purpose of being there, yet being helpless to do anything about it.

(6) When caring for the elderly, serious ethical questions must be explored until a value can be found that is personally acceptable and conducive to the maintenance of life and enhancing the quality that remains by dedicated and skilful care.

(7) The skills required to nurse the elderly effectively are:
   - verbal and non-verbal skills that enhance communication;
   - psychomotor skills that involve physical contact and are used to satisfy the physiological human needs;
   - group skills to enhance socialisation and potentiate remaining memory and reality.
   - management skills to create an environment that minimises the chances of confusion and enhances reality orientation.

Suggested Further Reading

Barton, M.A. 'Reaching the Patient (Nursing Elderly Patients with Dementia)', *Geriatric Nursing*, vol. 4, no. 4 (July/August 1983), pp. 234-6

Browne, Kevin, 'Confusion in the Elderly', *Nursing: The Add-on Journal of Clinical Nursing*, vol. 2, no. 24 (April 1984), pp. 698, 700-2, 704-5

Chenitz, C. 'The Nurse's Aide and the Confused Person', *Geriatric Nursing*, vol. 4, no. 4 (July/August 1983), pp. 238-41

Holden, U. and Woods, R.T. *Reality Orientation: Psychological Approaches to the 'Confused' Elderly* (Churchill Livingstone, Edinburgh, 1982)

Mitchell, Robert G. 'Confusion (Causes and Treatment)', *Nursing Times*, 13 April 1983, pp. 62-64

Wolanin, M.O. and Phillips, L.R. *Confusion: Prevention and Care* (Mosby, London, 1981)

18 THE DYING PATIENT

This chapter seeks to share with you our strong convictions that nursing the dying patient can be a rewarding and insightful experience. Understanding the stages of dying is only the beginning of a whole area of study we believe the psychiatric nurse is most appropriately qualified to undertake. It is included in this text because we feel it is an area offering potential personal growth through self-awareness, and contains within it some essential principles and skills which ought to be within the psychiatric nurse's repertoire.

It has been observed by Kübler-Ross (1978) that people pass through stages of dying. These stages are extremely important for nurses to understand if good care and skilled interactions are to be implemented with patients who are dying. The five stages most commonly observed are denial, anger, bargaining, depression and acceptance.

Although these stages follow a generally accepted sequential order, it should be pointed out that individual patients may not necessarily follow them in sequence. It is quite possible for a patient to experience denial, e.g. after depression, or anger after depression. Some patients may appear to have reached the final stage of acceptance, and still regress to depression or anger from time to time. It is an extremely useful guide to the process of mental adaptation to the concept of death, but the point we are stressing is that it is not an immovable, inflexible progression.

We are suggesting that it is the skilled nurse's job to enable the patient to work through these states whenever they occur, towards acceptance, at his own pace, with as little trauma as possible, and as constructively as possible. Each stage of the process is a normal healthy reaction, and should never be considered otherwise. However, to be fixed in any one stage is not only unhelpful, but may be counter-productive to the natural healing processes leading to a peaceful natural death.

The observant nurse used to dealing with the terminally ill patient is able to recognise each stage and be prepared for the behaviour associated with each. The person who may be involved with informing patients they have a terminal illness may be regarded as courageous, but because the mechanism of **denial** is usually the initial response to such news, seldom is this nurse confronted with more than stunned silence, or incongruent laughter. The disbelief of the reality of oncoming death is far more likely in most patients than sorrow or depression. **Anger**, on the other hand, is commonly directed at the nurse, professional carer or close relative. The feelings of the patient are actively focused on the unfairness of him dying, when others far less deserving are to remain alive. The sudden insight into the things undone and unsaid, the appreciation of all the wonderful people, places, aromas, sensations, tastes and activities that he is to be deprived of are unbearable to contemplate. Why him? What, after all, has he done to deserve this? It is not hard to imagine our own indignation and anger to appreciate this stage of the dying process. It is probably in this stage that most unresolved anxiety occurs. This does not necessarily reflect only his fear of physical pain, but his emotional pain. How difficult it must be to have the constant reminder every day that before long you will never see your children, your wife, your home again. This constant reminder is a continual torment, raising anxieties that cannot be quelled, raising anger that cannot in justice be directed at anyone, or anything. This mixture of anger and anxiety is extremely difficult to deal with, for the intensity of the injustice potentiates the anger, and the intensity of the anger prevents any action taking place. This in turn creates anxiety which maintains the inactivity. As anxiety is usually a self-limiting phenomenon, most people break out of this vicious circle and progress to bargaining.

Bargaining is the person's first attempt to control the events that appear to have overtaken him. Some method of action to buy time to undertake all the things undone, unseen, unsaid, is needed. The only course open to the patient is to make bargains with himself, his God, his beliefs that he will be better, not make the same mistakes, or make amends in some way if only he can be granted more time. Although this may sound somewhat unrealistic, almost like fighting reality with fantasy, it is in our opinion a very constructive stage. The realisation that time to act is the thing that really matters, to contemplate in fact what the time is really for, and how best each second can be maximised is the process that leaves the patient able to go on. Nurses are often involved in bargaining and in many cases nurses may be distressed by questions, almost desperate pleas sometimes, of: 'If I give up smoking now, nurse, will I live long enough to . . .,' 'Is there anything I can do to just hang on long enough to . . .'

It is our belief these questions should not be shrugged off, but dealt with seriously and honestly, no matter how painful that may be for both parties initially. Without honesty from professionals, how are the terminally ill ever going to be able to make plans of a realistic nature, and make purposeful choices?

Depression may be the beginning of a fatalistic, although angry, acceptance that whatever happens, or whatever the individual tries, death is inevitable. If the bargaining stage has been short lived, then the depressive stage may be longer. This could be due to the reflective thought and analysis that are usually dealt with previously, but now have to occur under the realisation of depressive finality. If, however, a lengthened bargaining process has occurred, the depressive aspects may be very short. It is our assumption that it is inevitable that reflective thought in either stage will more often than not result in the same conclusion: if death is inevitable for everyone, but I have the knowledge of how soon mine is to be, I have an advantage in being able to use what's left of my time constructively. I intend to waste none of it on regrets, but spend all of it purposefully, usefully, and to its full potential.

This, as Kübler-Ross suggests, is 'the final stage of growth'. This final stage of **acceptance** can be viewed as the most meaningful insight life has given the individual. Many patients share with nurses the realisation that it is only with the confrontation with oncoming death that they learned to appreciate life. To learn how to live, to live one day at a time, to appreciate everything, every experience as if it may be their last, is indeed a worthwhile insight. How many of us are able to say if we were struck down today that we have no unfinished business to complete? For instance:

— Would my children know I loved them?
— Would I have said sorry for the things I've done and left undone?
— Will the loved ones I leave behind understand how unhappy I would be if they grieved for me?

Perhaps when we consider the advantages the terminally ill patient may have in dealing with these issues — albeit having this thrust upon him — we would save our pity for him, in case we forget to learn from him.

The elderly patient may have very similar stages to progress through, although it is generally accepted that there is less anger and the first stage of acceptance is reached more readily. It may be presupposed that your entire life could be considered as the whole process through the stages: in youth and adolescence death is ignored, denied; the concept of death in middle age is met with anger and bargaining; in the elderly progressing towards death is a depressing finality, but with much more emotional contentment, stability and fulfilment of unfinished business, acceptance is more commonly seen. This analogy with life's progress through the stages of dying may perhaps clarify why the death of children, and young adults has such a profound effect on nurses. Yet especially in children, the anxiety, despair and anger we feel is not necessarily shared by the patient. The concept of fear associated with death is in some ways a learned behaviour, for until this century death was not such a taboo subject. Even today, many cultures and societies do not treat death as such a terrible and apprehensive finality. To transfer our anxieties onto children may be seen as an unnecessary burden on them and to discuss death openly and frankly may be a policy worth careful consideration.

Nurses dealing with terminally ill children are invited to reflect on these words written by Kübler-Ross (1978):

> It is hoped that all the children of our next generation will be permitted to face the realities of life. It is hoped that we will not 'protect' them as a reflection of our own fears and our own anxieties! It is hoped that we adults are beginning to have the courage to realize that it is our fear that we project onto the next generation. Once we have courage enough, we can acknowledge honestly that there are problems, and we can solve them if we have someone who cares and who facilitates the expression of our fears and guilts and unfinished business. If we can do this, we can empty our pool of repressed negativity and start living fully and more harmoniously.
>
> Children who have been exposed to these kinds of experiences — in a safe, secure and loving environment — will then raise another generation of children who will, most likely, not even comprehend that we had to write books on death and dying and had to start special institutions for the dying patients; they will not understand why there was this overwhelming fear of death, which for so long covered up the fear of living.

The Problems and Needs of the Dying Patient

The patient who is terminally ill requires skilled nursing of a very high standard. Although the physical care of each patient may be completely and effectively dealt with, it is not uncommon to see the psychological care that is, in our opinion, so important largely overlooked. Years of controversy surround the principal issue of whether the patient should be told when he is diagnosed as having an incurable disease. We would pre-empt this debate by asking how we will know if he even wants to know if we do not take time to find out? Most nursing approaches that fail do so because the nurse fails to appreciate the needs, values and wishes of the patient. Never is the factor more pronounced than in nursing the terminally ill patient. Nurses and doctors who consider it their role to cure appear to feel personally guilty, lacking in some way, perhaps a failure, when confronted by a patient they are unable to 'cure'. Often the error they commit is to defend their position by avoidance and pretence rather than facing issues and dealing with them effectively. They may not be able to cure, but they are most certainly able to help if they are possessed with sufficient personal resources and the requisite caring attitudes.

It is our hypothesis that the dying patient requires the following:

(1) Honesty from his carers.
(2) Permission to grieve for his impending loss.
(3) Support to work through the stages of dying.
(4) Information that is as accurate as possible to enable realistic plans and goals to be formulated.
(5) To be part of the decisions made about him, at least to be allowed to voice his opinions on issues that concern him personally, e.g. where he's to be nursed; whether his life should be prolonged (use of antibiotics); how alert he should be in contrast to how much sedative/pain relievers he may need/want.
(6) A knowledge of how his death/dying is affecting the emotions of other humans around him — not only his relatives and friends, but the professionals caring for him.
(7) To be able should he choose, to discuss in an open climate how he feels about his death. To have around him at his death the people he wants in attendance.

In simple terms, to die with dignity.

Implications for the Nurse

Should all patients be told fully about their illnesses when of a terminal nature?

Some patients already know, but simply want concrete affirmation. Some demand to know, others do not wish to know at all. In fact the latter category will employ denial whether you tell them or not, so it may not even matter. In the final analysis, all patients will know, whether 'officially' informed or not; it is usually only a question of timing.

So when should patients be told?

When they want to be told. If the nurse is a skilled listener, has formed an empathic bond with the patient and cares, the patient will indicate when he is *ready* to be told. If, on the other hand, the nurse does not form a meaningful rapport, that nurse will be constantly avoiding contact as she carries a dreadful fear of being asked, 'Am I going to die, nurse?' The nurse who really listens to her patient and understands him will know when this question is asked whether it is an honest request requiring a realistic answer, or whether it is a plea for reassurance and hope. Either requires a skilful answer, but it is our contention that the deeper the relationship, the easier that skill becomes. Attesting to this concept, Kübler-Ross (1978) cites an unidentified social worker, quoted in Dr George's Wahl's book, as saying:

> I know he wanted to talk to me, but I always turned it into something light, a little joke or some evasive reassurance which had to fail. The patient knew and I knew, but as he saw my desperate attempts to escape, he took pity on me and kept to himself what he wanted to share with another human being. And so he died and did not bother me.

This, we suggest, shows a typical example of how fragile our own emotions surrounding death may be. The patient in this case is so strong and the professional so weak that it would seem right to pity us from his position. Maybe this strange reversal of role epitomises the powerful influences that occur in the knowledge of one's own finiteness.

The nurse, to be successful at caring for the dying, should have fully explored her own feelings about death. How does she feel about her own mortality: does she pity the patient through a raging fear of her own death, or can she be peaceful and confident in the knowledge that dying is only a final stage of life? Looking closely at how we feel about death may not be pleasant, but is a realistic option that a self-aware professional may need to take. It may answer many questions about how we behave with the dying patient:

— Do we identify the death of a child with the prospect of losing our own children? Is this why we react so violently on these occasions?
— Do we falsely reassure the dying patient not to comfort him, but to comfort ourselves?
— Do we shun the subject of death so readily because it upsets people, or because the subject is so close to our only personal certainty?
— Do we feel we are in some way tempting fate to be open and honest about death, that in some way talking about it will hasten our own?

If even some of this strikes chords of recognition, then perhaps it is not difficult to understand why dying patients are 'screened off', or nursed in side wards, have minimum contact from very 'busy' nurses, and the chat we've been meaning to have with Mr Jones never materialises.

It may be helpful to you to know at this point that we are *not* implying criticism of nursing care presently employed with terminally ill patients. We *are* stating that in our past professional careers, we have used avoidance and pretence and are now so unhappy with our past performance in the light of new insight that we hope to enable others to see a better, more effective way of caring.

Often difficult situations make an honest and open relationship almost impossible. It is important that these situations are dealt with effectively to maximise effective care. One example is when relatives express a wish that the patient is not told of the terminal nature of his illness.

This situation is extremely difficult and may need some time to be resolved. Although it is unwise to generalise, we wish to emphasise that anything which interferes with the nurse/patient relationship may reduce the effectiveness of its value. The relatives need to be in full possession of the significance of their wishes.

They need to be told that to be dishonest to a patient will significantly reduce the quality of care that he will receive, not perhaps in physical care, but in the psychological support he could be offered. It may be pointed out that denying the patient information will rob him of his independence, the ability to plan, and to finish off his life's business. They should be asked how they will cope with direct questions from the patient, and how their dishonesty will affect the relationship. Finally, they may be asked what the nurse should say if asked about discharge, test results and similar difficult questions. Although this may seem rather hard on relatives, it should be remembered that they are in fact taking responsibility for an individual, so they should know what responsibilities they are accepting. In the light of lucid explanations and insight, the implications of their often ill-considered wishes may change. In the event of an adamant relative, a nurse may offer an undertaking not to inform a patient directly, but we believe it would be most unwise to guarantee non-disclosure, when in her professional judgement it may be in the patient's best interests.

It is our belief that this approach will generally prove effective in situations similarly difficult, such as with other nurses, senior professionals, medical officers and administrators. In principle, when a nurse is asked to be dishonest with a patient, a sacred trust may be broken, interfering with an empathic relationship which in turn will detract from good care. We believe that, when anyone interferes with good nursing practice, it must be challenged.

Principles and Skills of Nursing the Terminally Ill through the Stages of Dying

Denial

When information is given to patients which confirms the terminal nature of their illness, but reactions observed seem to contradict this, it is reasonable to assume some degree of denial is occurring. The nurse's interactions should not change during this stage, and she should continue to be honest, open and to work towards the patient. Sometimes difficulties exist when unrealistic goals are discussed with the nurse. This may make the nurse uncomfortable and potentiate avoidance, so other strategies need to be employed. Take the following examples:

Patient. When I go back to work, I shall have a lot to catch up on.
When the course of radiotherapy is finished, I'm going to try jogging again.
If I can just put on some more weight, I'll regain my strength and go home.

In theory the nurse should not reinforce the denial stage by playing along, but it is extremely difficult to dash a person's hopes and dreams to the ground, no matter how unrealistic. The examples above may engender an extremely high charge of emotion within the nurse. It would be easy for the sensitive nurse to be overwhelmed by a wave of sympathy or pity for the individual and resolve it by simply replying, 'Yes, that's a good idea.' It would, however, be wrong of us to advocate this, as it would be wrong to condone the abrupt or brusque response, 'Don't be silly, you'll never be able to do that.' Instead, we would suggest that an honest, yet empathic, reply is more sensible and therapeutic: 'I can see you feel hopeful of being able to do that, and I would love to share your hope, but under the circumstances I wonder how realistic it is?' This response has the advantage of not denying the patient's feelings of hope, but neither reinforcing his denial. It is not overtly sympathetic, which would distract the patient from himself to perhaps feeling sorry for the nurse. It leaves a little scope for the patient to shrug it off and continue denial if that is his need. Finally, and probably most powerful, it shows the patient that the nurse is not interested in pretence, that she is prepared to be helpful and professional no matter how difficult and uncomfortable that makes her feel. This is a healthy beginning on which to base a future close, open, trusting relationship.

Anger

The terminally ill patient has every right to be angry at the injustice in his life. After all, why should this happen to him? Why him? is the question that may continually torment him, for there appears no satisfactory answer to this inflicted frustration. There are so many things left to do; he *should* be angry at someone or something responsible for his misfortune. In logic there is no focus for this anger, so the patient either projects it outwardly on to people around him, or inwardly to himself. The outward projection of anger is a profoundly more healthy reaction, as the internalised anger tends to manifest itself as deep and intractable depression which may result in premature and unnatural death in the form of suicide. The skilled nurse will therefore have to deal effectively with this anger, as she needs to be able to absorb it and accept it usefully. The patient who learns the patience, tolerance and acceptance of his nurse also learns to trust her, disclose to her and share his final stage of growth with her. The nurse who has the qualities required to go through this stage with her patient receives as her reward not only the trust of her patient, but an insight into how close a nurse and patient can become. Contrary to popular belief, this does not make losing the patient more difficult, but less traumatic. For there is no guilt to feel, only sadness at the natural passing of someone who was close.

So how should the nurse facilitate the patient venting his angry feelings? Firstly she needs to identify it, and if she knows her patient well, she will identify anger in his tone of voice, facial expression, posture and the attitudes he is able to express. The nurse must somehow communicate her permission to the patient, to be able to say, not necessarily verbally, that it's 'OK,' 'I understand you're angry,' 'I understand your anger, and in some ways share it,' 'If it's directed at me, that's OK too,' 'You have a right to be angry and it's better out in the open than simmering inside.' Open statements which share the nurse's ideas should be openly discussed: 'I know you're feeling angry at everyone, I'm trying to understand and accept your bitterness, but unfortunately I'm human too, and I need you to tell me every so often that it isn't me personally and maybe release your anger in other ways.' Knowing you understand and are accepting his emotions may be very helpful to him at this point. You may be able to show him ways of directing this energy into constructive areas, such as writing about the things that make him feel angry, or talking to others about how caring for the terminally ill could be better. Useful strategies simply to help the patient dissipate his anger would include physical pursuits such as plasticine modelling, use of punch bag/pillow, ball games, art work (especially finger painting). If a patient says, 'I just feel like shouting or screaming,' the nurse may feel inhibited about encouraging this — after all, patients screaming in a ward would not help the confidence or peacefulness of other patients. Finding an appropriate place to facilitate this should not be completely dismissed, though, as this strategy may be most helpful for some patients. Most of these ideas will require tailoring to the individual patient and institutional needs: some patients may not be as mobile as others, some activities may only be appropriate for outdoors, and the latter requires either a soundproof room or a very isolated area.

Openly verbalising and accepting the need to pass through this stage may in itself accelerate the process.

Bargaining

Patients will often involve nurses in bargaining, i.e. 'If I stop smoking, will I have a few extra months, nurse?' The skilled nurse will attempt to make this rather vague statement more specific. A straight answer would probably be, 'no', or at best a 'maybe'. A more empathic answer demonstrating the skill of *concreteness* may be the most helpful reply here: 'Am I right in thinking you're anxious because you may have less time left than you need, and stopping smoking is the one thing you think you have some control over?' Pause. 'I'm not really sure about the smoking, but perhaps it would be helpful looking at how best your time could be spent.' These types of response may enable the patient to make productive steps forward in this stage and help the patient to see how best his *'bargain'* with himself can be made. The vain hope of 'more time if I . . .' can be made productive by converting it to 'If I do . . . first then I may have time left for . . .'

Striking bargains with themselves, their God, or whatever else they believe in is a necessary step towards acceptance. If the nurse is able to achieve something concrete from this stage, to develop plans and priorities, then we suppose she will do so through using the skills more fully dealt with in progressive responding (see pp. 53-68).

Depression

Unlike clinical depression, which has routes in pathological mental functions, this stage of dying is the culmination of an emotional journey, leading to an inevitable conclusion. Depression may be a short or a long stage, depending upon the personality of the individual, and the circumstances of his environment. The skills the nurse requires in this stage are fully discussed in Chapter 6 on depression but, additionally, the nurse needs to be able to communicate the knowledge that this depression is not pathological, but natural and normal. It is the patient's grieving process, for the loss he is about to have. It is the quiet reflective stage, where there is no hope of denial, just the depths of despair in the knowledge that before long life with all its values that it holds for that individual is to be taken away. The nurse needs to spend time with the individual showing she cares, reassuring the patient by reflecting his strengths, his qualities and his resources, showing the patient by her presence that he still has a lot to offer, that his wisdom, humour, smile, touch and conversation have a value to her and anyone else in contact with him. This can be emphasised by simply being with the patient, holding his hand, smiling, making eye contact and with empathic and reinforcing verbal messages, e.g.

'I know you feel down at the moment, but I do miss your smile.'

'You look really low today, it almost makes me feel sorry for you, but do you remember you said I should never do that?'

Or by gentle challenges:

'I remember you complaining a week or so ago that you had such little time, now you keep saying there's nothing left to do, and you don't feel like doing anything. I'm a little puzzled.'

This should not be an attempt to bludgeon him out of his depression, or get him to 'pull himself together', but to remind him gently and continually that you are with him, you trust and accept him, and you have confidence in him. He will work through this stage.

Acceptance

When the patient reaches acceptance, the nurse's task is nearly complete. This is a time for the nurse to listen to the patient in order to share in his growth. He has reached the point where each new day is a bonus to be lived to the full, in the knowledge that death is inevitable, and it need hold no terrors. The unfinished business is completed and all that is left is to appreciate fully each precious second of life. Perhaps we may learn from the patient that to value each moment as if it is our last is the secret of exploiting the full potential of our life span.

The stages are not arbitrary barriers which need to be fully broken down and the spaces between them fully explored; there is bound to be a blurring between stages. The nurse should always expect the unexpected: anger to occur in denial; some denial in bargaining and so on. The principal skill in helping the dying patient must always be an empathic acceptance and an awareness of needs.

Summary of Skills

The principles and skills of nursing the dying patient are to:

(1) Own your own feelings about death.
(2) Understand the stages of death.
(3) By not avoiding contact, achieve an honest, open relationship based on a mutual empathic understanding.
(4) Be able to make concrete the patient's vague plans, and thereby control anxieties within him.
(5) Avoid robbing the patient of his independence, over compensating for your own feelings, and giving false reassurances.
(6) Support the patient through the stages of dying by communicating the patient's resources, strengths and your own confidence in him.
(7) Through your experience and knowledge, facilitate the venting of his emotions by whatever strategies are available and appropriate.
(8) Continue to listen, accept and learn to understand the patient and grow from this learning.

Key Concepts

(1) The stages of dying are extremely important to understand if good care and skilled interactions are to be implemented with patients who are dying.
(2) The observant nurse used to dealing with terminally ill patients is able to recognise each stage and is prepared for the behaviour associated with each.
(3) Realisation that death is inevitable, and imminent, may facilitate appreciation of life.
(4) The concept of fear associated with death is in some ways a learned behaviour.
(5) To transfer our own anxieties on to children could be viewed as an unnecessary burden to them.
(6) Most nursing approaches that fail do so because the nurse does not appreciate the needs, values and wishes of the patient.
(7) The nurse, to be successful at caring for the dying, should have fully explored her own feelings about death.

(8) Anything that interferes with the nurse/patient relationship may reduce the effectiveness of its value.
(9) A person interfering with good nursing practice should be challenged, whoever they may be.

Suggested Further Reading

Caughill, Rita E. *A Dying Patient: A Supportive Approach* (Little, Brown, Boston, 1976)

Corr, Charles A. and Donna, M. *Hospice Care: Principles and Practice* (Faber and Faber, New York, 1983)

Kübler-Ross, Elizabeth *On Death and Dying* (Prentice-Hall, Englewood Cliffs, New Jersey, 1970)

______ *Death. The Final Stage of Growth* (Prentice-Hall, Englewood Cliffs, New Jersey, 1975)

______ *To Live Until We Say Goodbye* (Prentice-Hall, Englewood Cliffs, New Jersey, 1978)

Nursing Times Publication *Care of the Dying*, 2nd edn (Macmillan, London, 1978)

Stedeford, Averil *Facing Death, Patients, Families and Professionals* (William Heinemann Medical Books, London, 1984)

Thompson, Ian (ed.) *Dilemmas of Dying: A Study in the Ethics of Terminal Care* (Edinburgh University Press, Edinburgh, 1979)

19 THE BEREAVED

> Pain is inevitable in such a case and cannot be avoided. It stems from the awareness of both parties that neither can give the other what he wants. The helper cannot bring back the person who is dead and the bereaved person cannot gratify the helper by feeling helped. No wonder both seem dissatisfied with the encounter. (Murray Parkes, 1972)

Raymond's face contorted into a painful but controlled grimace, as if forcing inside him the emotions he was violently wishing to suppress. He reached out for the chair arm and sat down, as if his legs could not longer bear his weight. His head bent forward and his hands seemed to come up only just in time to catch it. Colour began to return to his knuckles which until now had been almost continually clenched. The charge nurse repeated his statement as if he were unsure that he had been heard: 'I'm very sorry, there was nothing we could do, your father was already dead when the ambulance arrived in casualty.' There was something similar to panic and confusion inside Raymond's head — he felt so many emotions he had not realised it was possible to feel at the same time. He felt like shouting angrily, but there seemed no point, he felt like crying, but what would that achieve? Perhaps it was a mistake, perhaps they'd got it all wrong, but he knew this was only a vain hope. He continued to feel angry, afraid, confused, yet dulled, somehow numb. He began to realise that he was behaving strangely, rocking backwards and forwards in the armchair, and now acutely aware that the charge nurse was still standing over him. 'What can I do?' he thought, 'I'm expected to do something, say something, but I can't, I don't want to, I don't know what to do.' 'I'm sorry, it's such a shock. I'll be OK in a moment, just give me a little time, I'll be OK. Thank you' was all he could manage, it seemed so feeble but it took tremendous effect just to get those few words out. 'I'll leave you for a while then,' said the charge nurse, quietly closing the interview room door. The charge nurse had undertaken this task many times before, but it never quite became routine, and he was, as always, relieved to leave the room.

Raymond's response to being informed of his father's death

could be viewed as reasonably typical, but every individual will react to this traumatic news of a death in a different way. Within the first few minutes of hearing news of a death of a close relative, any of the potential emotions of grief — shock, disorganisation, denial, depression, guilt, anxiety, aggression and acceptance (see p. 287) may be evoked. Any nurse who has been exposed to bereaved relatives will know the sense of helplessness and the anxiety that is always around in situations like the case illustration.

Being prepared for the variations in behaviour of grief-stricken people may help the inexperienced nurse cope more effectively. Probably the most unexpected response is that of anger and resentment directed at the nursing and medical staff. This response, although not common, usually follows the initial shock of the news, and is generally an attempt to resolve feelings of guilt that may be associated with the death. The fact that the bereaved was not present at the time of death, has in some way not fulfilled promises, said or done things they feel they should have may result in this guilt being projected on to the unfortunate person present. 'Why didn't you make it clear he may die?' 'Why didn't you phone me sooner?' 'Why did you let him die?' can be expressed most violently and can be very distressing to the unprepared nurse.

Frank denials and disorganisation can be difficult to deal with in ward situations: the relative who simply refuses to believe the news and insists on visiting the deceased; or the bereaved person who becomes so distraught, confused and distressed that the nurse is right to fear for their personal safety. To allow a person to leave the premises in a mental state as described may be foolhardly and all attempts to dissuade the individual from leaving should be made until they have recovered from the shock.

It is also appropriate to bear in mind that some other circumstances may parallel bereavement behaviour. A person may suffer similar emotional trauma and behavioural extremes when going through divorce proceedings, unemployment, when informed of some chronic illness process, or when burdened with sudden responsibility in adolescence. It should be remembered that it is just as feasible to grieve the loss of a spouse, a job, health or childhood as it is the death of a close person. It may then be reasonable to assume that many causes of reactive depression are associated with a loss of some important or valuable asset in the individual's life. Many middle-aged and elderly individuals grieve for their fertility and youth long before they grieve the death of someone close to them. The bereaved individual may be seen in many disguises and manifesting very different behaviours; the skilled nurse is the nurse able to detect the grieving process, understand it and deal with it appropriately.

The Needs of the Bereaved

As Raymond portrayed, the essential need of a bereft individual is time — time to adjust, and come to terms with a significant loss. Many people are tortured by anxiety feelings following the death of a spouse, largely due to fear of the unknown. Tasks and responsibilities that they now face, and have previously been dealt with by the deceased, are now barriers to their peace of mind. There now exists a vacuum, an empty place, which somehow has to be filled. There may well be much resistance to filling the deceased's place initially, which may create additional difficulties. For example, the widow with a young family to care for may need help from the eldest child to take some of the burden of everyday life away from her. Simple tasks like babysitting, washing up and minor domestic chores that her husband may have helped with may now be displaced on to the elder children. This may make her feel inadequate or guilty for asking 'too much' of her children. It is often these very practical issues, and the subsequent emotional intensity that they stimulate, that prevent the individual coming to terms with a loss. The mental equilibrium of the individual needs to stabilise sufficiently to enable a rational appraisal of the situation. To be able to accept that life is going to be different. That there will be difficulties to overcome, and to succeed in overcoming them, vacuums have to be filled. There will be new people to meet, different approaches to consider and substitutes to be made. To reach this rational stage effectively, the individual must have dissipated her anger for the unfairness of her loss, shed the guilt that is implicit in most bereavement situations, and begun to accept her anxiety as a real thing and focus it upon tangible problems. Sadness and depression take a great deal of time to ease, but they will be more speedily dissipated when tangible issues are worked on. When practical issues begin to be solved, the collateral influences on mood are removed and depression may lift much more quickly. For example, when a person is very anxious about the future without her deceased husband, whether she can cope, and additionally becomes upset and confused when she remembers past encounters, a vicious circle exists. Somehow this circle must be broken. First steps may be to ensure the person is having a reasonable amount of sleep, eating a reasonable diet and generally looking after herself. This may sound trite or obvious, but a meal, a hot bath, a change of clothes and a good night's sleep are good starting points for solving problems. Sorting out priorities, resources and possibilities may require some assistance from friends, relatives or neighbours, but generally these are fundamental beginnings for bereaved individuals to refashion their lives.

It is important to remember that the grieving process takes time, and that it is a natural process which cannot be artificially rushed. It may take many months, and possibly up to two years, for a bereaved person to return to 'normal life'. If people are given the right constructive help to deal with their emotions and practical problems, we believe this time period will be usefully spent and fewer people would suffer pathological grief syndromes later on.

Implications for the Nurse

The nurse should be able to appreciate the emotions and likely behaviour bereaved relatives of her patients may be going through. She should not shy away from difficult emotions with the bereaved, but facilitate these emotions being expressed and dealt with effectively. To be able to do this, the nurse may have to consider how she would cope with a personal bereavement and the difficulties she may encounter. Even for the nurse who has suffered a bereavement, it is useful to look again at the needs she had and how best these were fulfilled. We must, however, urge one caution with this approach — what may have been right for the nurse should always be tempered with empathy for the unique individual being helped. The nurse should not develop one inflexible or stereotyped approach, but be aware that individuals have different needs and require different responses. Many times we have been asked how a relative should be told of a patient's death. There is, of course, no simple answer: the skilled nurse will know how best to handle the situation. The charge nurse in the original illustration favoured the 'tell them and leave them approach'. This may be a good method for some individuals, but to observe relatives' reactions, see how much support, discussion, debrief or privacy they require and act accordingly would be a more flexible model. Similarly, there is no safe way of actually saying the patient died. Some people will be upset by euphemisms such as 'passed away' and most by a blunt 'Mr Brown is dead.' This perhaps is why 'I'm not sure how to break this news to you' is favoured by many. This allows for the relative to respond with whatever euphemisms they wish. 'Take one step forward all you soldiers who think you've got a father,' said the sergeant. 'Where do you think you're going to, Brown?' This old joke shows how one imaginative mind focused on telling bad news. We don't recommend this, but it does illustrate that the most difficult and serious tasks become trivialised by humour in order to make them more acceptable to us. It also points out that breaking bad news should be environmentally planned if possible. A quiet room with an easy chair, where there will be no distractions of phones ringing or people coming in and out, is far more suitable than the parade ground or, for that matter, the middle of a day room or dormitory. The environment should at least offer a vehicle for privacy and appropriate support if necessary. Preferably, nurses involved in breaking bad news to relatives should arrange to have a sufficient amount of time to spend with them should the need arise.

Principles and Skills in Caring for the Bereaved

Information Giving

The relative will usually require certain information following a death: whether there is to be a post-mortem, how to contact medical records for death certificates, collection of property and such like. It is unlikely that any relative in a distressed state will remember much of what is being said, so it is of great importance that the nurse considers what needs to be said verbally and what information should be in written form.

If at all possible, information should be given to friends, neighbours or other individuals not so closely involved. It should be the nurse's intention to help the bereaved, not to add to a burden by additional tasks at this time.

Occasionally relatives may ask very searching questions at this point: 'Did he die in pain? 'Did he ask for me?' 'Who was with him?' Some of these questions require answers, others are purely rhetorical. In any event, the nurse confronted with them may feel very uncomfortable, for she will undoubtedly not have the answers to all of them — some may be unpalatable, and she may be tempted to tell white lies. Almost stock phrases have crept into nursing vocabulary to cover these events, such as:

'He was made as comfortable as possible.'
'He didn't regain consciousness.'
'He didn't appear to be in pain, and died quite peacefully.'

These may not always be entirely honest, but are designed to ease the distress of relatives at a time when the harsh realities may be intolerable. We believe that nurses should always try to be honest, and preserve the integrity of a relationship whenever possible, but using these particular examples of euphemisms wisely and judiciously may in these circumstances be acceptable.

The relatives who refuse to believe in the death of the patient and become agitated and distressed may need very skilled handling. A firm but gentle approach is needed to restore a calm and genuine understanding of the situation. Generally this individual exhibits almost a panic reaction and requires similar nursing interventions. Firmly comforting the person with a guiding arm and directing them to a seat is usually effective as is continuing to talk in a calm, soothing voice, saying that 'Things will be OK,' 'There's no cause for alarm,' 'You simply need a little time,' 'We are here to help you' and similar supportive statements. With this type of response, it may be necessary to spend some considerable time counselling the person both before and after visiting the body, should this be the elected course of action. We believe relatives who do visit the body, and are helped to release some emotions at this time, are generally benefited in the ensuing grieving process.

Interactional Skills with the Bereaved

The bereaved relatives will require essentially the basic skills of counselling (see Chapter 2).

— Attend — show the individual you care, by listening attentively to what he has to say.
— Listen carefully to facts about the deceased so you may share with him important insights into his loss.
— Reflect — his emotions so he appreciates the complex emotional factors affecting him presently.

- Clarify — his confusion, contradictory beliefs, attitudes and emotions, so both you and he can see discrepancies in self-blame, and anger at the death.
- Summarise — in the hope that a clearer picture of the entirety of the emotional components will enable a focus of action to be formulated.
- Challenge or facilitate self-challenge when it is obvious he is being too hard on himself, and pursuing self-defeating strategies.

Customs and fashions change over the years, and one in particular surrounding death is the custom of viewing the body. At one time, nearly all funerals took place from the home, with the body lying in the front parlour. More recently, the custom has become leaving bodies in 'chapels of rest' in the undertaker's premises. This trend towards distancing the close relatives from the body has become general practice, and sometimes extends to relatives and friends not visiting the body at all. We believe this is a crucial factor in the development of pathological grief syndromes and the precipitation of unnatural taboos concerning the cultural aspects of death. We sincerely believe that every effort should be made to facilitate relatives and friends being given the opportunity to visit the body to say their final farewells in private. In the case of the patient dying in hospital or some similar institution (and incidentally, in our home city of York 95 per cent of all deaths occur in such circumstances), relatives should be offered a chance to see the deceased patient as soon as possible following death. It seems reasonable to have an opportunity to prepare the body in the customary fashion — wash, shave, change linen, brush hair and remove any drips, tubes or other medical artefacts — before visiting. It certainly should not be a facility exclusively available in clinical morgues or chapels of rest, but if possible viewing should take place in the natural setting where death occurred. Nurses escorting relatives to visit a deceased patient may skilfully 'model' emotional disclosure that may be beneficial to the bereaved. To illustrate this, the following life situation of one of the authors is described.

Entering the side room, I saw my father lying on a bed with a sheet pulled up to his neck. His face was blanched and a little contorted, as though his death had not been painless. He had obviously been dead for many hours. My brother stood by my side. His rela-

tionship with my father had not been as good as my own, and I knew he was feeling guilty and distressed over the death. I began by finding my father's hand and, holding it, I said, 'I'm sorry, father, I wasn't with you when you died, I should have spent more time with you and I feel very guilty now I look at your body lying there cold and lifeless, but I know you knew how much I loved you, and how much you were loved by everyone. I know you'll forgive me, so I'll say my final goodbye now.' My brother listened to this, and as if by my unembarrassed disclosure of emotion, broke down in tears, touched his father's hand and spoke to him in open and tender emotion that had not occurred between them for many years.

A nurse cannot, on such a brief meeting with relatives, have the same empathic understanding as a man may have for his brothers, so it would perhaps not be appropriate or possible to facilitate so much emotion with relatives who are after all largely strangers. It is, however, valuable to facilitate a monologue from the relative to the deceased patient if possible. In a similar vein to the illustration, the nurse may speak to the patient in the presence of the relatives before leaving, e.g. 'I've brought your sons to see you to say goodbye — I'd like to say goodbye as well. I've nursed you for some weeks now and you've not complained. We all feel guilty that we could not have helped you more, but I think we did our best. We'll miss your smiling face. I'll leave you with your loved ones now.' This might appear to you rather bizarre, embarrassing or even ridiculous — it is designed to facilitate the release of emotions within the bereaved which may prove to be a healthy start to the grieving process. The nurse undertaking this modelling skill may well feel uncomfortable, she may even receive some odd looks from colleagues and relatives, but the potential good this may achieve is a priceless gift to the bereaved person who may benefit.

Following a visit to the deceased, the relatives should be seen again before they leave, to ensure they are coping adequately. The nursing skill here is listening to the emotional content of the bereaved and responding accordingly. Some relatives may be so distressed and unable to cope that they require referral to other agencies. Nurses should endeavour to have resources available for these eventualities: social worker, community nurse, family doctor, telephone numbers of friends or neighbours who may be helpful. National organisations such as CRUSE may be helpful in offering specialised counselling for the bereaved. Once the patient has died, the nurse's overall responsibility shifts to the care of the relatives.

This care may only be minimal or transient, but none the less it should be proficient — professional and efficient.

Summary of Principles and Skills

(1) The nurse needs an awareness of the stages of grieving in order to prepare herself for the potential emotional components of the interpersonal exchanges encountered in bereavement.
(2) The nurse must be able to absorb anger directed towards herself or the institution should this arise.
(3) The nurse must have an ability to be patient, to allow emotions to be released and to listen and show empathy.
(4) She should use her skills of non-verbal behaviour, especially touch, tone of voice and posture to help the bereaved individual, especially if shocked, agitated and distressed.
(5) Information given should be clear, and preferably written. It should be given to the person most likely to understand and employ it.
(6) The nurse should not avoid the bereaved, but give all the skills she has to them. This may include modelling 'debriefing emotions' with deceased patients and relatives.
(7) The nurse should have 'contingency resources' for referring distressed bereft individuals for continuing care.

Key Concepts

(1) Once the patient has died, the nurse's overall responsibility shifts to the care of the relatives.
(2) It is important that the nurse does not shy away from difficult encounters with the bereaved. Every individual may react to traumatic news of a death in a different way.
(3) The nurse should not develop one inflexible or stereotyped approach, but be aware that individuals have different needs and require different responses, and being prepared for this variation in the behaviour of grief-stricken people may help the inexperienced nurse cope more effectively.
(4) The potential emotions of grief are shock, disorganisation, denial, depression, guilt, anxiety, aggression and acceptance.

(5) It should be remembered that the grieving process takes time and it is a natural process.
(6) It may be helpful to remember that some other circumstances may parallel bereavement behaviour, such as when going through a divorce, unemployment or chronic illness.
(7) It is often the very practical issues and the subsequent emotional intensity that they stimulate that prevent the individual coming to terms with a loss. For example, 'What am I going to do about bills, the funeral, my job, the children,' etc.
(8) Relatives who do visit the body may require help to release some emotions at this time.
(9) In connection with the latter, it follows that some relatives may be so distressed and unable to cope that they require referral to other agencies.

A Behavioural Proposition for Dealing with Intractable and Pathological Grief: Grief Therapy

Grief is a common component of human behaviour. It would be unusual if not impossible to go through life without at least one experience of grief.

It can be argued that, additionally, there are degrees of grief. For example, perhaps the loss of a pet in the formative years of life may seem the end of the world to a child, while in later life the adult may well be upset, but be more philosophical in regard to the event. Losing your mother at the age of 96 may well be more acceptable than the sudden death of a spouse in a road traffic accident. The degree of grief relates directly to the suddenness, closeness and intensity of loss for each individual in any situation.

The psychiatric nurse will be familiar with death through both her professional contact — the patient and his relatives — and unfortunately through the inevitability of being human, and her personal experiences and thoughts. Whichever is uppermost in the nurse's mind is unimportant, however. What is imperative is that she has an awareness of and an openness to her feelings about death. Before any therapy is attempted for the grieving patient, the nurse/therapist must have a depth of understanding and an awareness of her own mortality and her own reactions in grieving situations, or at least an ability to control them.

Grief therapy, although one of the most potent of all

behavioural strategies is, in our opinion, one of the most traumatic and potentially hazardous. It would serve no good purpose whatsoever to have the nurse in a shattered emotional state alongside the patient.

The basic concept that grief therapy is founded upon is that each individual progresses through a process of grief as briefly mentioned earlier in the chapter. This process can be expressed in commonly recognised stages. It is thought that those people who remain in a grief-stricken state and subsequently exhibit symptoms of mental illness are those who have not progressed through these stages adequately.

These are the most commonly accepted as being the stages of grieving in more detail:

(1) *Shock:* the initial response to being told of a death. These may include physiological responses such as nausea, vomiting, fainting or psychological traumas such as withdrawal, apathy, confusion or disinhibition.
(2) *Disorganisation:* an inability to think clearly, to arrange the simplest plan. This disorganisation often takes the form of ritualistic 'searching' behaviour.
(3) *Denial:* this is the complete disassociation of the knowledge of the death, an inability to believe, despite the facts. This is often like total amnesia for the event.
(4) *Depression:* usually the result of denial breaking down, the finality of the knowledge sinking in, often accompanied by feelings of unworthiness, helplessness and poverty of ideas.
(5) *Guilt:* a component that no death can escape. Not only feelings of blame for the event, but also that the bereaved has survived.
(6) *Anxiety:* often connected with coping without the deceased, not being able to control events, including fears for self.
(7) *Aggression:* from irritability to anger, not only directed to yourself or significant others (i.e. doctors and nurses) but also to the deceased for having deserted you.
(8) *Acceptance:* believing that all has been done that can be, saying a final goodbye, and committing the deceased only to a memory — continuing life.
(9) *Reintegration:* restarting and eventually, perhaps, replacing, finding substitutes for the deceased and relegating the past and concentrating on the future.

The therapy proceeds on the premiss that each of these stages needs to be worked through, but first it is important to be sure that therapy is appropriate. The therapy is traumatic and as such may have risks attached, and it is therefore suggested that it be used only in severe cases of intractable grief. The natural grieving process is one that can take anything up to two years, so at least that period should have elapsed before therapy is contemplated.

The process of therapy should be explained to the patient in detail, making no pretence that it will not be painful and will require total co-operation with the nurse. There must exist a relationship of trust and one of high motivation on the part of the patient to be free of grief.

Dr Ron Ramsey, who has researched and treated many patients in intractable grief syndromes, maintains that a specific contract should be drawn up, the main areas being as follows:

(1) The patient must commit himself to complete the therapy.
(2) During the therapy he will not commit suicide.
(3) He shall not physically assault the therapist.

Once this is achieved, the process somewhat artificially takes the patient through the six most troublesome stages of grieving to move the patient quickly to the end process of reintegration and consequently resolving the grief.

The first stage the patient is asked to consider is denial. This is done by confronting the facts. The nurse may use artefacts to aid this stage, such as the death certificate, paper notices, letters of condolence, etc., asking questions such as:

'How long has your child been dead?'
'Do you believe your child is dead?'

and subsequently statements for the patient to repeat:

'My child is dead.'
'I will never see her again.'
'She has gone forever.'
'Her body is in the ground.'

Asking the patient to read the death certificate, notice in the paper and letters out loud may also be necessary.

This brings about a cathartic reaction in the patient and reinforces the facts to him. Although this appears very cruel and traumatic, its effect is to release the emotion, and is clearly important in the patient's treatment. It may furthermore be necessary to help the patient now physically to discard personal items used by the deceased — to throw away items such as soft (even favourite) toys, or clothes, perhaps even a wedding ring in the case of a deceased spouse. This helps to consolidate the knowledge that they are not coming back, that he or she is not just away, but dead. As may be imagined, this stage may be very distressing, and for both patient and nurse it requires tenacity and perseverance.

It should also be noted that if the patient blindly obeys without the release of emotion — sobbing, agitation and some resistance — the nurse should be suspicious that the patient has not indeed passed through denial, and continued effort must be maintained until such time as the nurse is sure the patient has accepted the death. Once this denial has broken down, the patient will be left in a state of depression, and the nurse must try now to support the patient through this stage.

A common misconception regarding supporting a depressive patient is that the nurse should be sympathetic. In fact, related to behavioural principles, sympathy is a positive reinforcer: most patients find sympathy rewarding, and therefore the great danger is to fix the depressed behaviour by this reinforcement. Certainly in grief therapy something much more productive than sympathy is required.

The nurse should in fact highlight the main areas of the emotional state for the patient — to heighten awareness — then move onto a more productive phase.

Empathic responses may help here, such as:

'You feel sad now because you now realise you have lost your child for good.'

'You feel helpless, perhaps even unworthy because you can't bring him back.'

This empathic feedback will help maintain the trust and rapport between the nurse and the patient, which could have been damaged during the first stage. The patient should be encouraged to verbalise his feelings, but with positive supporting statements added to them, i.e.:

'I do feel helpless' ... then ... 'Yet this is quite normal, and I will get over this. I am capable of coming to terms with these feelings.'

'I do feel sad' ... then ... 'But I will get better.'

When the nurse is confident that the patient is happy with these statements, progress should be made into the third stage, guilt.

It should be explained to the patient that all humans are fallible, that in fact to be perfect is impossible. There is no bereaved person who does not feel remorse in some way; even a saint will feel guilty after the death of a close one. He will still feel he could have done more, said things differently, expressed his emotions openly.

This perhaps is the one thing that will help the patient unlock the guilt he still has — 'It's not too late.'

It is our experience that the locked-in emotions of guilt are probably one of the most important factors in grief syndromes. The key to this lock is to facilitate the verbal expression of the things left unsaid. The nurse should seek some focus of contact with the dead person, a photograph, the graveside, whatever the patient has left that will help him to be in touch finally with the deceased.

Prompts can be used, in fact modelled by the nurse at this point to facilitate this release, e.g.

'I'm sorry for the things I could not do when you were alive.'

'I loved you very much — perhaps I didn't tell you just how much I loved you.'

'I'm sorry I wasn't able to say goodbye — but I'll say it now.'

'I miss you very much, but I have to get on with my life now — so goodbye.'

These verbalised emotions addressed to a photograph are in fact very powerful indeed, and allow the final breakthrough for the patient. It is always amazing just how much relief the patient accomplishes from a session such as this.

If possible during this session, the final stages should be attempted. Using the same technique, any residual anger or aggression can be dissipated, by using statements such as:

'You hurt me so much when you left me.'

'I hated you when you died, leaving me with so much unsaid, so much undone, left me to cope.'

These verbalised expressions are usually enough to take the patient up to the final stages of acceptance, leaving the nurse only to complete the treatment by reinforcing how much better he is feeling now he has resolved his grief, ending on positive statements for the patient to practise such as:

'Although I'll always remember you, you have to be part of my past now, I have my life to restart.'

'My husband/child/mother needs me now, I have to begin again.'

There is no finer satisfaction than reaching this stage, and comparing the withdrawn and pathetic soul at the beginning of the therapy to the hopeful, refreshed patient at the end. During the therapy, the patient and the nurse have lived through tremendous traumatic emotions, and at times they will both have had their doubts, but, in practice, the therapy is so powerful and successful that it will have proved to be most worth while.

It is impossible to state how long this therapy will take. For some patients it may take several days only, for others much longer. This therapy should not deter neighbours, chaplains and voluntary organisations, e.g. CRUSE (national organisation for bereaved families), helping individuals through bereavement counselling with the patient in less formal settings prior to hospitalisation; we do not deny their importance, or detract from their success. However, so often in our experience patients with *intractable grief syndromes* are undiagnosed, and consequently unhelped. Patients suffering pathological grief are often admitted as simple depressives and it is only when an empathic bond is built with the patient that the potential benefits of this therapy are realised. For this reason, it is our opinion that the therapist most able to carry out this technique is the ward-based nurse, community psychiatric nurse or similar therapist in the patient's home. In any event, the person needs to be thoroughly conversant in behavioural principles and sound counselling techniques.

Conclusion

This chapter intended to stimulate your interest in helping the bereaved relative or the patient suffering grief in other, perhaps more covert, manifestations, i.e. divorce, amputation, etc. It is hoped that the text, and the sharing of our personal insights and experience, have influenced you to undertake an intelligent and sensitive approach to bereaved people. Having introduced the concepts of grief, we ended the chapter with a behavioural programme specifically constructed to help patients suffering from *pathological* forms of grief. We cannot stress strongly enough that the introduction to grief therapy is not an open invitation to practise it. It must be clearly understood that grief therapy should be used only in states of protracted and pathological grief states by an individual who is trained in behavioural techniques. It is our view that it would be most unwise to begin this therapy without consultation with the responsible medical practitioner, an established empathic relationship, and the informed consent of the patient. If these criteria are met, it is our belief that the therapy can produce remarkable benefits for the patient, and should not be denied to those in need.

The dying patient and the bereaved will always represent a consistent part of the psychiatric nurse's practice, and it is hoped that this chapter has in some small way helped you to help this patient group further.

Suggested Further Reading

Dunlop, Richard, S. (ed.) *Helping the Bereaved* (Charles Press, London, 1978)
Murray Parkes, Colin *Bereavement: Studies of Grief in Adult Life* (Penguin Books, Harmondsworth, 1976)
Schiff, Harriet Sarnoff *The Bereaved Patient* (Souvenir Press, London, 1979)
Worden, J. William *Grief Counselling and Grief Therapy* (Tavistock, London, 1982)

PART III:

EXTENDING KNOWLEDGE AND SKILLS

20 COMMUNITY SKILLS

Thomas has been in and out of psychiatric hospitals for many years. He has had many therapies and therapists. He expresses quite convincingly that the community psychiatric nurse (CPN) who visits him will be his last. His life has had many painful experiences, he is unable to deal with life's stresses, he finds great difficulty in forming relationships with women, and generally feels life is hardly worth living. Although Thomas had a good job as a teacher and meets interesting and stimulating people, he remains isolated and wholly unable to trust himself to be open, and the subsequent risk of being let down again.

Elsie is reaching her sixties, and has had several children, now all grown up. Her husband left her years ago, and she now lives alone in a council flat. She is permanently anxious and frequently depressed. When the CPN visits, she is nearly always tearful following a crisis with her family, or agitated as she is about to enter one. The root of her problems seems to be her inability to control her conflicting feelings. Her children abuse her kindness by demanding support from her at one period, then ignore her and have no contact with her for several months. One of her children is constantly in trouble with the law, and another frequently dumps all her children with her and runs off.

Elsie is left feeling constantly afraid of excessive demands and being unable to cope, or despondent because she feels rejected and deserted. She appears unable to communicate these feelings due to contrasting anger and guilt.

Joan is in her mid-thirties, married with a teenage daughter. Previously Joan had had a homosexual affair which, when discovered, caused extreme reactions within her marriage. Her husband, understandably perhaps, became rather suspicious, resentful and bitter. Joan paradoxically became extremely jealous and smothered her husband. As if she expected some ironic revenge to be meted out, she felt insecure and anxious, expecting him to leave her. After many admissions to hospital with anxiety, and exhibiting intense jealous reactions, it appears that these symptoms have run their course, and Joan seems to have dealt with both her jealousy and anxiety, and now feels resentful towards her husband for what she suspects has been his enjoyment of her difficulties. She has become bitter in the awareness that he has used her infidelity as a weapon against her, and deliberately increased her insecurity and jealousy to make her more dependent upon him. It is apparent that the family and marital tensions have reached a critical point.

Role of the Community Psychiatric Nurse

It may be apparent in viewing the brief case histories above that in each case the CPN has a difficult, yet different, role to play. Thomas requires a friend's support, a therapist's advice, and a counsellor's understanding; Elsie needs someone to show her that she can cope, and that she is needed, to reinforce the realities of life so she can realistically help her family, and also rationalise and understand their ungratefulness. Joan, her husband and her daughter require a skilled family therapist, an arbitrator, a defuser and a social worker. In later stages of distress, the CPN may find herself having to intervene in highly emotive issues that would not normally be the province of the nurse. As if this role were not demanding enough, she must also be able to deal professionally with the administration and monitoring of medicines, have the skills, knowledge and resources of a social worker, and the practical managerial application of a charge nurse.

Implications for the Community Nurse

It can be easily seen that the role of the CPN is multi-faceted. Taking this a little further, it is not hard to imagine that the nurse requires a considerable repertoire of skills and resources to fulfil that role. The nurse employed in such a role must therefore be able to offer an eclectic approach — an approach unique almost for each unique situation — and be resilient enough personally to withstand the pressure of such a totally demanding occupation. The main pressures upon the CPN, or any professional working alone, need to be fully understood by both the nurse and her employing authority to ensure that it does not impair effectiveness.

Isolation

The CPN is an autonomous professional, often working on her

own with no personal feedback from other colleagues. Although CPNs may work in teams, and have team meetings, the actual interpersonal exchanges between nurse and patients will be isolated from other observers. In a hospital situation, although interactions may be personal and unobserved, a collective opinion is none the less formed within the confidentiality of the staff room. These opinions take the form of how difficult, unreceptive, or even downright awkward some patients appear to the majority of the staff. This subjective information is at least of some help or comfort to the inexperienced and insecure members of staff who may otherwise believe that they are 'doing it all wrong'. This collective subjective feedback is not available to the community nurse, so other strategies have to be used.

Trust

The CPN must have confidence in her own abilities, and sufficient experience in successful therapy to be able to trust in her own personal resources. She should not be so arrogant as to believe she will always be right, or always know best, but neither should she be so self-doubting that she is hesitant and procrastinating. The community nurse's job is based on a clarity of action, a sensitivity of needs and a discriminating ability to judge situations correctly. This difficult balance can only be achieved if the individual has a highly developed sense of trust in her own senses and knows not only that she is able to deliver the appropriate approach, but to sense when she is unable to.

Self-analysis, Evaluation and Self-awareness

Having no accurate objective feedback of her own effectiveness, other than her patients' progress, the community nurse needs to reflect on her work performance and self needs from time to time.

It is most important that she analyses what she is trying to achieve with each patient, what she is actually achieving, and to what extent the outcomes are dependent on herself. To reflect actively on her own needs to achieve progress, knowing she is succeeding and that she is coping with the job, is by no means an insignificant ability that she requires to develop. The autonomous nature of the job dictates that the nurse is self-directed and self-aware, but, more importantly, that the direction is accurate and the self-awareness realistic. Being industrious and energetic towards an inappropriate goal is obviously counter-productive, but many caring individuals may fall into this trap because they are blinded by the fact that they are 'busy' and always 'rushing about' organising. Similarly the nurse's self-awareness may be depressing and demotivate her, she may feel that 'Whatever I try fails.' The problem here is that without other collateral information from other professionals, it is difficult to bring reality into the situation. The failure has become 'personalised' rather than realistically assessed. It may require someone to point out that whatever and whoever tries in these circumstances, they are *bound* to fail. It is imperative to stress this particular aspect of self-awareness at this point: self-awareness may potentiate a depressed mood because it lowers the defences and allows more insight. People concentrating on self-awareness may find greater difficulty in using mental mechanisms such as projection and rationalisation (Freud, 1958). It is for this reason that self-awareness should be tempered with reality constructs, i.e. human beings are human; it is impossible to be perfect; faults recognised can be changed, but not all at once; and faults recognised should not be punished, simply rectified steadily. Our fundamental belief, then, is that if guilt or depression results from self-awareness, the appropriate dose of reality has not been mixed with it.

Debrief

A skill absolutely essential for the community nurse to learn is how to debrief. It is always very difficult to discuss with another person the most intimate fears of our own limitations; to be able to admit to feelings of insecurity, inadequacy, embarrassment or simply not knowing something we believe it is expected that we should know. It is, however, one of the few simple ways of maintaining an individual's mental health. To harbour these negative feelings, to foster them and allow them to infiltrate the nurse's confidence will eventually undermine her efficiency and personal well-being. Unfortunately many nurses feel debrief is simply 'dumping' problems on to someone else. We on the contrary believe that this disclosure, which after all requires considerable courage, honesty and trust, does not place a burden on the listener, but allows her to share the problems. It facilitates a reciprocal arrangement so that common feelings of high intensity and considerable anxiety can be identified and dealt with by mutual support.

It is our belief that the autonomous professional should endeavour to practise debrief skills on a regular basis with a colleague, supervisor or friend, if she is interested in her own well-being and personal efficiency. We believe this should be at least a monthly programmed meeting and may be made more powerful when these meetings are group facilitated in working terms. Debrief meetings have the added benefit of allowing a cohesive group team to emerge directed towards honest appraisal, self-awareness and personal effectiveness, which in turn is patient orientated. It is in the supervising nurse's interest to schedule these meetings within the work programme, to facilitate them in a non-authoritarian, confidential and trusting environment. The group may be facilitated by an outside agent (professional group facilitator, psychologist, counsellor) initially if this is thought to be beneficial, or depending upon the method of group interaction desired (drama therapy, group discussion, T-group, group counselling). Whichever method is used and whether an outside agent or a group member facilitates the group, they should seek to be ongoing, non-threatening and relaxed to be most successful. Any group meeting for debriefings would be advised to meet frequently initially, and then vary meetings according to need. It is becoming more frequently accepted that debrief groups are a necessary part of the effective working life of a stressful occupation. Organisations, from multinational companies to small pressurised sales type businesses, recognise the need for debriefing sessions more and more. Social workers, teachers and counsellors are becoming increasingly committed to setting up professional support groups. It seems to us that in this particular area community nurses may learn from their example.

Debrief skills require the nurse to disclose facts concerning her behaviour in certain situations and how she felt about them. It is a two-way process, in that the disclosure must be listened to accurately without judgement or condemnation. The process of relaying this information to another in an atmosphere of support may be sufficient to enable the nurse to work through her anxieties. However, there are times when she may require more than listening and support. The frustration of working and making decisions on her own can sometimes cause a saturation of ideas which may in turn reduce motivation. In such a case, a group of people coming together for debrief is particularly useful, in that experience and ideas can be shared. The listeners in a debrief group must be careful not to give advice, at the same time not letting this deter them from sharing ideas, in order for the discloser to look at her situation from a different perspective. The skills of self-disclosure and information giving 'borrowed' from the counselling model could be useful in helping a group share experiences without being directive.

Before terminating a 'debrief' relationship, whether it is just two people or a group, it is important to allow the discloser to state how she feels 'now', having had an opportunity to share her experience. This may in fact bring out more issues that need to be dealt with, so if time is a constraint current feelings need to be shared at least 15 minutes before the end of a session so that the person concerned is not left emotionally confused. Although not always appropriate, the end should aim towards a positive outcome, which may vary from everyone feeling 'great' to a 'Let's see what develops and bring it back to our next meeting,' emphasising the importance of a continual support system.

Skills of Community Psychiatric Nursing

The previously described counselling skills will be a sound base for practising psychiatric nursing in the community. The formation of rapport from an empathic base cannot in our opinion be faulted as a starting point, but there are some significant differences between hospital and home nursing.

Control of Environment

The patient in his home is no longer as dependent upon the nurse. Often he is more self-directed and independent, and the contrast here to his behaviour in hospital can often be striking. The nurse is not able to control the environment as she may wish. When a patient invites the nurse to sit down, it is into a chair, in a room and at the time of day that the patient decides upon. Practical problems emerging from this may be distractions such as the television remaining on, or friends, spouse or neighbours interrupting. The patient may decide to sit away from the nurse and make meaningful communication more difficult: in short, barriers to good communication may be out of the nurse's hands. If the nurse's relationship is strong enough with the patient, these barriers may be discussed and dealt with relatively easily; if not, then the nurse needs to work very hard indeed to establish a deeper relationship.

The nurse working in the patient's home must be sensitive to and respect the individual patient's cultural norms. For example, some patients may be quite offended by nurses asking to use the toilet. They may be embarrassed, for if the bathroom is upstairs, it may be considered strictly private. Although this example may seem strange to some nurses, breeching this type of cultural conditioning may result in the patient being out the next time the nurse calls. Being able to interpret and understand non-verbal signals in socially sensitive situations such as a patient's home is an invaluable skill. This skilful sensitivity will prevent many damaging behavioural interactions occurring.

Another contrast necessary to appreciate when involved in patients' homes is the closeness or intimacy of involvement that it often precipitates. Homes are currently sacrosanct, with only 'special' people generally invited inside, unless on errands of business. The CPN is in the position of having one foot in both of these particular camps. The skill in this situation is using the special nature of being invited into homes to its maximum advantage, and simultaneously maintaining a professional purpose. In other words, the CPN will be the friendly professional, not a professional friend. Counselling skills concentrate very keenly on the patient finding his own solution to problems with the nurse taking a catalytic role, and in the patient's home situation (such as those seen in the case studies) problems may be so acute that the nurse may feel advice, persuasion and solutions are quite legitimately her prerogative and necessity. Although we appreciate the pressure upon the nurse to resort to this approach, we strongly urge caution, for quickly offered instant 'solutions' are often grasped by the patient, but seldom result in positive outcomes and are therefore not realistic solutions for the patient.

An example of this type of situation would be the following illustration of Joan's case:

Joan. I think what it really amounts to is I don't love my husband any more. In fact, I don't really like him. Do you think I should leave him, would you write to the council for me, and help me get a solicitor?

Joan requires much more here than an instant answer. Is she asking the nurse for reassurance for a course of action she has decided upon, or is not sure about, or is she hoping the nurse will say, 'No, you shouldn't'?

The skilled nurse will know her patient sufficiently well to be able to share her doubts about the question:

'I'm not really sure why you're asking me, have you decided already, are you unsure, or do you want me to say no?'

Or she may offer a simple challenge:

'I'm not really sure that it matters what I do or think, I'm wondering if you've really thought it through yet yourself?'

The nurse may decide that offering new perspectives on the issues may be useful:

'I think you know that whatever you finally decide, I will support you as much as I can, but there are perhaps other factors to consider. There is your daughter, financial issues and your job. Perhaps you haven't thought this through yet?'

Or she may want to contrast leaving with staying:

'Well, Joan, what are the things that make you want to leave, and the things that make you want to stay? Let's see if you can list them, then we can go on to what things that will help either course of action be better.'

This is leading to a 'forcefield analysis' approach (see p. 63) and may be followed up with open suggestions of resources which may be helpful: marriage guidance, social services, single parent family associations.

It should be stressed that these options are not given as advice, but simply as information and resource knowledge for Joan to choose freely.

It may be felt by the nurse that Joan's problems involve the whole family so fundamentally that she needs to see Joan regularly with both her husband and daughter. To observe how they interact, how communications become unclear, and how emotions are repressed within the family group may open up other options for solving their difficulties. The skills required here are basically family therapy skills, which are closely related to those used in counselling. Other approaches that may be considered may include behavioural based therapy, or a transactional analysis approach (see Suggested Further Reading for further information on these approaches).

Elsie's case requires the CPN to be familiar with the principles and skills of behaviour therapy. Certainly the nurse needs to establish a rapport, but it is important that her non-verbal communication and her desire to be helpful do not reinforce her helplessness. Helping Elsie deal with her anxiety may involve teaching her to be able to relax (see Chapter 3) and perhaps helping her reward herself positively for her decision making behaviour. Being able to say 'no' to excessive demands made upon her and subsequently not feeling guilty for refusing requests may be a significant advance for her. Taking a behavioural approach while simultaneously helping her see herself more clearly by using counselling skills may be the most appropriate nursing interventions.

Helping Thomas may represent the most intensive and continuous therapy. Thomas seems to be testing each therapist until eventually his prediction of them failing with him comes true. Somehow the skilful nurse has to be able to get through to him that it is his responsibility to become well, and that this should be important to all parties. Not playing games with him, and expressing to him the anxieties and practical problems with his case may be ways of challenging him helpfully. To raise Thomas' self-awareness of his previous dependence on his therapists, and his subsequent feelings of disappointment and rejection may make the nurse/patient relationship more honest and open. The nurse needs to be able to evaluate realistically how he can be helped, what he expects of her, and what goals he hopes to achieve. The main skill demonstrated with Thomas will be the skill of immediacy (see p. 59) operated from the core conditions of warmth, genuineness and empathy (see p. 26). The relationship formed between Thomas and the nurse is to be the most therapeutic tool in his care. To experience a relationship where he is free to explore his feelings and be exposed to honest feedback of his presentation of himself may be powerful medicine. In a climate of trust he may be able to take risks in exposing his feelings in the knowledge that he will receive accurate feedback in a non-threatening and non-punishing way. He may find this difficult at first or in fact give up. As long as this is reinforced as his decision to give up, that it is his responsibility for his own future that he has decided, then even this may be a positive step forward. Should he maintain the relationship with his nurse it will require the nurse to use her judgement of his stability, for at some time in the future she will need to encourage Thomas to transfer his learning to the real situation outside therapy. At this stage in Thomas' development, he may require tremendous support and reinforcement, but care must be taken not to encourage him to be dependent, or to be so sympathetic as to reinforce any failures he may encounter.

In Thomas' case, the nurse does not set out to be the paragon, to be all understanding or the perfect role model: indeed, this may spoil the effect. The nurse represents honest feedback for a learning purpose and one aspect Thomas needs to learn is that human behaviour is human, fallible and, on occasions, disappointing. Taking risks in relationships can have negative results, but generally the pay-offs outweight the disappointments. If the nurse can teach Thomas this, and allow him to look at his own behaviour and previous experience openly and honestly in relation to this, then some advances in his well-being may be anticipated.

Key Concepts

(1) She must be able to deal professionally with the administration and monitoring of medicines, have the skills, knowledge and resources of a social worker and the practical managerial application of a charge nurse.
(2) The nurse requires a considerable repertoire of skills, an eclectic approach — an approach unique almost for each unique situation. This is especially important as the CPN may find herself having to intervene in highly emotive issues that would not normally be the province of the nurse.
(3) The autonomous nature of the job dictates that the nurse is self-directed and self-aware, and it is for this reason that the CPN must have confidence in her own abilities and sufficient experience in successful therapy.
(4) A skill absolutely essential for the community nurse to learn is how to debrief. This skill is particularly stressed because the actual interpersonal exchanges between nurse and patients will be isolated from other observers and this may result in there being little support or objective feedback for difficult cases.
(5) The community nurse's job is based on a clarity of action, a sensitivity to needs and a discriminating ability to judge situations correctly.

Summary

The community psychiatric nurse may have many different roles to play, but primarily her role will be to maintain an empathic rapport in order for the patient's needs to be satisfactorily fulfilled. The nurse must be aware that the patient may be more self-directed and be in the process of restoring some independence, and it is vital that this is not taken away by well meaning advice, which reinforces dependency.

If the nurse operates from a position of understanding, she will be sensitive to the cultural uniqueness of the patient, be able to read his non-verbal cues accurately, and respect him as a person. It is important to remember that the balance between being a friend and a professional is a tenuous one, and it has been suggested that the nurse should seek to be a friendly professional, not a professional friend. Once the appropriate climate of helping has been established, by which we mean the correct balance between the nurse's support, the patient's independence and the demands of society as represented in the community by friends, neighbours and significant others, the nurse can be more effective. It is the nurse's role at this point to use her skills to enable the patient to make appropriate choices and wise decisions. We suggest that simple challenges, offering new perspectives, and using techniques such as forcefield analysis and immediacy skills (see Chapter 2) are probably the most useful in these situations. To help the patient successfully, the nurse should have a sound knowledge of resources available in the community, accurate information that may be helpful, and understand the principles of the more common therapies such as transactional analysis, family therapy and counselling.

Finally, in order for her to continue as an effective helper, the community nurse needs to seek strategies that will maintain her sensitivity, yet not rob her of confidence, and seek objective appraisal of her ability and skills, yet do so in a supportive climate. For this reason we strongly recommend support groups and debrief sessions.

Conclusion

Community psychiatric nursing is perhaps one of the most rapidly growing areas of the psychiatric service. It is our hope that this short chapter may be useful to readers interested in this new area. Our aim was not to create an exhaustive piece of work to be used as a reference text, but simply to outline the interactive skills and implications for nurses operating outside the confines of the traditional psychiatric hospital. It is true, of course, that not all CPNs will operate as autonomously as we suggest. Some will be heavily involved in mental health education, running groups, and as part of the primary health care team. An important part of any professional's work is in relating to and complementing other allied workers in the field, whether they belong to voluntary agencies or statutory bodies. The omission of these from the chapter has not occurred because we consider these areas less important, but simply because this volume cannot hope to cover them in any depth. In consequences what is presented here is intended as an introduction to a growing body of knowledge and skills and a foundation for development.

Suggested Further Reading

Butterworth, Charles Anthony and Skidmore, David *Caring for the Mentally Ill in the Community* (Croom Helm, London, 1981)

Carr, P., Butterworth, C. and Hodges, B. *Community Psychiatric Nursing: Caring for the Mentally Ill and Handicapped in the Community* (Churchill Livingstone, London, 1980)

Jansen, Elly (ed.) *The Therapeutic Community outside the Hospital* (Croom Helm, London, 1980)

Reed, John and Lomas, Gillian (eds.) *Psychiatric Services in the Community (Developments and Innovations)* (Croom Helm, London, 1984)

Sladden, Susan *Psychiatric Nursing in the Community: A Study of a Working Situation* (Churchill Livingstone, London, 1979)

21 HUMAN SEXUALITY

A nurse must be sensitive to all the needs of an individual, including sexuality. In order to care for this aspect comfortably and skilfully, the nurse must first of all attempt to explore her own sexuality.

To facilitate this exploration we intend to give a brief outline of the following:

(a) Psychological aspects of sexuality.
(b) Sociocultural aspects of sexuality.
(c) The physiology of sexual encounter.
(d) Potential problem areas throughout the life cycle.
(e) Sexual problems associated with:
  the mentally handicapped;
  the physically handicapped;
  the mentally ill.
(f) Gender identity and sexual expression.

Introduction

Before reading further, explore your personal feelings towards the following statements by indicating whether you:

	Strongly Agree	Agree	Not sure	Disagree
Homosexuals should be allowed to teach in primary schools.				
Sexual intercourse between the mentally ill should be prohibited.				
Masturbation should be viewed as a very healthy activity.				
Nurses should be prepared to talk about any aspect of human sexuality, e.g. oral-genital sex, rectal intercourse.				

The above statements reflect some of the attitudes commonly associated with a degree of prejudice. It may be interesting for you to examine these statements again after studying this chapter.

Sexuality involves the whole person, whereas the word 'sex' connotes a physiological act. Human sexuality includes the biological, sociocultural, psychological and ethical components of sexual behaviour. A common factor to all definitions of human sexuality is the recognition that it is an intrinsic part of our being. J. Fonseca (1970) coined the phrase 'the quality of being human. All that we are as men and women.' It influences our thoughts, actions and interactions and is involved in all aspects of physical and mental health. A major part of human sexuality is in fact sexual expression. The freedom for sexual expression is partly reflected in the World Health Organization's (1974, p. 16) statements concerning the elements of sexual health. These are:

(1) A capacity to enjoy and control sexual and reproductive behaviour in accordance with a social and personal ethic.
(2) Freedom from fear, shame, guilt, false beliefs and other psychological factors inhibiting sexual response and impairing sexual relationships.
(3) Freedom from organic disorders, disease and deficiencies that interfere with sexual and reproductive factors.

In recognising the elements of sexual health, the nurse must, if appropriate, attempt to facilitate this aspect of health in the individuals she cares for. In order to do this effectively, the nurse must be able to listen skilfully and communicate in an accepting non-judgemental manner.

The ability of the nurse to communicate and relate to the patient will depend upon the degree of her own self-awareness and acceptance of the patient as a 'person'. The following is an account of a dialogue overheard in a male admission ward:

Patient. Just because you think homosexuality is abnormal doesn't mean to say I am.

Nurse. Listen, I don't blame you for being 'gay', it's just that it gives me the 'shivers' to think that ....

Here the patient is talking quite freely about his own sexuality, the nurse hints that it is abnormal – hence the patient's reply. The nurse immediately becomes defensive but, in doing so, insinuates that there is something to be blamed for, then conveys her own negative feelings towards homosexuality. This type of communication is not conducive to progressing towards an effective therapeutic relationship. So it seems reasonable to expect the nurse to initiate some effort towards increasing her own knowledge base relevant to this highly emotive area. In doing so she may enhance her own sexual awareness.

Psychological Aspects of Sexuality

Many theories attempt to explain the evolution of sexuality in a developmental context. One factor common to them all is the fact that sexual and psychological processes are intimately related and that it is difficult to understand one apart from the other.

The following is a brief résumé of some of these theories. We are suggesting to you that this is not by any means comprehensive and is only aimed at giving relevant directions. Further study should take place for a fuller understanding.

Sigmund Freud related much of his theory to unconscious processes in patients who suffered conflicts, many of which he believed stemmed from various stages of sexual development. He described a *sex instinct*, a strong basic physiological need. This need is expressed by the *libido* (Latin for lust) which is the psychological and erotic longing of the sexual instinct. Freud (1930) describes the process of sexual development from the newborn through to the adult. He states that a sexual energy exists and is expressed through certain body pleasure zones, which he terms the psychosexual stages, or oral, anal, phallic and genital.

Oral Stage

This is a major source of infantile gratification and pleasure. It contrives and varies in its importance at any stage of life, e.g. thumbsucking, smoking, eating and drinking, and the use of the oral area as a pleasure giving and receiving agent during the act of sex.

Anal Stage

Aspects of gratification include: pleasure obtained from defaecation; increased muscle control leading to increased independence; control over parental emotions. The anus is an erogenous zone.

Phallic Stage

The child's increased awareness of his or her own genitals, and the pleasure associated with their manipulation.

Latent Stage

From about four years of age the child's sexual impulses become secondary to intellectual and social growth.

Genital Stage

From the onset of puberty, the erogenous areas are focused onto the genital region. The sexual impulse now becomes directed outwardly rather than inwardly as in the previous stage.

Freud explained that many problems in adult life were a direct result of excessive or insufficient gratification during psychosexual development. Some examples include:

Problems related to excessive or chronic abuse of food or drink:	Oral stage
Passive homosexuality:	Anal stage
Sexual inhibition, exhibitionism:	Phallic stage

In contrast to the psychoanalytical theory, the behaviourists claim that sexual action is not the result of some intricate psychological process, but is rather a measurable psychological response to a stimulus. Much of adult sexuality has been developed by continual learning or conditioning throughout childhood.

Human sexuality, according to Maslow (1970), is one of the basic human psychological needs in the sense of survival of the species. It is also, however, intrinsic to the other higher order needs. Sexual pleasure in the self-actualised individual is not just a passing pleasure but a kind of basic strengthening.

The relevance of these theories is appreciated by taking whatever is appropriate in order to enhance your understanding of any particular individual. By forming an eclectic viewpoint, relevant issues arising from psychological theory can be utilised. It will guide you towards understanding the complex concepts of 'self', 'self-esteem' and 'self-image', all of which are fundamental issues for the humanistic psychologist but also for the psychiatric nurse, if she is to apply her skills effectively from a sexual person to another sexual person.

The Sociocultural Aspects of Sexuality

The Kinsey reports (1948, 1953) were the first major significant social comments on sexuality. As Houston, Bee and Rimm (1980) put it, 'suddenly "everyone" was normal – you could almost hear the sigh of relief!' Following the results of over 18,000 interviews, Alfred Kinsey made statistical comments concerning the sexual activities of Americans, subdivided into social class, black, white, age, male, female, and many other categories. They made a significant impact then and even now they are generally accepted as an indication of human sexual behaviour today. Even to summarise its major conclusions is beyond the remit for this book, but further reading is highly recommended.

Studying sexuality of other cultures besides our own may help in accepting an individual's right to hold certain values, those values being the 'norm' depending on the religious and cultural background. Hogan (1980) states several examples to illustrate this:

- the Kerabi bachelors of New Guinea practise homosexual anal intercourse as a part of puberty rites;
- the Toda of India permit women to have several lovers and husbands;
- Hopi Indians keep boys and girls aged 10 to 20 apart.
- Polynesians see love as the 'life force'. There are no words in their language for sexually obscene, indecent or impure, nor are there words for illegitimate, adultery, bigamy or divorce.

And so the list goes on, providing interesting insights into the way others live. Contrasting these behaviours with those of modern society leads us into the area of describing the changing pattern of sex stereotypes and sex roles. From the women's civil rights campaign to the women's liberation movement, people have been fighting against sex stereotypes and roles for years. Nevertheless society still chooses to 'mould' boys and girls into certain ways of behaviour. It is, however, more acceptable today in certain subcultures to 'cross over' to a degree – certain pop stars illustrate this well – but this attitude is hardly comparable to the attitude of society generally. Changes in divorce rates, education, occupations, particularly in relation to the role of women, are all well documented. An appreciation of these changes and the possible direction our society will take may be useful for you as a 'male' or 'female' nurse to examine the present position in relation to your own attitudes to the male and female role and the expectations of others around you, including family, friends, colleagues and patients.

One final comment is required in order to complete this outline of relevant sociocultural factors of sexuality, and that concerns religion. The effect of religion on sexuality is hardly going to be an obvious one when, to many, religion and sex are probably two of the most private areas of their lives. However, an appreciation of how religious belief can affect sexuality can be found by reading the general comments Kinsey (1948) makes on human sexual behaviour and the religious. He comments that certain individual religions of the West, mainly Catholicism, Judaism and Protestantism, generally condemn such things as masturbation, abortion and homosexuality. The exploration of these facts linked with the principles of morality should generate beneficial discussion.

The Physiology of Sexual Encounter

It is important for the nurse to recognise the physiological processes involved in sexual encounters in order to understand the problems of sexual functions, be they physical or psychological. Much of the information concerning human sexual response has been due to the work of Masters and Johnson (1966). They used basic medical research methods to study sexual response in the laboratory. The sexual response cycle (see Figure 21.1) is the same for men and women in that both follow the same sequence of events, although they may vary in length of time and intensity. The excitement phase, plateau phase, orgasmic and resolution phases are not separate, but overlap each other.

Excitement Phase

Female. Vaginal lubrication, within 10 to 30 seconds of sexual stimulation, is the first sign of effective excitement. This lubrication is a sweating reaction. Many other changes occur, including an

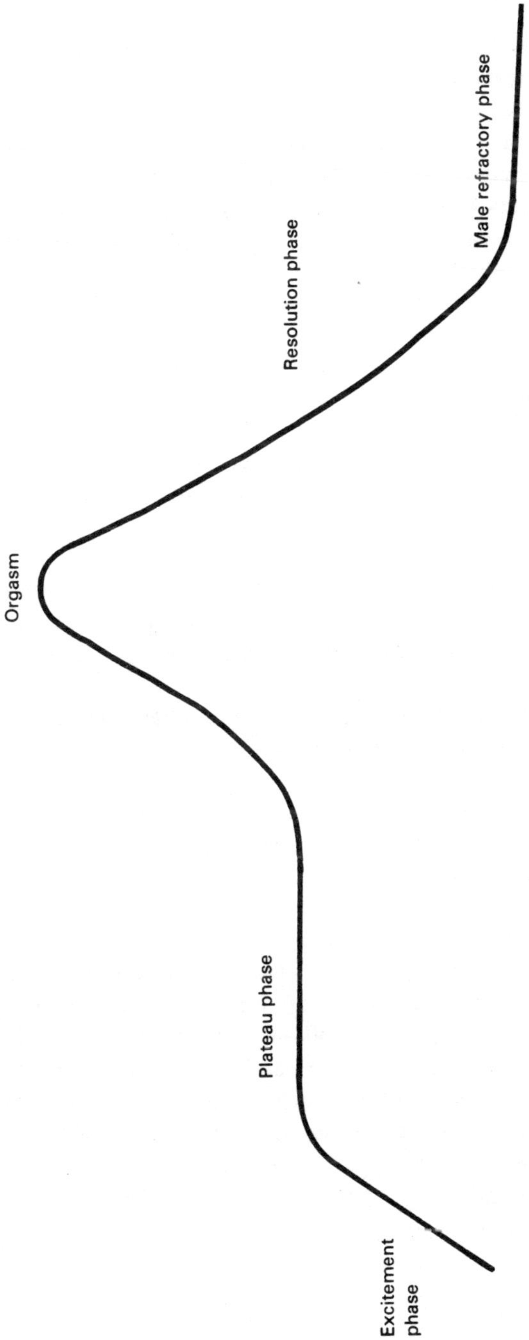

Figure 21.1: Sexual Response Cycle

increase in the size of the labia and clitoris; muscle tension increases and localised vasocongestion also occurs.

Male. First physiological response is penile erection due to the spongy tissue being engorged with blood. Other changes affect the scrotum and testes and muscle tension increases generally.

Plateau Phase

Female. The outer third of the vagina becomes engorged with venous blood, decreasing the opening by a third, which is called the *orgasmic platform.* There are colour changes in the labia and the clitoris retracts.

Male. Slight increase in the diameter of the coronal ridge. Spermatic cords shorten, pulling the testes higher.

Orgasmic Phase

Female. Muscles tense, rhythmic contractions begin in the orgasmic platform. Uterine contractions may occur. Muscular contractions round the pelvic floor force the blood out of the engorged blood vessels.

More recently than Masters and Johnson, it has been found that orgasms vary in women depending upon the type of stimulation. Many orgasms are as a result of clitoral stimulation, but it has also been found that stimulation of the 'G', or Grafenburg, spot inside the vagina can produce a different response, often one of greater intensity (Richards, 1982).

Male. The testes, prostate gland and seminal vesicles are involved as they collect sperm and seminal fluid and expel it into the prostatic urethra. It is at this stage that the subjective feeling of orgasm occurs. Ejaculation usually follows almost immediately, caused by contraction of the urethra and muscles of the penis. It is commonly thought that multiple orgasms in men are not possible. However, by learning to control the muscles responsible for ejaculation, it is possible to achieve the first stage of orgasm without ejaculation, thus allowing further stimulation before resigning to the refractory phase (Dale, 1982).

Resolution Phase

Female. The clitoris returns to its normal position 5 to 10 seconds after orgasm or indeed orgasms. The labia return to normal size, as do the inner vagina and uterus. Some women experience an urge to micturate shortly after orgasm. This is thought to be due to a female ejaculatory response arising out of the release of ejaculatory fluid from the walls of the uterus (Richards, 1982). There is a general relaxation of all muscles and slowing down of vital signs.

Male. After ejaculation, half of the erection is lost immediately, followed shortly by the rest. The scrotum and testes return to their unstimulated state. A refractory period follows the male resolution phase, whereby erection is not possible. The older a man becomes, the longer this refractory period is.

Having reviewed the normal sexual response cycle, it may now be useful to look at how problems can occur which affect these. The following is a list of the most common sexual dysfunctions and we recommend that the nurse uses the references to research these in order to gain a fuller understanding of the sexual response cycle and its common dysfunctions:

- frigidity or female orgasmic dysfunction;
- vaginismus;
- dyspareunia;
- impotence or the inability to achieve effective erection;
- premature ejaculation;
- ejaculatory incompetence.

Potential Problems throughout the Life Cycle

Before embarking upon the sexual problems of the handicapped and mentally ill, consider the problems of the so called 'normal' population from childhood to old age.

Potential problem areas affecting the child:
- psychosexual developmental problems;
- masturbation;
- sexual assault;
- sexual precocity;
- guilt about sexuality;
- parental nudity and sexual activities;

— incest;
— pornography.

Potential problem areas for the adolescent:
— onset of puberty;
— body image;
— identity crises;
— peer influence;
— masturbation;
— homosexuality;
— pregnancy.

Potential problem areas for the adult:
— marital and extramarital relationships;
— sexual dysfunctions;
— sex technique;
— ignorance;
— anxiety failure;
— menopause;
— male climacteric;
— the growing family;
— changing role of partners.

Potential problem areas for the elderly:
— change in sexual response;
— slower erection, poor vaginal lubrication;
— physical ailments and constraints;
— society and self-ignorance of the sexual activities and needs of the elderly.

Sexuality and the Mentally Handicapped

A major philosophy of care of the mentally handicapped is to provide a normal environment and activities of daily living outside the institutional setting. These people have the same need for love and the same degree of differences in sexual interests that characterise the 'normal' population. Sexuality and sexual expression of the retarded is generally controlled and restricted by society, which is probably operating on myths and misconceptions about retarded persons' behaviour. Their problems may involve inappropriate masturbation, pregnancy or sexual acting out, but many can be taught to develop an appreciation of sensuality, to make responsible choices and to handle feelings in a socially acceptable manner. Discussion aimed at exploring your feelings and attitudes to the mentally handicapped may be useful, especially in the areas of marriage, pregnancy and contraception.

Sexuality and the Physically Handicapped

A nurse should be aware that the loss of physical function does not mean loss of sexuality. Many paralysed individuals live in a world of frustration, anxiety and isolation, much of which is due to the ignorance of the paralysed person or his/her partner, or their inability to adapt their life-style. There are varying degrees of paralysis and loss of sensation. Although sexual intercourse is usually difficult, there are many alternative ways of expressing your sexuality to such an extent that the physical frustration no longer becomes a sexual frustration. It may be the nurse's role to counsel an individual or couple who find themselves in this predicament, a situation where not only the nurse's skills are put to the test, but also her degree of sexual self-awareness. She must listen accurately without her own feelings of discomfort preventing her from doing so, and must not show embarrassment to the couple, as it is probably difficult enough for them to communicate their problems without having to consider the nurse's feelings as well.

Sexuality and the Mentally Ill

The relationship between sexuality and mental illness, be it as a contributing factor or an aspect of living that is affected, is generally accepted. With this in mind it may seem surprising that in the past the sexuality of a patient, particularly a patient in hospital, was hardly acknowledged by the staff responsible for his care. Patients were often left in ignorance because the nurse was either not aware of the sexual needs of patients, or ignorant to such an extent that she was not sure what they are, or too embarrassed to deal with any sexual issues if she was confronted with them. There are several major areas that the nurse must be familiar with in order to cope effectively with the sexuality of psychiatric patients. These are:

— the effect of mental illness on an individual's sexuality;
— the effect of the institution on an individual's sexuality;
— the effect of psychiatric treatment on an individual's sexuality;
— the effect of the nurse on an individual's sexuality.

The Effect of Mental Illness

Mental illness affects individuals in so many different ways that it is difficult to generalise on the effect of mental illness on sexual functioning. However, there are some generally recognised patterns peculiar to certain symptoms. Schizophrenia is a manifestation of a set of symptoms that affects the total personality. Its effect on one individual is different from that on the next. Sexual functioning varies from early onset of the symptoms, showing lack of interest in sex, to hypersexuality or bizarre and unreasonable sexual behaviour when certain symptoms such as delusional and hallucinatory experiences influence the thought pattern of the individual. This type of behaviour can have a drastic effect on any previously stable sexual relationship and often the nurse may need to reassure the partner about the nature of the patient's sexual activity, particularly if it is overt and inappropriate.

Patients who experience severe mood changes from depression to mania will also experience a reciprocal change in sexual drive, i.e. increased sexual drive with mood elevation and vice versa. In severe depressive states sexual drive, interest and expression are totally lacking. However, the reverse is true in mania, for, as the mood elevates, the individual's sexuality and the sexuality of others become increasing stimuli for focusing attention upon. As the mood elevates to the state of mania, much of this attention may be based on poor judgement and result in inappropriate behaviour, and the nurse needs to be aware of this in order to protect the patient.

Kaplan (1981) states that any severe emotional state affects sexuality adversely. The connection between stress and decreased sexual interest is not clearly known. There are several mechanisms postulated, varying from a pure redirection of psychological and endocrine changes to the effects on the autonomic and central nervous systems. Whatever the cause, the effect still remains, and it depends upon how much the patient values sexuality as part of his 'being' that will determine the intensity of concern. For if this concern is great, exploring this area may reduce a contributory factor for the causation of anxiety in the first place, or, at the very least, the patient may be reassured that this effect is only a temporary symptom of his general state.

The Effect of the Institution

The institution can take responsibility for individual care too far, to the extent of depersonalising and regularising a patient's behaviour so that he has little choice, and when he does have a choice he finds it difficult to make a decision. This pattern can also relate to staff attitudes towards sexual behaviour within the hospital setting. Patient's sexuality can often be ignored in a single sex ward, mixing with female patients may be discouraged, masturbation is usually discouraged and no facilities except the toilet areas are given for personal sexual expression. Dormitories are often impersonal, sexual intercourse between patients is prohibited, and often treated with anger and disgust.

Are these the attitudes of caring individuals? We believe that certain questions must be asked to explore ward and hospital attitudes to the sexual needs of the patient:

- Should sexual activity be allowed on the ward?
- Should facilities be provided for this to occur?
- How practical are 'conjugal visiting' rooms, i.e. a room set aside for a patient to be alone with his partner without fear of disturbance?
- Which patients are to be allowed to express their natural drives?
- How are we to facilitate this?
- Do we provide appropriate sex education for the long-term patients?
- Do we offer sufficient opportunity for contraceptive counselling?
- How willing are we to facilitate the use of contraception?

Akhtar (1977) implies that some sexual activity might be tolerated but identified certain limitations. He states that sexual activity between in-patients should be discouraged if one or both are either:

(1) legally minor;
(2) a non-consenting adult;
(3) mentally handicapped;
(4) delusional or in other ways grossly disorganised in affect and behaviour;
(5) receiving significant amounts of psychotropic medications;
(6) acting out.

Whether these guidelines are sufficient or extreme will depend largely upon the attitudes, facilities and skills of any particular nursing team. We believe that each individual relationship should be assessed on its own and limitations set if potential harm is possible to the individuals concerned or their 'significant others'.

The Effect of Psychiatric Treatment

A major component of many psychiatric treatment regimes is the provision of medication to counteract the symptoms of certain disorders. Many of the drugs involved have side effects relating to sexual functioning, some of which are summarised below.

Phenothiazines, e.g. chlorpromazine, thioridazine. Many of these agents produce impotence or ejaculatory difficulties, including absence of ejaculation and painful ejaculation. Amenorrhoea, galactorrhoea and loss of libido are other commonly expressed side effects.

Tricyclic antidepressants, e.g. Amitriptyline and Tofranil. As the depression resolves, sexual activity usually resumes, but continued use of these antidepressants has been known to cause impotence and ejaculatory difficulties. Delay in orgasm has been experienced by some women.

Hypnotics-sedatives. These are generally known to have a depressing effect on the central nervous system, consequently reducing the effectiveness of sexual activity.

Chlordiazepoxide (Librium). This has been associated with a delay or failure to ejaculate.

The Effect of the Nurse

The nurse as a therapeutic agent will often be a focus of sexual interest from the patient. This may vary from personal advances — asking for a date, telephone number, enquiring about love life — to aggressive acting out behaviour — making seductive comments, physical contact or exposing genitals. How the nurse deals with these situations will depend upon the relationship already established and the skill and confidence of the nurse. It is important to understand that, due to hospitalisation or distorted perceptions, the sexual needs of patients are often frustrated, and consequently they will seek channels to express their needs. If one of these channels happens to be directed towards the nurse, then she must deal with it in a manner that is acceptable to her as a person and to the therapeutic relationship. This may involve the nurse being honest and expressing to the patient that she understands the meaning of his behaviour, but is unable to accept its focus any longer. Clear limit setting in order to protect the professional relationship may be necessary. This could involve the nurse being firm, but without degrading or patronising the patient. For example, a reply from a nurse to a patient who has just fondled her breasts whilst she was making his bed could be 'I can understand your frustration, Mr Richards, but your actions make it difficult for me to care for you professionally, so I must ask you not to do that again.'

This reply clearly communicates to the patient that his behaviour was not conducive to the situation and depending how the nurse replies, on her use of tone of voice, gestures and use of her skills later will depend whether or not a positive relationship based on respect can be developed from this situation.

It is clear that the sexuality of the patient and the sexuality of the nurse cannot be ignored, especially in quite intimate relationships that are often developed. When the sexuality within the professional relationship becomes dominant, it can act as a barrier to effective helping. The people concerned may become so involved with each other that objective care becomes extremely difficult. In order to avoid these situations, the nurse must be clear and honest to the patient concerned when any signs of sexual overtones become barriers to the helping relationship.

Gender Identity and Sexual Expression

It is often taken for granted that to be normal requires a male behaving like a heterosexual male and a female behaving like a heterosexual female. The question then arises: how should a heterosexual behave? When we start exploring gender identity and sexual expression it becomes apparent that there are many variables, all of which are 'normal' to the individual concerned. Society generally has difficulty in openly accepting individuals who stray from the so-called 'norm' of sexual expression, and many are subjected to added pressures as a consequence. But no one is free from the possibility of needing psychiatric nursing skills, so it is necessary to have an awareness of the variations that do occur in order to begin trying to understand the different forms of sexual expression. This awareness is all we shall facilitate — much further study is required to comprehend the complexity of any individual's world.

Heterosexuality

This is sexual attraction for the opposite sex. It is generally the predominant form of sexual expression and is readily accepted by society. However, it is subjected to many pressures, mainly contracted relationships through marriage, which are under pressure to be predominantly monogamous, the responsibility of rearing children, and the trauma of divorce for one in every three marriages.

Homosexuality

Sexual attraction for the same sex. This is probably the most popular form of sexual expression to be subjected to gross generalisations. A homosexual relationship can be as varied as the next in the context of dynamics, roles and sexual activity. It is estimated that the gay population in certain countries could be one in ten, and in certain cities throughout the world much higher. It is also estimated that as many as eight out of ten people experience some form of homosexual attraction at some time in their lives.

Bisexuality

'The best of both worlds', i.e. sexual attraction for the opposite and the same sex. It has been postulated that this in fact is the most common form of sexuality, for as Jung states, 'we are both anima and animus — in us we have both the spirit of man and the spirit of woman. We are not male or female, we are human.' It seems unlikely that the population is made up of pure homosexuals and heterosexuals. It is probable that a gradient exists between the two extremes, bisexuality being the midpoint.

Transvestism

A transvestite is a person who derives pleasure or increased sexual arousal from wearing the clothing of the opposite sex.

Transsexualism

This refers to a person who psychologically identifies with one sex but belongs physically to the other sex. It is likely that this person will experience much pain psychologically and physically before he or she achieves the desired gender identity. With education, counselling, training and surgical intervention, the desired identity can be achieved.

Variations of Sexual Aim

Many of the following involve some disordered psychopathology in the individual concerned.

Gerontophilia: sexual assault of an elderly person.
Necrophilia: sexual contact with a corpse.
Zoophilia (or bestiality): sexual contact with animals.
Fetishism: the act of deriving sexual pleasure from an inanimate object.
Voyeurism: a person who derives sexual pleasure from viewing others' sexuality.
Frotteur: a person who becomes sexually aroused by rubbing up against someone. Often occurs in public and crowded places.
Exhibitionists: derive sexual pleasure from exposing their genitals to surprised victims, often in public places.
Sadism: the act of achieving sexual excitement from inflicting pain on their partner.
Masochism: the act of achieving sexual excitement from experiencing personal or mental pain.

Incest, Rape and Paedophilia

The nurse should study in detail these three areas in particular, as they will frequently come across not only the people responsible for these acts, but also the individuals who have suffered by them. The consequences of all three are very different, but they are equally traumatic to the people concerned. Probably one of the most difficult situations a nurse may have to deal with is to attempt to counsel a 30- or 40-year-old man who has admitted sexually assaulting a six-year-old girl. A nurse must be in touch with her own feelings and must recognise when negative feelings compromise the care that she gives. In this situation, the quality of unconditional positive regard (see p. 25) is certainly tested, and it is important that the nurse is honest to herself and her own limitations.

Conclusion

If we are to care for individuals as unique and total human beings, then we as professional helpers must overcome the tendency to neglect this basic need of sexuality. Throughout this chapter all we have endeavoured to do is give relevant facts and opinions in order for you to *begin exploring your feelings in respect of your own and others' sexual identity.* This is essential if you as a psychiatric nurse wish to employ your skills to individuals at two major levels. The first, and generally applicable, is to be sensitive to the sexual needs of the individual; the second involves listening to people with problems concerning their sexuality. In this latter situation, the patient may require more specialised skills associated with sexual therapy. The psychiatric nurse is in a prime position to know when this is applicable and to use the appropriate referral methods when necessary. There are many different types of sexual therapy available, some of which are listed below:

- rational-emotive approach to sex therapy;
- sexual therapy of Masters and Johnson;
- behavioural techniques;
- the new sex therapy (Helen Kaplan);
- group counselling.

If the nurse is to specialise in dealing with problems associated with sexuality, we recommend that further training and experience in this area are sought, especially before embarking upon using specific therapies. However, we believe that the qualities and skills of the psychiatric nurse provide a most appropriate foundation to develop and use these techniques.

Finally, we as helping professionals must continue to deal with the general ignorance and discomfort that exist around the topic of sexuality. It is only when we become aware of our own sexuality and associated attitudes and values that we can then develop sufficient skills in order to help individuals maintain or regain sexual health.

Key Concepts

(1) Sexuality involves the whole person; it includes the biological, sociocultural, psychological and ethical components of sexual behaviour. It influences our thoughts, feelings and interactions and is involved in all aspects of physical and mental health.
(2) Forming an eclectic appreciation of relevant psychological theory will guide the nurse towards the complexities of 'sexuality and self', 'self-esteem' and 'self-image', all of which are fundamental for the nurse if she is to apply her skills effectively as a sexual person to another sexual person.
(3) An appreciation of the changing roles of men and women in society may help the nurse to examine the present position in relation to attitudes and expectations of the male and female role in relation to nursing, patients, family, friends and colleagues.
(4) It is important for the nurse to recognise the physiological processes involved in sexual encounters, in order to understand the problems of sexual functions, be they physical or psychological.
(5) Sexual activity between psychiatric in-patients should be accepted once the individual relationship has been assessed on its own merit and limitations set if potential harm is likely to occur to the individuals concerned or to their 'significant others'.
(6) Either due to hospitalisation or distorted perceptions, the sexual needs of patients are often frustrated, and consequently they will seek channels to express these needs. How the nurse deals with this will depend largely upon the relationship already established and the skills and confidence of the nurse. It must be handled in a manner that is acceptable to the nurse as a person and to the therapeutic relationship.
(7) A nurse must be in touch with her own feelings and must recognise when negative feelings compromise the care that she gives.

Suggested Further Reading

Belliveau, F. and Richter, L. *Understanding Human Sexual Inadequacy* (Hodder and Stoughton, New York, 1971)

Bentley, N. 'Plugging the Gap', *Nursing Times*, 13 January 1982)

Glover, Jean *Human Sexuality in Nursing Care* (Croom Helm, London, 1985)

Greengross, Wendy *Entitled to Love, the Sexual and Emotional Needs of the Handicapped* (National Marriage Guidance Council, London 1976)

Kaplan, H.Singer *The New Sex Therapy* (Penguin Books, Harmondsworth, 1981)

Ladas, A.K., Whipple, B. and Perry, J.E. *The G Spot and Other Recent Discoveries about Human Sexuality* (Corgi, London, 1983)

Lion, E. *Human Sexuality in Nursing Process* (John Wiley, Chichester, 1982)

Tiefer, Leonore *Human Sexuality, Feelings and Functions* (Harper and Row, London, 1979)

22 CREATIVE SKILLS

Art

Art work is often considered to be a very specialised area, and many psychiatric nurses may well think it completely out of the normal scope of their skills. Although we would not wish to over simplify, or in any way demean the skill and expertise of the trained and practising art therapist, we do believe that this is an area where nurses may profit from the pioneering work of other professionals. It is our belief that this approach would be more widely available to enhance the treatment of mentally ill people if some simple aspects of art therapy were more universally adopted by skilled and thoughtful nurses.

At the risk of repeating ourselves, we would say that the psychiatric nurse is uniquely placed to offer this type of activity. There is a wide range of needy people who would undoubtedly benefit from these techniques. If simple rules are followed, it is a safe but different communication method between the patient and his emotions, and by a side effect — the nurse.

We recommend, however, that before any such therapy is attempted, the nurse is quite sure exactly what she is doing. Consequently we offer the following brief guidelines:

(1) Wherever possible, allow any art work to be introduced to the patient in a non-threatening environment. A suggestion for this would be simply to present paper and paints, or whatever art materials are being used, in a spare moment and simply ask, 'Would anyone care to do some painting/modelling/drawing?' To suggest that this is 'therapy' or is in some way a treatment, or is structured, may well affect the volunteer rate, and raise unnecessary anxieties in some patients.

(2) There should be no compulsion or unnecessary 'encouragement', especially in initial introduction. Most sessions will build volunteers gradually when the more timid patients begin to realise that the sessions are 'fun'.

(3) Remember you are not an art therapist and as such any interpretation of the *content* of the session should not be made. It is

sufficient for the participants to enjoy the work, and when they feel comfortable, you may be able to facilitate some discussion, and consequently sharing of meaning, feelings and themes may then be appropriate.

(4) During sessions, patients may become anxious about what they should be doing, especially if they feel they are competing. Be there to support them and answer their questions.

(5) A few useful hints about running an art group:
   (a) Explain first quite clearly what you require of them, and if there are no specific goals, be clear about this by saying, 'Have some fun and splash some paint about.'
   (b) It may be better to offer coloured paper, as white paper may intimidate the patient and discourage him from starting.
   (c) Explain that it is not necessary to fill the whole paper.
   (d) Explain that no one will be expected to talk about their work if they do not want to, and what they do with their painting/model/drawing afterwards will be up to them.
   (e) Participate yourself if possible, as by modelling and demonstrating you may be able to break the ice in later discussions naturally, so that no anxieties are raised.
   (f) If you do participate, and are very able, it may be a good idea not to produce an exquisite piece of work that may discourage the less artistic in the group.
   (g) Explain that it is not a competition and you do not have to be an artist to participate.

The latter holds true not only for patients, but equally for the nurse/therapist. The benefits of art groups are manyfold, but few are to do with the content of the art itself.

No doubt by now you are intrigued to know what this is all about? We have suggested that the nurse/therapist should not interpret or analyse the work, so what is the purpose of the group? For many psychiatric patients the main benefits are as follows:

(1) The art group is an activity that is fun. At worst it will help alleviate boredom, at best it will be an absorbing and stimulating part of his life that he will anticipate with great pleasure.

(2) 'Through spontaneous painting, the patient expresses himself, frees himself from repressed wishes and drives, fulfils desires,

and creates a bridge between himself and the outside world' (Assael, 1978).

(3) Art therapy is a powerful form of non-verbal communication, and facilitates an increase in the empathic relationship between the nurse/therapist and patient.
(4) Emotions previously unseen or unrecognised may be expressed through art work, and more easily discussed.
(5) Subsequently self-awareness and insights are often raised for both patients and nurse/therapist, especially in areas of their own relationships.
(6) If nurse/therapists are observant, they will use their observational skills during art groups to discover many facts about their patients, and their interactions with their peers.
(7) Lastly there is, in our opinion, a very definite therapeutic value in art work, being, by its very nature, creative and expressive. It may facilitate lost skills of movement, concentration and purpose. Certainly through a planned and co-ordinated programme it can create group cohesion, and enhance social skills for all its participants.

Over the last few years, art therapy has been used extensively in all fields of psychiatry. Nurse/therapists usually quick to catch on to a new theme or idea seem to have been rather slow to encompass this strategy into their skills repertoire. We offer this short review of the areas where it has proved useful in an attempt to illustrate what may be achieved.

Donnenberg (1978) used art therapy in a drug community with young adolescent offenders and concludes that its use enhanced group cohesion, helped identify the stages of development during treatment, and increased mutuality and expression within the group. Halbreich (1978) used painting as a complete dialogue between therapist and schizophrenic patients by simply painting something in one colour and encouraging the patient to add — or respond to it by painting on the same paper in another colour. The interchange in this situation was therefore entirely non-verbal and it is suggested that this technique enhances the nurse's empathy with the patient. It certainly can be seen that this technique may well be extremely useful for the more mute and inaccessible patients, who may refuse to speak, but may enjoy the distraction of art.

In a very specialised area, Carozza and Hiersteiner (1982) used art therapy for their work with incest victims. This requires very high expertise and it is not suggested that the psychiatric nurse should try to use this unsupervised, but, nevertheless, it exemplifies tremendous possibilities and potential. In one particular case, very highly emotive, frightening and embarrassing feelings were expressed through an art group, when verbal descriptions were out of the question.

Clearly much potential good can be done by encouraging the expression of non-verbal behaviour through art. We advocate that psychiatric nurses research the area before contemplating any elaborate therapeutic programmes, but by following the initial guidelines, we are confident that many nurses will be able to add another most powerful tool to aid their armoury of qualities and skills.

Suggested Further Reading

Dalley, Tessa (ed.) *Art as Therapy* (Tavistock, London, 1984)
Feder, E. and Feder, B. *The Expressive Art Therapies* (Prentice-Hall, Englewood Cliffs, New Jersey, 1981)
Mitchell, A.R.K. 'Art and Dramatherapy as Part of a Multidisciplinary Team', Conference Paper, College of Art and Design, St Albans, 1982
Pavey, D. *Art Based Games* (Methuen, London, 1979)

Dramatherapy

Background

Much of the present dramatherapy or psychodrama in current use is derived from early work undertaken by Dr Moreno, a Viennese psychiatrist in the early part of this century. Most of the techniques used today are attributed to his early work, which he undertook when it was by no means as fashionable as it is today. His pioneering work must be acknowledged, for many of the refreshing and 'new' approaches we meet in psychiatry in this field are rooted in his earlier work, including many aspects of group psychotherapy. Some of the work of Carl Rogers, especially the concept of dealing with the 'here and now', was originally provided by J.L. Moreno (1946).

Much has been written about dramatherapy and there are some fine books in print dealing with the subject. We cannot, and do not hope to, compete with this literature; our purpose in including a short section on dramatherapy is simply to put it into the context of psychiatric nursing skills. No book on such a subject would be complete without at least introducing its readers to the very relevant area of dramatherapy.

Theory

Dramatherapy is, in our opinion, an important resource which may be used as an independent therapy with suitable patients or as a complementary therapy for many other patients when appropriate. Psychotherapy and psychoanalysis seek to explore the patient's thoughts and feelings by intensive listening and skilled responding to the patient's communication, the latter taking a more theoretical and interpretive account of the patient. Psychodrama or dramatherapy seeks to study and provide insights to and for the patient through *actions* and words. Often words and simple non-verbal behaviour do not give sufficient insight into the real problems, needs and issues surrounding the patient. Dramatherapy seeks to fill the gap in the information, and in certain situations solves some problems in the process.

The Uses of Dramatherapy and its Application to Psychiatry

Dramatherapy uses many techniques designed to construct or reconstruct situations and the associated feelings, and act them out in a safe and structured environment. The simplest form is perhaps the role play reconstruction in social skills training. Here a patient who is anxious or unable to enter certain social situations can artifically reproduce the scene and be mentally and physically escorted through the process. The individual can explain the thoughts and emotions he feels step by step and rehearse more effective ways of dealing with the negative aspects of the situation as they occur. It could be realistically argued that assertion training, desensitisation, skills training and most experiential educational methods are all based on dramatherapy. The essential difference in many of these examples is purely the accent of 'client centredness'. In behavioural techniques, the therapist has in her mind a desired outcome, and uses positive reinforcement and the shaping process to mould the patient towards these goals. The dramatherapist is generally more interested in the process of insight rather than the direction it takes the patient.

Its application to psychiatry arc perhaps obvious, but it may be stressed at this point that it is not suitable for all psychiatric patients. Any process as powerful in releasing repressed or suppressed emotions must carry with it certain dangers or potential problems. There are unfortunately some patients whose conditions are characterised, quite fortuitously perhaps, by a lack of insight. Any method of therapy which seeks to break down that lack of insight may well be damaging to that individual's well-being.

Patients categorised as 'psychotic', especially those suffering from schizophrenia, should only be involved in dramatherapy, or for that matter group therapy, after very careful consideration of possible consequences of such action by the team responsible for their care (see Langley and Langley, 1983, esp. p. 59). Similarly, some patients may be temporarily unable to tolerate a close introspection of themselves, and should not be considered for a dramatherapy group. It should be realised that even despite careful section of patients for dramatherapy, an undesired reaction may occasionally occur within a group session. It is for this reason that only trained dramatherapists or nurses who have undergone a thorough instructional course under the supervision of a dramatherapist should undertake such a group, especially if it is intended to conduct therapy as an independent method. There are, however, simple techniques used in dramatherapy that may be of great benefit to the nurse in her armoury of eclectic techniques, and for this purpose we describe some of these below.

Role Play

This is perhaps the simplest technique, although it is extremely powerful. Usually the patient will act out using any props he may need by improvising or imagining, and playing out a scene. The nurse's role is usually to play a counter part in the situation, and she is advised by the patient on the type of response he would normally expect. For example, the alcoholic patient who has difficulty refusing an invitation from a friend to go to the pub may ask the nurse to play the friend, while he rehearses saying NO. This simple technique helps the patient relieves the feelings he has to deal with in the situation he fears may bring about his downfall. The nurse may well pick up useful information at the same time about the patient's ability to recognise and deal with his emotions during this role play. Individuals criticise this technique as being artificial and somewhat ridiculous. Indeed we would agree it may well be a little embarrassing at first, but we know of very few people who have tried this method who can still wholeheartedly say that there is no value in it. Despite its artificiality and atmosphere of the unreal, very much of the content of the role play does become real. The emotions expressed within it are mostly very real to the person acting out his situation, and the information extracted from it is generally very useful for personal growth (a useful insight into this may be gained by reading Chapter 9 in *Using the Creative Arts in Therapy*, edited by Bernie Warren). A third person wherever possible should be used to observe the role play, as she can then make notes about the various ideas, feelings and behaviour that she sees as potentially significant. This is then fed back to the patient in a tentative questioning manner in order for him to try to make some sense of it all. For this to be effective, the feedback should be as objective as possible and we suggest notes and verbal feedback take a literal format. For example:

'I noticed when you spoke, Mr X, your voice trembled ...'

'I noticed you clenched your fist when ...'

'I saw you ...'

'You said ... after ... '

'I heard you say ...'

Avoiding statements such as 'You were obviously very puzzled when ...' which indicate an interpretation on the observer's part. It would be necessary, however, to enable the patient to match up in some way his non-verbal and verbal behaviour and actions to his emotions, and for this purpose it is suggested that open questions be asked, such as 'I wonder how you were feeling when ...' or 'Perhaps you could explain to me what you were feeling when ...'

Following the role play and feedback, the nurse may follow either a behavioural or counselling philosophy to bring about the patient change, depending on which approach is most suitable for the patient.

Another simple technique that follows on from role play is role reversal. This is simply using the same format as above but with the patient playing the part of the other person. This is designed to initiate some insight into how others may feel in situations, and to provide further information that may help the patient communicate more effectively. Role reversal can also be played out with just the patient playing both parts. This requires a little more versatility but can be extremely effective in providing meaningful insight into the process of the interchange and how others react immediately to the patient's verbal message. It is a good idea, however, to help the patient change roles, to insist he changes chairs when playing both parts. The actual process of bodily movement into a different chair appears to facilitate the complete change of roles. Role reversal is extremely useful in family therapy, e.g. to have a young adolescent for the first time actually try to imagine completely how his parents feel, what they would say and how they would say it, can be very beneficial. When this is coupled with the parents observing this and seeing how their son or daughter sees them, real insights can be achieved. It is, of course, vitally important that all parties involved have ample opportunity following any role play situation to express their feelings and thoughts fully, and that the debrief is handled skilfully.

Empty Chair and Happy Chair

These are two very simple techniques that can quite safely and easily be incorporated into the nurse's repertoire. The empty chair is in fact a very useful 'safety valve' technique. In group or individual therapy, if patient feel that emotions are running high, either positively or negatively, then they may be encouraged to release them safely and swiftly by expressing them to an empty chair. Usually a particular chair is designated and in group situations this facility is made known to the group at the beginning of the session. Anyone at any time may approach the chair and express his feelings. It is recommended in early sessions that the identity of the subject of the feelings is not exposed, so no one's feelings are hurt or anyone embarrassed.

The happy chair is designed in much the same way, except that sitting or standing on this chair indicates to the group that the person is unhappy, feels rejected, embarrassed or has a negative feeling. This invites the group to respond positively to that individual in any predetermined acceptable way. Mostly this will be in an upsurge of clapping, whistling and shouts of 'good old ...' The amount of demonstrative affection the group is able to give will be entirely up to the individuals within it, but the skilled facilitator is usually able to ensure that the experience of sitting in the happy chair is in fact a happy one. A side effect of this situation which generally helps the group is the trust it generates within itself. People forming a group usually care for and nurture the separate members of the group, and this procedure helps to reinforce this fact.

Guided Fantasy

This most popular technique in dramatherapy allows the patient to experience his own mental imagery in a very relaxed and positive fashion. It is for some individuals very close to a light hypnosis, and can be extremely useful in allowing a patient to become closer to some personal insights in his life which he may have been hiding from himself. The process begins with simple relaxation exercises, ensuring that all the participants are relaxed and comfortable. This can often be facilitated by immediately preceding this event with a very physically exerting warm-up exercise, or dancing. Once the group or individual is relaxed, some soft music may be played in the background, and the therapist begins to guide the participants through a journey. The journey may be to a particular place, through a particular time, or to see a particular person. The subject of the journey will be constructed in the context of the individual travellers. It is important not to go too quickly or the effect of the imagery is lost; similarly, it is important not to be too specific in describing the journey, as this may conflict with an already constructed image and spoil the effect. To be as loose in descriptive terms allows the potential symbolism of the journey to be client-centred. Useful devices within a simple journey may be for the patient to meet someone 'significant to him', for him to 'say something to this person' and 'remember the most important thing this person says'. The patient may be invited to receive a gift from the person and return with it, or the person may do something before he leaves. The things the patient experiences on his journey, the people he sees and what he hears should not be unduly influenced by the guide, so that when the patient recounts the journey, it will be full of meaning for him from his mental imagery. Often following the guide's return trip, the patient will be asked to share what he wishes with another person, or a small group. The significance or symbolism he wishes to attach to the journey is for him to imply.

An example of a simple journey is as follows:

'Imagine you are facing a door, look closely at the door, see the handle and lock — open the door and before you is a long corridor — proceed along the corridor, taking notice of what you see. At the end of the corridor is a light; as you get closer you can see more clearly. Even closer, you begin to smell familiar fragrances. You can feel the temperature outside, and now see quite clearly the scene before you. Continue walking — as you walk you are aware of all the sounds around you, you can feel the texture beneath your feet, and hear the sound of your footsteps. There appears to be a building

of some kind in the distance. Can you make out what it is? I think you may just be able to see a figure beside the building, can you make out who it is? As you get closer you can see more clearly the building and the figure. The person seems to be holding something for you. You may take it if you wish. Examine it. The person seems to be saying something now. It appears to be important. You may feel you want to reply; there seems to be a need to express something between you.

'It's almost time to return now, take another look around, smell the fragrances, feel the sensations surrounding this place, say good-bye to the person and prepare to return. Begin your journey back. You may just be able to make out the corridor now. Enjoy the walk back, take note of what you can see. You're just about in the corridor now, proceed along it to the door. Open the door, recognise the room you're in and open your eyes when you feel ready.'

Some individuals will simply find this a beautiful relaxing experience, while others may find it turns into a significant walk into their subconscious. In situations where the patient may be frightened, or likely to imagine a particularly unpleasant journey, the therapist may feel she has to build in simple safeguards. Some ideas in this area might be to suggest they take a very close and trusted friend with them; to reassure them continually that the place is friendly; to describe in clearer and specific detail a 'springtime' walk, and to build in more pleasantness in the journey. The person is smiling and so on. The skilled therapist should know her patient sufficiently well to be able to build in safeguards as they are appropriate.

There are, of course, many more techniques that may be used by nurses in their eclectic repertoire; we simply do not have space in this small volume to include them. We do, however, recommend most strongly that the interested reader pursues the excellent material available (see below).

Suggested Further Reading

Highly recommended is:

Langley, Dorothy M. and Langley, Gordon E. *Dramatherapy and Psychiatry* (Croom Helm, London, 1983)

Other useful volumes suggested are:

Blatner, Howard A. *Acting In: Practical Applications of Psychodramatic Methods* (Springer, New York, 1973)

Hodgson, John *The Uses of Drama: Acting as a Social and Educational Force* (Methuen, London, 1972)
James, N. *Introduction to Dramatherapy and the Role of Staff Members* (Napsbury Hospital, St Albans, 1979)
Jennings, Sue (ed.) *Remedial Drama: A Handbook for Teachers and Therapists* (Pitman, London, 1979)
Remocker, A. Jane and Storch, Elizabeth, T. *Action Speaks Louder* (Churchill Livingstone, London, 1982)
Scoble, S. 'Dramatherapy with Psychotic Adults', *Journal of the British Association of Dramatherapy*, vol. 1, no. 4 (1978), pp. 13-16

Music and Dance

Music and dance are often forgotten amongst the mass of interactive therapies now presently available to the nurse/practitioner. However, we feel that this book could not be complete without at least a short explanation of these two powerful influences upon human behaviour. We do not feel qualified to go into great depth on the specific and elaborate styles of therapies currently being practised, as our experience in these special areas is not particularly extensive. We would nevertheless like to offer you some practical insights which we have come to through our flitting exposure to these therapies.

Movement and Dance

Most healthy individuals have at some time been invited to, or participated in, dance activity. The wild frenzied 'letting it all hang out' type dance, in contrast to the rather controlled and skilful conventional dance steps appear to be poles apart. Nevertheless, both of these activities share common factors with very similar activities such as gymnastics, or almost any type of physically active sport or recreation. Whichever is your particular favourite, this activity gives an expression in physical behaviour of the mental process within you. No experienced psychiatric nurse would argue with the very practical nature of encouraging the frustrated or aggressive individual to participate in some socially accepted physical activity. Similarly, dance and movement therapy are designed and structured to enable the patient to find suitable expressions for his emotions.

For most people, dancing becomes an extremely entertaining activity. It allows an expression not only of the mood or personality, but may also facilitate the expression of certain skills. There can be no doubt that the accomplished dancer is credited with enviable skill, yet the movements involved are paradoxically rather meaningless. Perhaps even more noticeable is the fact that although it is a pursuit of considerable energy, most people agree that dancing is a form of relaxation. This could be because it is such a basic form of communication that there is only a release of mental energy rather than a need to expend it. The subject simply acts what he feels in the dance rather than having to think of ways of expressing it. Generally all forms of dance are socially accepted, and consequently there are no cultural restraints on the expression of mood within dance, and no one is likely to be offended. The nurse involved in dance therapy may be able to increase her valuable insight into the patient's emotional state by observing the non-verbal behaviour and posturing during therapy, and the patient may be able to communicate his emotions much more easily in a non-threatening situation such as dance therapy.

Music

Music and dance are difficult to separate as distinct theapies, but it may be beneficial to make one significant distinction. When the patient chooses the type of music he wishes to dance to, he is using the music to accompany his feelings: the music he chooses will match his mood. Conversely, if music is chosen for the patient, a quite different effect may be observed. The patient who was previously irritated and may have chosen a rather loud and lively piece may now become quiet and relaxed when asked to dance to a soft and gentle sound. The point we make is that music may be used to potentiate the expression of the present mood, or to facilitate possible changes in it. This can only be reinforced by individual experience. If you care to imagine for one minute you are listening to specific pieces of music, can you connect emotions very directly to them? Try the national anthem, for instance, or 'Land of Hope and Glory', which are particularly stirring tunes surrounded by many highly emotional thoughts. Setting the scene for a romantic evening or choosing music for yourself when you are about to be busy will invariably involve some musical accompaniment suitable for the occasion. The simple fact is that if you want to feel a particular emotion, say sadness, you will almost inevitably choose some music that reminds you of a sad event or time. Conversely, if you are happy and wish to remain so, the music chosen will be one associated with happiness to sustain that mood. In therapy this has several practical applications. Firstly, in reality orientation, playing records which help the patient focus back to a particular time will stimulate memories associated with that time. War songs are perhaps an obvious example, but, perhaps more subtle, the wedding or funeral march may equally strike very emotional memories. The use of music in positive conditioning (see Chapter 3) can be very powerful, and associating a specific piece of music with the patient's calm state may induce relaxation if replayed when the patient becomes anxious.

In its simplest context, music is just pleasant; it is entertaining, occasionally creative and potentially soothing. Without music our world would be deprived of a wonderful source of sensory stimulation that a lot of people consider joyful. (Appendix II in Langley and Langley, 1983, is recommended for some useful aids to appropriate musical selection.) In contrast, one final consideration we would like to point out is that nurses sometimes forget that it is possible to spoil the effect by over exposure. To be constantly bombarded with sound, no matter how beautiful, may irritate an individual to the extent that all sounds are perceived as unwelcome noise. In practical terms, for music to be linked with therapy or simple pleasure, it is most important that it should be separated from everyday sounds. Preferably music rooms where patients can choose what they hear should be available, but at least music should not compete for attention with the television, conversation and domestic noise.

Implications for the Nurse

The main implication for the nurse in music and dance therapy is to be aware of just how powerful these techniques can be. There is, we feel, a general feeling amongst nurses that these areas are not very exciting, or that they are surrounded in mystery and therefore not particularly appropriate to them. We wonder if some of this attitude comes from the nurse's reluctance to join in some of these therapeutic pursuits with patients. Music is reasonably dignified and most nurses would have few reservations about becoming involved; dance, on the other hand, may be a different matter. 'Dancing around a hall with a group of patients somehow does not seem very dignified, not that there is anything wrong with it, it just seems odd.' We have often heard this dialogue amongst nurses, and we can to some extent reflect back to our days of studenthood and perhaps sympathise. Nevertheless, embarrassment should be no disincentive to ensuring that the patient has every opportunity to express himself. In the long run, the patient will respect the nurse who risks looking foolish to help him, far more than the nurse who steps back and by her example denies him an additional therapeutic experience.

We believe music and dance therapy will play a significant part in the treatment and rehabilitation of patients in the future, and it is therefore our hope that nurses will shed their anxieties and reluctance over something different, take an interest in it and use it positively to their patients' benefit.

Suggested Further Reading

Dance

Bernstein, P.L. (ed.) *Eight Theoretical Approaches in Dance/Movement Therapy* (Kendal, Hunt, Dubuque, Toronto, 1979)

Warren, Bernie (ed.) *Using the Creative Arts in Therapy* (Croom Helm, London, 1984), Ch. 7

Music

Storms, G. *Handbook of Music and Games* (Hutchinson, London, 1981)

Warren, Bernie (ed.) *Using the Creative Arts in Therapy* (Croom Helm, London, 1984), Ch. 8.

General

Axline, Virginia, M. *Dibs: In Search of Self, Personality Development in Play Therapy* (Penguin Books, Harmondsworth, 1981)

Jennings, Sue (ed.) *Creative Therapy* (Pitman, London, 1975)

23 MANAGEMENT PRINCIPLES AND SKILLS

Many nurses tend to believe that nurse management is the same as administration, and state quite openly that they trained to be a nurse, not an administrator. We firmly believe that all nurses would benefit from learning management principles and skills, even if very few will ever become nurse managers and subsequently administer.

Administration is a part of management studies which helps senior nurses formulate policies, calculate manpower, devise plans and collect data. It is not, however, what we wish or intend to discuss in the chapter.

Management as applied to nursing involves the skilled use of resources to effect a high degree of nursing care. This is the area where all nurses of all grades should be skilled if they are to maximise the therapeutic potential for their patients.

This chapter seeks to identify resources available, principles for their use and strategies particular to nursing situations. We end with a short section on leadership, which we hope will be useful to those nurses responsible for teams.

Resources

It is necessary to identify resources, as they are often hidden, and if the nurse is unable to see what is available to her, she will inevitably fail to maximise them. Resources can be broken down into people, time, equipment, environment and finance. In order to see the elements in more detail let us take each separately.

People

The people involved in the care of patients are often more widespread than originally thought. For instance, in a hospital environment the laundry worker, porter, cook, seamstress, domestic and storeman may seem insignificant to the ward nurse, but in fact in terms of influence and power, these people have the potential both to enhance or sabotage the nursing care given to each patient. Good relationships, thoughtful appreciation and sound communication are basic principles to bear in mind when considering people resources.

Close to the patient, the nurse may see herself in isolation as the person who knows the patient's wishes, hopes and expectations best. This is as it should be, but she will at best be able to help the patient fulfil only some of these. Doctors, physiotherapists, occupational therapists and psychologists are but a few of a constant file of professionals, also skilled and specialised in fulfilling particular aspects of the patient's needs. To understand the role of each professional and non-professional helper should be an aim of all nurses who wish to manage their patients' care effectively. Looking at people resources even further, two other factors emerge. The first is to acknowledge that the specialist who offers a particular resource is also a person. She has a unique interpersonal relationship style and consequently each person has a personality potential as well as a special knowledge. The skilled nurse will try not only to find the best specialist, but also the best personality match whenever this is possible. The second factor to acknowledge is the timing of the person resource. Each person who may potentiate a therapeutic effect will do so only if it is offered at the appropriate time. A social worker invited to discuss after care with a patient is only an appropriate resource if the patient is ready to accept the idea of discharge at that moment. Even more subtle timing may be seen in the terminally ill patient. Religious or spiritual advisers may be very powerful person resources for the patient, but, if poorly timed, the results may be seriously harmful to the patient's progress.

Occasionally the sex of the person is significant: a few years ago both of us were involved in the care of a patient who from time to time became very deluded. His delusion normally took the form of a religious persecution and within it he held the belief that all male nurses were homosexual and conspiring to persecute him for his religious beliefs. Although at most other times we had a good relationship with him, it would have been foolhardy for either of us to attempt to persuade him to accept an intramuscular injection. Even though he occasionally, during these deluded periods, became violent and aggressive, the most appropriate person resource was a female nurse. More often than not she was successful without any untoward incident, where we would undoubtedly have failed.

Availability of manpower is of course a major factor in people resources. So often in British hospitals, staff are overworked and thin on the ground. For this reason alone, the nurse should be skilled at managing people resources. During periods of manpower shortage, the maximum effectiveness of individuals should surely be the principle to the forefront of our minds. If each person is operating at maximum efficiency in areas where she is effective, the task, in this case patient care, will be achieved. If the task is still not achieved, this proves only that resources are insufficient and not that management is poor.

To summarise briefly, people resource management is identifying the right person to help the patient at the right time, bearing in mind that person's skill, knowledge, personality, sex and availability.

Time

Time is seldom considered as a resource with anything other than a cursory examination. In fact time is one of the most squandered of all resources available to the nurse. The nurse who learns how to manage her time effectively will have the advantage of being seen to be in control and never in a real flap. Once it is accepted that time can be accounted for, allocated and controlled, the nurse will run out of it less.

Drucker (1967) suggests that time is such a valuable resource that we should control it more carefully than physical resources. More materials can always be found, but time cannot be manufactured — once it's been expended it is lost forever. We suggest the most practical way of controlling your time is firstly to measure it. Take account of what you spent it on today: be totally honest and make a list. Better still, take a note pad to work and divide it into half hour periods and note down exactly what you have spent time on. It is likely that your list will include many periods sitting scratching your head wondering what's next. Ordering your priorities will take even more time, and talking to colleagues and planning care another large slice. Using the telephone will undoubtedly crop up frequently, sometimes to give information, and other times to pass it on. In most organisations there will be some statutory slot for a 'handover', some system of shift change over, or organised communication. Somewhere on the list will be writing reports, filling in forms and evaluating nursing care and patient progress. These areas we are fairly sure will figure prominently in your lists. We are not suggesting that anything on your list is a complete waste of time, but what we are suggesting is that it may be organised in a more efficient way.

If you take your time seriously, and make a list, then we are pretty sure the conclusions drawn will be helpful. We are convinced that most nurses will organise their time effectively once its waste is drawn to their attention. Additionally, we suggest that you also consider the following questions addressed to your lists, as thought provokers:

(1) Did I spend that long because it needed time or because I like doing that?
(2) Was that time spent effective for good patient care?
(3) If I put all those little bits of time spent on the same thing together, would it have been quicker/more efficient? (e.g. ten telephone calls to various departments throughout a shift, as opposed to ten minutes all together)
(4) Could I have combined these two jobs together to save time?
(5) What are my priorities in the list?
(6) How much time did I spend during the day on each priority?
(7) What time have I spent on low priorities that I could transfer to high priorities?
(8) Is there something on the list that crops up again and again and seems to achieve nothing?
(9) Which items rob me of valuable time?
(10) What do I want to change?

Equipment

Equipment is a valuable resource, often abused by nurses of all grades. To have an item of equipment in a ward area tends to fall into the following categories:

(1) Necessary — without this equipment the nurse would not be able to function — items such as tables, chairs, beds and kitchen equipment.
(2) General medical — this equipment would probably be found only in a hospital, but is considered necessary for most areas — oxygen/resuscitation equipment, sphygmomanometer/syringes, needles.
(3) Special therapeutic — this is the equipment that makes the

difference between an area that houses patients and one that has a therapeutic value — items such as paints, paper, record player, games and such.

These categories are simply an aid to the nurse to evaluate how important each item of equipment is to *her.* To every individual, each item we have suggested may be swapped to a different category. What is important is that all nurses have a clear idea of which piece of equipment falls into which category. We believe that without such a clear idea, very wasteful equipment collection policies are soon implemented. To illustrate this, all the observant nurse needs to do is to look in store cupboards and determined how much previously valued equipment is lying unused. All these items may be 'on order' in other units desperately needed. It is very easy to become 'I'll order it just in case' minded.

When recommending the ordering or purchasing of equipment, the skilled nurse, aware of resource scarcity, asks herself the following questions:

(1) Is it necessary, special or general?
(2) Can it be borrowed when required, or is it vital that it is 'owned' by the ward?
(3) Will it be used?
(4) Is there something more valuable we need first?
(5) Can it wait?

Once these questions are answered thoughtfully, a more logical case to purchase or order may be evident. Any item of equipment may be considered a luxury by someone else who doesn't value it. A heart-lung machine is a necessity to a thoracic surgeon, but may be seen as extravagant by a patient on a waiting list for a walking frame. Before leaving this section we feel it should be stressed that we are not advising psychiatric nurses to 'make do and mend'. In fact it is our experience that nurses are perhaps too good at this — we are simply saying that careful judgement is required. This should not deter the nurse from insisting on equipment that she requires, but it should certainly sober her judgement when requesting expensive items.

Environment

Resources within our environment are often missed. Sometimes the simple conversion exercise is overlooked in the struggle for perfection. Examples of this are numerous: one charge nurse stated that he could not take female patients on his ward because he did not have the correct facilities. By reorganising a dormitory area and making a second toilet block female only, the integration occurred without any structural changes. Linen cupboards can be changed into offices to facilitate a music or therapy room. It is not necessary to be constrained by the ward itself. In most hospitals there are areas not in constant use that can be used for activities that take too much space in the ward. Recreation halls, occupational therapy departments and gymnasiums are seldom in use all the time. Moving patients into these alternative environments creates additional stimulation, and gives space for such creative therapies as drama, music and movement, yoga, keep fit and suchlike.

Alcoholic and drug addiction units await large financial commitment from bureaucratic sources. Millions of pounds are spent creating new 'glossy' units to help these particular individuals. Is it because without these special environmental facilities they cannot be helped? Essentially the only differences between these units and the present arrangements are that like diagnosed individuals will spend whole days together. Surely then, with some thought, could not alternative group meeting places be found within existing structures? We are not suggesting that new units should not be built. We would not suggest that it is not a worthwhile project, as they have many advantages. The point we seek to make is that there are many environmental resources untapped, if the nurse looks for them. Nurses should not be strait-jacketed into waiting for 'the new unit to open'; if a need exists it should be served as quickly as possible. This usually means seeking resources that exist already. We have seen admission units create mother and baby units with no more resources than a 'desire to serve', therapeutic communities set up in run-down old houses, and alcoholic specialties in side wards and dormitories. Will and imagination are the only management tools required to manipulate the environment.

Finance

There remains a myth that without money no progress is possible. We use the word 'myth' because it is our experience that commitment, positive attitudes and personal skills are far more important in progress than money ever will be. It is unfortunately a fact of life that to purchase staff, equipment and premises, money is required. The availability of finance, however, is in most cases dependent upon the original premiss that staff involved need to show commitment to the enterprise requiring support. Most nurses in Britain are now beginning to realise that finance will not always, and in some cases seldom, be supplied by central government. Voluntary agencies, charities and benefactors are a source of income that remains largely untapped. If these people and organisations are impressed by a need, an idea, or an enterprise that is by its very nature highly altruistic, funds are usually forthcoming. In smaller, possibly even more frustrating, areas of financial insufficiencies, a more imaginative tactic is required. In the past few years, one of the authors had the irksome task of managing a rehabilitation unit of four wards. The most active of the four, involved in predischarge work, continually submitted requests for an electric cooker. The request was by no means unreasonable, as patients about to go back into the community should at least have some practice at cooking their own meals. The problem was not so much the cost of buying a cooker, but the necessary electrical installation work required. The solution to the problem was achieved by asking what the patients were actually going to cook on it. The discussion with the patients it appeared that breakfasts and suppers were the main need. This was quickly catered for not by the purchase of a cooker, but by the purchase of a toaster and an electric ring. All they required to cook could be easily achieved without expensive wiring. Although this example may seem trite, it does illustrate how divergent thinking can sometimes circumnavigate the need for additional finance. Management is after all about managing with what is available. A clothes line across the bathroom is not as appealing as a tumble drier, a bicycle is not as comfortable as a limousine, but if we each cut our cloth according to our needs, a prime principle of management is achieved.

Management Contrasts

Task versus Patient

Systems organisation in nursing presently operates on two main ideas. The first is the currently unacceptable 'task' orientated system, and the more widely accepted 'patient' orientated system.

The task system has several advantages for the management of a ward. It is generally efficient and succeeds in completing the work schedule, everyone knows what they are responsible for and they are easily identified should substandard or unfinished work be later discovered. The system operates on a task list, and nurses are delegated to a series of nursing duties, i.e.

Staff Nurse Jones	Take report. Check O_2 and resuscitation equipment including aspirators. Give out medicines. Doctors' round Group therapy. Handover.
Student Nurses Brown and White and Black	Supervise patients dressing. Supervise patients washing. Give out breakfast. Escort patients to Occupational Therapy.
Enrolled Nurse Green	Supervise students early morning. Assist S/N Jones with drugs. Prepare patients for ECT. Escort to ECT. On return assist S/N Jones with doctors' round and group.

This is a very simple management system which has inbuilt communication, supervision and accountability. Its great disadvantage, which makes it largely unacceptable for current practice, is its lack of continuity and the dehumanising effect it may have on nurses operating within it. The nurse delegated a task to carry out may well not understand why she is doing it and she may not relate personally to the patients involved in the process. It is largely mechanistic, valuable interactional processes may be ignored, information specific to individuals may be missed, and, more important, the nurse's interpersonal skills are largely wasted.

Patient orientated systems are now widely used, and take as their basis a more continual and humanistic approach. Based on a nursing process system, each nurse is allocated a number of patients and it is the nurse's responsibility to respond to the needs of these individuals throughout their contact with them. An organised plan of care is decided and written in a Kardex system, so accurate information is always available. Untrained nurses are allocated to teams so that their progress can be monitored and their work supervised by a trained nurse, the team leader. This system has many advantages: it is easy to divide patients into high, medium and low dependency and allocate staff accordingly; nurses are involved with a smaller group of patients and have a continual input into total patient care. Rather than doing a whole task for all the patients, they are involved in all the care for a group of patients.

The disadvantages are of a practical nature. In periods of staff shortage, the groups of patients become so large that some tasks may be missed or forgotten. This is no 'grand design' strategy, so individual care is largely left to the initiative of each supervising nurse. A criticism levelled at this system is that it is wasteful of resources: on a surgical ward, every nurse may need a dressing trolley at the same time. In the psychiatric setting, its potential effect can disintegrate if individual care plans send patients from a nurse's group in different directions: Nurse Brown is responsible for total care of patients A, B, C and D. Patients A and B require ECT; patient C is scheduled to go to the Occupational Therapy Department and patient D is to attend the Psychology Department.

It may occur to you that, as in all systems, advantages and disadvantages can be potentiated and minimised respectively only if the manager is versatile and flexible. It occurs to us that any system has inherent faults; the intelligent and skilled nurse takes from each what she needs for her circumstances.

Positives versus Negatives

Contrast the nurse who constantly voices her indignation at her colleagues who are always late, sloppily dressed, uncaring, untidy, unprepared, lazy, ill-tempered and boring with the nurse who compliments her colleagues for their positive attributes. How many times have you been 'caught' doing something wrong and chastised for it, yet can you remember being 'caught' doing something really well? The principle is simple. It is unlikely that you will change someone's faults very quickly if at all, although you may stop them doing something, but what do you replace that something with? Taking the contrasting view, most nurses have some positive strengths. They are good at something, they show a talent, a flair for a particular task — isn't it more productive to potentiate that than condemn the negative?

The ideal nurse, we suppose, is perfect at everything, but in reality nurses are like every other individual, with skills ranging from below to above average ability. The skilled manager will identify all these and maximise the above average ones and largely ignore the below average. If a nurse is encouraged, rewarded and commended for valuable service, she will continue to improve and work hard. If she is continually harassed, punished and reprimanded for the inadequacies she largely cannot control, her entire work performance will suffer. An acquaintance of ours illustrates this point quite clearly. He was considered rather slow, showed little initiative, and was generally dissatisfied with his job. It was only when he was asked whether he knew a suitable venue for the staff Christmas party that he volunteered to organise it and subsequently showed his brilliant talent at social and recreational organisation. When this talent was recognised, rewarded and potentiated, his work improved generally, his initiative was considerably increased and his commitment to the unit became total. His ability was generalised into areas within the rehabilitation team, with him organising day trips, bazaars, holidays, shopping trips and such. The learning exercise for everyone is that if you don't use people's talents you lose them; if you ignore people's potential, they cease to function altogether.

Decision Making versus Problem Solving

An ability to make decisions is an attribute most nurses would wish to own. Indecisiveness in the nurse is a difficulty that may question her other skills. However, making decisions is not a difficult process, providing there are at least two possible courses of action. To shave or not, to go out or stay in, to buy a car or a bicycle, are hardly difficult or earth shattering decisions. More serious choices involving more complex issues may take longer, and deserve more thoughtful consideration. It would not be appropriate to decide whether to sue for divorce with the same cursory thought as it would take to decide whether to eat at eight or nine o'clock. Taking these decisions becomes more difficult whenever the choice has to be accurate. These more complex issues are within the realms of problem solving, for decision making is only a small part within the model of problem solving.

To take a familiar model of problem solving as an illustration of the process, we shall look at a management problem with Gerry.

The unit officer has to decide what action to take about Gerry's persistent lateness. Although he is always very apologetic, he continues to come late. Sometimes ten minutes, sometimes half an hour, but on some occasions he's been as late as two hours. It has been decided that some action has to be taken.

Decision choices:

(1) Formal discipline — a series of these will result in termination of employment.
(2) Transfer him to another unit — this will simply get him out of your hair.
(3) Continue to reprimand him — this has proved to be ineffective.
(4) Ignore it — ostrich strategy tends to breed resentment or even encourage modelling behaviour within other staff.

The choices appear difficult until we apply a problem solving approach.

Problem: Gerry's lateness.
Goal: Gerry reporting on duty on time.
Assessment: Factors affecting Gerry's lateness.
Buses don't run early morning.
Stays up too late at night.
Girlfriend works late hours.
Very tired in morning.
Plan: Adjust hours to accommodate difficulties: i.e. Gerry works late shifts permanently.
Implementation: Monitor punctuality.
Evaluation: Solves problem. Gerry reports on duty on time. The organisation is satisfied. ? How does Gerry feel about it?

Gerry was a particularly bright young man with lots of ideas, a very caring nature, and he was a skilled nurse. Taking any decision from (1) to (4) would have solved very little and possibly resulted in losing Gerry's expertise. Looking closely at what the problems were, what outcomes were needed made the original preselected decision obsolete, and the final decision more effective. Note that in the evaluation stage, some feedback is needed from Gerry, too. In reality Gerry became very unhappy working constant late duties, and eventually returned to normal shifts, by which time his punctuality had greatly improved.

To summarise: for decision making to be effective, it has to occur within a problem solving framework. Decisions themselves can be good, bad or indifferent. When the decisions that are taken address the problems accurately, and provide realistic and workable solutions, then and only then can we congratulate ourselves and claim to have the quality of a good decision maker.

Delegation/DIY

'If you want a job doing well — do it yourself' and 'There's no point having a dog and barking yourself' are contradictory in content. They do, however, represent two generally accepted viewpoints which are central to the issue of delegation/DIY.

One of the most difficult things a nurse in a team has to learn is that there is neither the time nor the necessity to conduct all nursing practice herself. She has learned through her training and by making endless mistakes that she is reliable and competent and she has no difficulty in trusting herself. In the event that she does make an error, it is hers to own and deal with. Once an established professional in a team, even when working autonomously in the community, a time occurs when the nurse has to accept that some of the workload needs to be relinquished if she is to remain effective. Charge nurses and ward sisters who continue to operate independently of others breed resentment, inadequacy and frustration. As difficult as it may be to delegate tasks that you feel competent to perform yourself, it is important to understand how the other individual feels when you continue to show no trust in their abilities.

The skill of delegation is not to divorce yourself from responsibility, nor to accept all responsibility with no control. The skill is to be able to assess the ability of others, to select appropriate tasks individuals can competently complete, and to monitor and supervise the implementation of your directions. In situations where nurses are expected to delegate tasks, they are temporarily becoming trainers and supervisors as well as practitioners. It is a compliment that their judgement is appreciated, that they are considered not only competent as professionals, but they also have the insight and personal resources to accept additional responsibility for someone else's performance.

This responsibility may hang heavy, but this is how it should be, for a good delegator needs to balance her judgement and trust and her suspicion and control finely. Bad delegators commonly ask impossible tasks of their subordinates, putting them under intolerable pressure and consequently putting themselves at risk when things go wrong. Equally poor delegators direct too little to others and consequently reduce their effectiveness by trying to do everything themselves. The effective delegator is the person who finds herself and the team constantly occupied in a purposeful way. Everyone's talents are being used to the full without risk to the patient.

Contingencies

Every good manager knows that no matter how good her plans are, 'sod's law' still decrees that anything that possibly can go wrong will go wrong. It is for this reason that when a plan is about to be implemented, a contingency plan should be set up alongside it. The skilled nurse tends to do this almost automatically, mostly because in the process of becoming skilled an awful lot of mistakes have been made. It is through these past mistakes that a repertoire of contingency plans is accumulated. The experienced nurse may say that it's just common sense to plan for the possible eventuality, but, although common sense is sometimes a rare commodity, it is what management is mostly about.

Contingencies are the well thought out 'what ifs?' If Joe Bloggs vomits on the coach, what can be done? If Arthur Brown gets lost at the fair, what action is available? Who shall I report to? What should I do first? What are my back up plans — the contingencies? In nurse education, every teacher knows she must always have contingency plans for the material that runs out too quickly, the unexpected question from the class, or the last minute rescheduling of a timetable. For every seemingly faultless implementation of a plan, there lies a manager with an endless supply of well thought through contingency plans. When they are at their most effective, no one is aware they have been used. A ship doesn't sail without life rafts, a fighter pilot without his parachute, and likewise a plan should never be implemented without the contingencies worked out.

Leadership

The successful leader should have the ability, qualities and skills previously discussed. She should be aware of resources available to her, know the strengths and weakenesses of her team, be able to make sound decisions that help solve problems that arise, and be able to delegate prudently. Having said all this, many people may have these abilities, but do not make good leaders. If these are the basic ingredients, what else is necessary? It is our view that the successful leader has, in addition, all the following qualities in various percentages.

She is a planner; she sees the whole nature and direction of the tasks and gradually moves forward towards what she sees as the overall goal of the team. She is intuitive in this planning, due to both experience, awareness and intelligent insight, and she is able to judge accurately what will and will not work. Intuitive is the only appropriate word to describe this ability, because it is a natural quality: it is not hard work for her to judge, foresee and plan. As if this is not enough, we see many other essential ingredients in this successful leader, for it is probably even more important that she is a brilliant communicator. There is no one in her team who is not aware of what she should be doing. Everyone knows what the overall outcome will be, and a complete trust in the leader is established. This communication skill is not one directional, for the wise leader knows that each one of her team not only has good ideas, but has a need to share them. Furthermore, even the ideas that are not so good have a kernel of quality which may be valuable if sifted out.

The leader will have ideas from many sources: her team, herself, other groups, individuals and her patients. It is her job to sort these out, to direct them appropriately into strategies that help the movement towards shared goals. She must be able to modify them and make them acceptable and usable both to the organisation and her co-workers and team. She must be consistent in her approach and prove to be consistently correct in her decision making or else her credibility as leader will suffer. This applies just as much to the 'democratic' leader as it does to the autocrat, for there is always someone who will need to apportion blame whenever things go wrong. Finally, she must be seen to be strong, reliable and fair.

Probably more important than having an awareness of what makes such a paragon, perhaps we might have a brief look at how each of us may employ a systematised approch to becoming such a leader.

Firstly, we believe whether you adopt a democratic or autocratic style of leadership will largely depend on individual personality and temperament. We would suggest, however, that much greater pressure is applied to autocratic styles, as other individuals within the team may feel more threatened, contribute less, and therefore the leader may be scapegoated more easily. Leadership by example, i.e. demonstrating in yourself all the skills and qualities you expect in your subordinates, is a very powerful model, but it is also very demanding and fraught with danger. Any mistake, misdemeanour or substandard performance by the leader gives precedence for subordinates to do the same. In a purely democratic style, the leader depends largely on her skills of oratory, logic and reason to demonstrate how each suggestion or idea could be used to fulfil the aim of the organisation. Trust in each member's intrinsic ability to be honest, work orientated and sensible is necessary before this style can be initiated in its pure form. It is also interesting to note that many leaders believe themselves to be democrats until they are put in a tricky situation which requires them to take responsibility for a decision that only they, with their particular knowledge and experience, can make. Their style then changes to the 'benevolent autocrat'. In this style the leader *knows* what the only course of action must be, then takes this to her team and sells it to them. We recognise this particular device as one which we have both used on numerous occasions in the past; it is only veiled autocracy.

If these are the main and popular styles we would suggest that none is perfect. It seems better that each individual should take from each style as the occasion determines. We suggest a reasonable compromise exists in the following scheme.

Listen to all arguments and discussions without contaminating them with your own, and then introduce your own ideas to the discussion. Logically and rationally rule out the unacceptable, refine the promising and then communicate your intention to act on your findings. Your reasons for taking particular actions should be clearly stated to avoid confusion. Subsequently, it should be stressed that this idea will be tried as soon as possible, but with a prearranged time period it will be evaluated by free discussion and then adjusted. The advantages of this system are it has an open approach, it takes ideas from many sources, it refines them, communicates intention, acts and has built in safety in the form of evaluation and adjustment (see Figure 23.1).

It is important to have *shared objectives* if a leader is to be effective. For every member of the team to have the same firm idea

Figure 23.1: A Circular Model of Communication and Action in Management

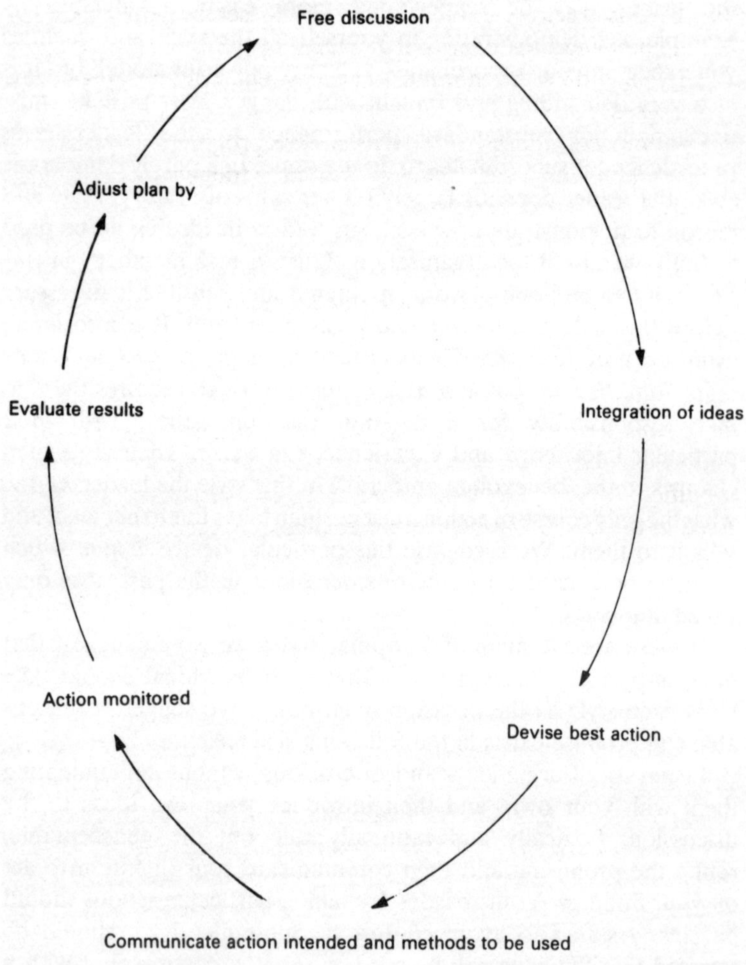

of what they are trying to achieve will have a very powerful effect. When issues become vague, and arguments and disagreements rage, the leader will be able to focus this energy productively on to the goal.

Therefore, it would seem reasonable to have a series of set objectives to attain in a set period of time, to encourage observable task achievement. For example: Ward X at their weekly meeting decide the following objectives:

(1) By next week — three teams will be set up to begin low, medium and high dependency planning.
(2) By the end of the month — each patient will be dependency assessed.
(3) Within two months — individual care programmes will be in operation for each patient within a framework of high/medium/low dependency.
(4) *Broad aim* — within six months each patient will be actively engaged in a progressive rehabilitation programme on an individual basis. He will be continually assessed by his respective nursing team so as to operate at his optimum potential.

Once these types of objectives are set up, everyone knows where their efforts are to be directed. Progress can be measured, and in the light of progress new objectives formulated, or old ones modified. When difficulties arise, if these objectives are firmly fixed in the leader's mind she can use them as a focus to encourage positive action.

Methods of achieving objectives will be monitored and supervised by the leader using her discretion. Some members of the team will be effective in working towards objectives, and some will be less effective. The leader's role here is to *observe, listen* and finally *demonstrate* when she is sure it is necessary. Leadership by example is very appropriate here. It is very powerful, as it shows the leader's skills as a practitioner as well as a supervisor. Equally its appropriateness must be valid, as interfering in the work of another professional must be well timed or it may breed resentment. If she is aware of how other members are successfully achieving objectives, her role is to share this success with all the other members of each team. This will not only be helpful to the recipients, but will be praise and encouragement to the originators of the methods. The successful leader in a supervising role will be patient, rewarding, reassuring and stimulating.

By the very nature of its task, leadership carries with it its difficult components: correcting people's mistakes, maintaining standards and making difficult administrative decisions which may be unpopular. We would not advocate a whingeing, weak, apologetic style of admonishment, or bad news bearing, but neither would we say the cold calculating approach is necessary. It has been our experience that the effective leader, despite making 'hard' decisions, tends to remain respected and popular. This is because her decisions are based objectively and fairly on the task that has been agreed and she is prepared to discuss, reason and, if necessary, justify her actions. It is not necessary for a good leader to pretend to be either super cool or super perfect: she will have emotions, and these need to be disclosed on occasions. To share how unhappy she is, or how difficult it was to make a decision is not a weakness, and it does not hurt to show subordinates that she is human. Similarly, admitting mistakes and readily accepting criticism are not necessarily harmful. The technique of leadership in this area is to demonstrate how useful the criticism has been, and how great an education was the mistake. This is not advising anyone to be ungenuine, simply to learn how to turn defeats into victories. We believe that most people would agree that individuals capable of retrieving something from a disaster are to be admired and looked up to — perhaps an apt description of a leader.

To Summarise

The Ideal Leader/Manager

Demonstrates she is consistent, patient, strong and fair.

Continually encourages and praises. Listens, discusses and proposes. Makes accurate problem solving decisions.

Occasionally observes, evaluates and adjusts, reprimands and admonishes.

Is aware of resources in people, time, equipment, environment and finance.

Calculates the strengths and weaknesses of her team.

Accepts criticism, her mistakes, and that she is human and uses each to its maximum potential.

Interferes only when necessary and does so by demonstrating a better way.

Shares her ideas, information and resources with her team.

Delegates appropriate tasks to competent personnel.

Does not become high handed, big headed, lazy, take her work home, or get an ulcer.

Is not an autocrat or democrat, but simply a person using her skills and qualities, intelligence and emotions to their maximum potential in a goal orientated approach.

Conclusion

Within this chapter we have tried to show that management principles and skills are important for every nurse. We have discussed aspects of resources that the nurse should be familiar with in order to be effective. The use of time, personnel, equipment, environment and finance are all resources that may be maximised if they are utilised efficiently no matter how scarce they appear to be. Drawing together and comparing some contrasting situations and approaches of task/patient orientation system, positives/negatives, decision making/problem solving and delegation/DIY was intended to provoke some thought within you on how you are currently operating, and whether other approaches may be helpful. Contingencies and leadership are the final components of this chapter, as these are the tools of the implementor. The effective manager requires to plan contingencies and possess the qualities and skills of leadership if she is to be effective.

It has occurred to us that some of you may be puzzled that a book essentially on psychiatric nursing should end with a chapter on management. For those of who have read the text and feel this way, we offer this as an explanation. The nurse who has acquired knowledge and skills and is unable to focus and direct them appropriately is not dissimilar to the 'perfect' nurse who is consistently off sick — of limited use to the patient. As this book has been written to facilitate what we hope is better care for the patient, it seems appropriate to us that we end with a section on the skills required to potentiate such a noble desire. So in fact we end this book on the same note as we began, thinking once more of the people we seek to help — the psychiatric patients.

APPENDIX I: MENTAL DEFENCE MECHANISMS

Anxiety can be a very uncomfortable emotion. In extremes it can threaten our well-being and cannot be tolerated for long. Consequently, people are motivated to do something to alleviate the discomfort of the anxiety. Freud (1958) observed and described certain types of behaviour, sometimes used unconsciously by people aiming to reduce personal anxiety levels, which he called 'mental mechanisms'.

People strive to avoid or reduce anxiety and maintain self-esteem. Defence mechanisms provide a protective armour while we are learning more mature and realistic ways of solving our problems, e.g. being able to rationalise failures that would otherwise cause us to despair, and to sustain us until we can work out better solutions to our conflicts.

Below are some examples of these defence mechanisms. A more detailed description of these can be found in the suggested reading.

Repression

Complete blocking from awareness of anxiety producing impulses. A form of amnesia for certain events, e.g. dangerous or embarrassing moments, an accident during childhood or other traumatic emotional situations.

Projection

Behaviour seen when unacceptable thoughts and feelings are unconsciously denied and are attributed to other people, e.g. if you are convinced that those around you are cruel or unkind, any harsh treatment you give them is not based on your bad qualities. Or, blaming your tools for your bad workmanship.

Displacement

Behaviour towards a person or object which has been substituted for the original person or object, e.g. bad day at work, person in charge directed his frustrations and anger on to you, all your pent up emotions are taken home with you, resulting in being bad tempered with your family and slamming doors.

Regression

Behaviour which is immature and more appropriate to an earlier stage of development, e.g. a new baby is brought into the household, the older child is unable to come to terms with this, thus regresses to a former behaviour pattern, i.e. enuresis and temper tantrums.

Rationalisation

Unconsciously finding 'good reasons' for your behaviour, e.g. I won't visit today as I'm sure she will have plenty of visitors and anyway the mood I'm in won't help cheer her up.

Sublimation

The resolution of unacceptable urges or tendencies by substituting unconsciously for socially acceptable behaviour, e.g. aggressive impulses channelled into sports such as rugby or motor car racing.

Compensation

Substitution of a more acceptable or denied form of gratification, e.g. the childless woman who is sterile takes up employment in a nursery.

Conversion

Behaviour that occurs when psychological difficulties are translated into physical symptoms, e.g. the student who is due to sit an important exam that she is inadequately prepared for develops paralysis in her writing arm the night before.

Suggested Further Reading

Freud, A. *The Ego and the Mechanism of Defence* (Hogarth Press, London, 1968)

Hilgard, R., Atkinson, L. and Atkinson C. *Introduction to Psychology*, 8th edn (Harcourt Brace Jovanovich, New York, 1983, pp. 433-8

Houston, John P., Bee, Helen and Rimm, David C. *Invitation to Psychology*, 2nd edn (Academic Press, New York, 1982)

APPENDIX II: TECHNIQUE FOR REALITY ORIENTATION

Reality orientation must take into account:

(1) Patients are withdrawn and easily distressed. The aim is to avoid stress in therapy by avoiding situations which will provoke it. So if a patient cannot remember quickly, an answer should be provided. 'Do you know my name? — It's Marie, can you say that? — Marie — That's fine.'

(2) All sessions commence with the routine of names, dates, time and weather. Also place, time and age can be used later on. The patient is to say, spell and write them.

(3) An elderly patient has a very short memory and poor attention span. He needs constant stimulation to keep his interest.

(4a) Constant repetition is essential. 'John, today is Wednesday, can you write Wednesday, John, write Wednesday in your book.' When a response is correct it must be reinforced by praise.

(4b) It is also advisable to extend the repetition to the ward. Patients should be reminded of the time, place and event consistently by all the staff. 'It is twelve o'clock, Mary, time for lunch' or 'It is three o'clock in the morning, John, you should be asleep' are appropriate remarks. These and others of a similar nature act as a stimulant for failing memory and orientation.

(5) The patient may be withdrawn, but he is not a child. His knowledge and memory are confused perhaps, but can be reawakened.

(6) Friendliness, politeness and knowledge of the patient are vital and assist in re-establishing his confidence. Each session should begin with a 'Good morning,' a handshake and a 'Goodbye' at the end. Courtesy always pleases and relaxes people.

(7) Patients and therapists should address each other by name. Signs of authority do not help. Ordinary clothes

rather than uniforms also ease the atmosphere.

(8) When a patient has assimilated and responded to a relearning situation, he should be allowed to progress, otherwise boredom may cause a reversal.

(9) As soon as possible the patients should be involved in group activities, as social interaction is essential to their rehabilitation. Interpersonal relationships should be encouraged, even in the early stages.

(10) All the senses should be used — interesting smells, tastes, sound and the feel of things should be introduced.

(11a) In the early stages, the use of a weather board, calendars, writing materials, large letters and pictures should provide stimulating repetition. Books, maps, charts, pictures of the seasons, money and a teaching clock are useful additions. Imagination on the part of the therapist provides many other avenues.

(11b) In the advanced group, occupations, interests and way of life are topics for discussion. For the ladies — pieces of material can be used to discuss suitable dresses; for men — books, pictures and mementoes of the two world wars are useful, and scents, coal mines, pigeons and greyhounds are also of value. Films, photographs, models or 'antiques' provide additional stimulation.

(12) Most vital of all is a friendly involved therapist who is capable of using her imagination and initiative.

Basic to the therapy is the need to capitalise on the patient's long-term memory store. Their prime of life — roughly 1920-45 — is the period they remember best. By making them comfortable with discussion of that era, it is possible to 'bring them up to date' by easy comparisons of then and now. — Una P. Holden, neuropsychologist, Leeds, 1980.

Suggested Further Reading

Allan, Chris and Bennett, Andrea 'What Year is it?' (Reality Orientation), *Nursing Mirror*, vol. 158, Clinical Forum iv-v (April 1984)

Holden, V.P. *Thinking it Through* (Winslow Press, Winslow, Buckinghamshire, 1984)

_____ and Woods, R.T. *Reality Orientation* (Churchill Livingstone, Edinburgh, 1982)

REFERENCES AND GENERAL FURTHER READING

Akhtar, S., Crocker, E. and Dickey, W. (1977) 'Overt Sexual Behaviour among Psychiatric In Patients', *Diseases of the Nervous System*, vol. 38, pp. 359-61

Altschul, A.T. (1977) 'Use of the Nursing Process in Psychiatric Nursing', *Nursing Times*, 8 September, pp. 1412-14

_____ (1980) 'Team Approach to Psychiatric Care', *Nursing Times*, 1 May, pp. 797-9

Argyle, Michael (1975) *Bodily Communication*, Methuen, London

Assael, M. (1978) 'Spontaneous Painting: Means of Communication', *Confinia Psychiatrica*, vol. 21, Parts 1-3, pp. 10-24

Barker, Philip (1982) *Behaviour Therapy Nursing*, Croom Helm, London

_____ (1985) *Patient Assessment in Psychiatric Nursing*, Croom Helm, London

Barton, Russel (1959) *Institutional Neuroses*, John Wright, Bristol

Beck, A.T. (1980) *Cognitive Therapy and the Emotional Disorders*, Meridian Books, New American Libary, New York

British Association for Counselling, 37a Sheep Street, Rugby

Carkhuff, R.R. and Truax, C.B. (1979) *Towards Effective Counselling and Psychotherapy: Training and Practice*, Aldine, New York

Carozza, Phyllis M. and Hiersteiner, Catherine L. (1982) 'Young Female Incest Victims in Treatment: Stages of Growth Seen with a Group Art Therapy Model', *Clinical Social Work Journal*, vol. 10, Part 3, pp. 165-75

Connor, M., Dexter, G. and Wash, M. (1984) *Listening and Responding: A Manual for Tutors*, College of Ripon and York St John, York

Dale, S. (1982) *Multiple Orgasms for Men*, Forum, London

Donnenberg, D. (1978) 'Art Therapy in a Drug Community', *Confinia Psychiatrica*, vol. 21, Parts 1-3, pp. 37-44

Drucker, Peter F. (1967) *The Effective Executive*, Heinemann, London

Egan, Gerard (1975, 2nd edn, 1982) *The Skilled Helper: A Model for Systematic Helping and Interpersonal Relating*, Brooks/Cole Publishing, Monterey, California

_____ (1984) Unpublished work, York Counselling Summer School Lecture Series

Ellis, A. (1962) *Reason and Emotion in Psychotherapy*, Lyle and Short, New York

English and Welsh National Boards for Nursing, Midwifery and Health Visiting (1982) *Syllabus of Training: Professional Register Part 3 (Registered Mental Nurse)*, London and Cardiff

Fonseca, J. (1970) 'Editorial Comment', *Nursing Outlook* (November)

Freud, Sigmund (1917) 'Mourning and Melancholia' in *Standard Edition of the Complete Psychological Works of Sigmund Freud* (1958)

_____ (1930) *Three Contributions to the Theory of Sex*, 4th edn, Nervous and Mental Disease Publishing, New York, pp. 35-45

_____ (1958) *The Standard Edition of the Complete Psychological Works of Sigmund Freud*, The Hogarth Press and the Institute of Psychoanalysis, London, vol. 12

Gentry, W. Doyle (ed.) (1975) *Applied Behaviour Modification*, Mosby, St Louis

Ginott, H.G. (1964) 'The Theory and Practice of Therapeutic Intervention in Child Treatment' in M.R. Haworth (ed.), *Child Psychotherapy: Practice and Theory*, Basic Books, New York

Halbreich, U. (1978) 'A Non-Verbal Dialogue as a Treatment of Schizophrenic Patients', *Confinia Psychiatrica*, vol. 21, Parts 1-3, pp. 58-67

Heath, J., Law, G. and Cross, I. *Nursing Process — What Is it?*, NHS Learning Resources Unit, Sheffield, 1982

Hogan, R. (1980) *Human Sexuality — A Nursing Perspective*, Appleton-Century-Crofts, New York

Houston, John P., Bee, Helen and Rimm, David C. (1980) *Invitation to Psychology*, international edn, Academic Press, Harcourt-Jovanovich Subsidiaries, New York

______, ______, ______ (1983) *Invitation to Psychology*, 2nd edn, Academic Press, New York

Kaplan, H. Singer (1981) *The New Sex Therapy*, Penguin Books, Harmondsworth

Kinsey, A.C., Pomeroy, W.B., Martin, C.F. and Gebhard, P.C.H. (1948) *Sexual Behaviour in the Human Male*, W.B. Saunders, Philadelphia

______, ______, ______, ______, (1953) *Sexual Behaviour in the Human Female*, W.B. Saunders, Philadelphia

Krumboltz, J.D. and Thoresen, C.E. (eds.) (1969) *Behavioural Counselling*, Holt, Rinehart and Winston, New York

Kübler-Ross, Elizabeth (1978) *To Live Until We Say Goodbye*, Prentice-Hall, Englewood Cliffs, New Jersey

Langley, Dorothy, M. and Langley, Gordon E. (1983) *Dramatherapy and Psychiatry*, Croom Helm, London

Mace, D.R., Bravermann, R.H.O. and Burton, J. (1974) *Teaching of Human Sexuality in Schools for Health Professionals*, WHO, Geneva

Maslow, A.H. (1970) *Motivation and Personality*, 2nd edn, Harper and Row, New York

_____(1971) *The Farther Reaches of Human Nature*, Viking, New York

Masters, W.H. and Johnson, V.E. (1966) *Human Sexual Response*, Little, Brown, Boston

Mitchell, A.R.K. (1974) *The Nature of Depression*, NAMHO, Penguin Books, Harmondsworth

Moreno, J.L. (1946) *Psychodrama 1*, Beacon House, New York

Mowrer, O.H. (1960) *Learning Theory and Behaviour*, John Wiley, New York

Murray Parkes, Colin (1976) *Bereavement: Studies of Grief in Adult Life*, Penguin Books, Harmondsworth

Norbeck, J.S. (1980) 'Psychiatric Nursing with Children' in P.C. Pothier (ed.), *Psychiatric Nursing: A Basic Text*, Little, Brown, Boston

Pavlov, I.P. (1927) *Conditioned Reflexes*, translated by G.V. Anrep, Oxford University Press, London

Piaget, J. *Child Psychotherapy: Pratice and Theory*, Basic Books, New York

Poteet, James A. (1978) *Behaviour Modification: A Practical Guide for Teachers*, Hodder and Stoughton, London

Pothier, P.C. (ed.) (1980) *Psychiatric Nursing: A Basic Text*, Little, Brown, Boston

Ramsay, R.W. (1975) *Grief Therapy*, Sixty Minutes, CBS News, USA (video)

Richards, B. (1982) 'The Grafenburg Spot and Female Ejaculation', *British Journal of Sexual Medicine* (December)

Rogers, Carl (1967) *On Becoming a Person: A Therapist's View of Psychotherapy*, Constable, London

Roper, Nancy, Logan, Winifred W. and Tierney, Alison J. (1980) *The Elements of Nursing*, Churchill Livingstone, London

Sundeen, S.J., Stuart,G.W., Rankin, E.D. and Cohen, S.A. (1976) *Nurse Client Interactions: Implementing the Nursing Process*, Mosby, St Louis

Warren, Bernie (ed.) (1984) *Using the Creative Arts in Therapy*, Croom Helm, London
Watzlawick, P., Beavin, J. and Jackson, D. (1968) *Pragmatics of Human Communication*, Faber, London
Wolfe, J. and Lazarus, A. (1966) *Behaviour Therapy Techniques. A Guide to the Treatment of Neuroses*, Pergamon Press, Oxford

INDEX

acceptance
  in dying patient 274
  in grieving 287
activities of living 117
aggression
  and attention seeking 171
  dealing with 168
  preventing 171
Akhtar 319
Alcoholics Anonymous 222
Altschul 127
anger
  in dying patient 271
  in grieving 287
anxiety
  non-verbal behaviour 182
  nurse's own 180
  physiological reaction 176
  psychological effects 177
  verbal responses to 181-2
approach skills 9-11
Argyle 37, 41
art therapy 327
  and non-verbal communication 329
  benefits of 328
  guidelines 327
  in drug community 329
  with incest victims 329
  with schizophrenics 329
Assael 329
assertion training 100-3
  case illustration 102
  eye contact 101
  the procedure 101
  touch in 101
assessment 113-27, 134
  nursing history sheet 118
  nursing priorities 118
  potential problems 127
  reasons for 114-17
  skill of 9-11
  sources of information 116
attending skills
  in deluded patients 238
attitudes 70
  for the psychiatric nurse 11-15
  learned 70
  prejudices 18

bargaining
  in dying patient 273
Barker 79
Barton 204
Beck 155
behaviour modification 78, 87
behaviour therapy 78
behavioural principles 76-86
  applied 83
behavioural skills 70-110
behaviourism 70
  consent boundaries 76
  consent guidelines 73-6
  consent in 72
  ethics in 72-6
  in society 70
bereaved 277
  development of pathological grief 283
  emotional disclosure 283
  in divorce 278
  information giving 281
  interactional skills in 282
  needs of 279
  potential emotions 278
  reactive depression 278
  telling bad news 281
  unemployment 278
bereavement, interactional skills in 282
bisexuality 322
breathing exercises 93
  see also desensitisation

Carkhuff 26
Carozza 329
child 243
  communication skills 246-50; boundary setting 248; conveying acceptance 250; creative communication 249; crises skills 247; exploratory skills 249; reasoning skills 249; teaching skills 247
  emotional involvement 252
  family groups 251
  family involvement 251
  hospitalisation and effects of 244; and subsequent needs 245

listening to the 246
overdependency 251
parent groups 251
psyschiatric problems of a 244
classical conditioning 77
client-centred 24-5
community psychiatric nurse 296
confidence 297
isolation of 296
role of 296
self-analysis 297
self-awareness 297
self-evaluation 297
community skills 295
control of environment 300
debrief skills 298
instant solution 301
patients' homes 301
compulsion 185
confidentiality 31-3
Connor, *et al.* 63
contracts, in grief therapy 288
contract therapy 191
counselling, definition 23
counsellor, qualities of 23
creative skills 327
CRUSE 284

Dale 314
dance therapy 337
debrief skill, in community 298
decision making, in management 350
deluded patients 236-42
distraction in 240
non-verbal communication in 238
delusion 236
definition 236
grandiose 237
ideas of reference 237
nihilistic 236
paranoid 236
systematised 236
unworthiness 236
dementia 255
denial
in dying patient 270
in grieving 287
dependent patients 219-27
and voluntary treated 224
drink, as substitute nurse 225
skills and principles 224
depression 141-58
behaviours in 143
communication in 143
continuum of 141
feelings in 143
in bereavement 278
in dying patient 273
in grieving 287
negative thinking 155
physical problems in 150
potential problems in 149
psychological problems in 149, 152
sleep patterns in 143
thoughts in 143
use of non-verbal skills 154
verbal skills 155
see also suicide
desensitisation 88
breathing exercises muscle relaxation 93
hierarchy of fear 91
programme 91-4
symptom substitution in 89
disorganisation 287
disorientation 255
distraction 164, 170, 247
divorce, as bereavement 278
Donnenberg 329
dramatherapy 330
and role play 322
and role reversal 333
empty chair 334
guided fantasy 334
happy chair 334
theory 331
uses of 331
Drucker 343
drugs, and sexuality 320
dying patients 263-76
acceptance 274
anger 271
bargaining 273
denial 270
depression 273
nurses' feelings about death 268
requirements 267

Egan 27, 42, 49, 63, 136
elderly
emotional disturbance 256
ethical considerations when nursing the 258
intellectual impairment 256
memory disturbance 255
physical problems of 256
psychological problems of 257
skills 259-60; group 260; management 260; non-verbal 259;

psychomotor 260; verbal 260
social problems 258
Ellis 95
empathy 27-8
advanced level 27-8
primary level 27
environment, in management 345
evaluation 132-4, 135
goal achievement 132
meaningful 133
nurses' performance 133
questioning 132
exploratory responding 44-53
active listening 44
clarifying 51-2
paraphrasing 45-7
reflecting 47-50; negative feelings 48-9; positive feelings 48
summarising 52-3
extinction 82, 85
burst 82
in operant conditioning 82
in the ward situation 83

fear inventory 190
fight/flight reaction 174
flight of ideas 159
response to 163
flooding 96-7, 191
Fonseca 308
free floating anxiety 174
Freud 175, 309

Gentry 79
genuineness 28-31
mutuality 29
non-verbal communication of 42
self-awareness 28
Ginott 248
Goffman 205
graded exposure *in vivo* 191
grief, stages of 287
grief therapy 286-91
contracts 288
development of pathological grief 283
intractable grief syndromes 291
guided fantasy 334
guilt, in grieving 287

Halbreich 329
hallucination 228-35
definition of 288
effects of 230-1
reinforcing reality 233
types of 229
Heath *et al.* 119
heterosexuality 322
Hiersteiner 329
Hogan 311
homosexuality 322
Houston 311
hypomania 160
hysteria 195
conversion symptoms 195
convulsion in 197
demands on the nurse 199
la belle indifférence 196
mental mechanisms 195
physical consequences 197
secondary gain 196
stocking paralysis 197
hysterical paralysis 196

ideas of reference 237
illusion 229
implementation 130-3, 135
general principles 130
team approach 131
inadequacy 212
institutionalisation
and nursing skills guideline 208
and rehabilitation 206
and respect 206
and staff expectations 204
interactive skills 11, 21

Kaplan 318, 324
Kinsey 312
Krumboltz 79
Kübler-Ross 263, 266, 268

lability 256
Langley and Langley 332, 339
Lazarus 79
leadership
and shared objectives 355
autocratic and democratic 354
by example 355
ideal leader/manager 358
qualities of 354
the benevolent autocrat 355
libido 309
limit setting 248
listening skills, in deluded patients 238

maladjusted 212
malingering 199
management 341-59
and contingencies 353

and finance 346
and leadership 353
decision making 350
delegation and responsibility 352
environment 345
equipment 344
ideal manager/leader 358
patient orientation 348
people 341
positives and negatives 349
problem solving 350
qualities 354
resources 341
task orientation 347
time 343
manipulative patients 212-18
antisocial behaviour in 216
disloyalty selfishness 217
elements of 213
self-mutilation 216
stealing 216
suicidal gestures 216
telling lies 216
Maslow 118, 126, 205
hierarchy of needs 126
Masters and Johnson 312
mental defence mechanisms 189, 360
modelling 86, 188, 191
Moreno 330
movement and dance 337
Mowrer 94
Murray Parkes 277
muscle relaxation 93
see also desensitisation
music therapy 338

negative reinforcement 80-2, 85
non-verbal attending 41-3
eye contact 42
open posture 42
warmth and genuineness 42
non-verbal communication 10, 12, 33-43
in caring for deluded 238
non-verbal sensitivity 35-41; eye contact 36; facial expression 36; gesture 38; posture and body space 36-8; tone of voice 40; touch 39
non-verbal responding 43
silence 43
Norbec 246, 250

observational skills 111, 113
physical observations 115
obsession 185
obsessive compulsive behaviour 185-6
and relaxation 187, 191
assessment in 189
effects of hospitalisation 186
family involvement in 186, 192
ritualistic hand-washing 187
operant conditioning 77
overactive patient, problems and needs of 161

pathological grief, *see* grief therapy
patient-centred 53
see also client-centred patient orientation, and management 348
Pavlov 77, 95, 97
personal ethics 13
personal equipment 12
personal satisfaction 13-15
personality disorder 212
persuasion 164
phobias 89, 174
alternative theoretical considerations 94
case illustration 94
formation; behavioural explanation 90
phobic reaction 89
planning 127-30, 134
goals of care 128
nursing action 129
nursing care plan 127
objectives of care 128
positive conditioning 97-9
case illustration 97
the procedure 98
positive reinforcement 79-80, 84
Poteet 79
Pothier 246
pressure of speech 159
problem solving 61-7
assessment 62, 66
evaluation 63, 67
forcefield analysis 63-6; facilitating factors 63; restraining factors 63
implementation 63, 67
in management 350
planning 62, 66
progressive responding 53-69
challenging 54-62; confrontation 58; data-based hunches 59-60; discrepancies 58; immediacy 59; information giving 61; owning problems 57; rules 61-2; self-disclosure 60-1; skill of 55; summarising 58

psychological care, of dying 267
psychopath 212
punishment 81, 85

qualities
effective living 13
for the psychiatric nurse 11-15
personal equipment 12

Ramsey 288
rationalisation 175
reality orientation 260, 362
relaxation 183
reminiscence therapy 260
response prevention therapy 187, 191
restraint 168
Richards 315
Rogers 24-5, 28
role play in dramatherapy 332
role reversal and dramatherapy 333
Roper *et al.* 117

satiation 87
schizophrenia and art therapy 329
self awareness 15-20, 30
congruence 16
personal defences 20
role awareness 17
self honesty 19
sensitivity 11
sexuality
alternative forms of 323
and mental handicap 316
and mental illness 317-21; effects of psychiatric treatment 320; effects of the institution 319; effects of the nurse 320; mood changes 318; schizophrenia 318
and physical handicap 317
physiological response 312-15; dysfunction 315; ejaculation, female 315; ejaculation, male 314; excitement phase 312; Grafenburg spot 314; orgasmic phase 314; plateau phase 314; resolution phase 314; sexual response cycle 312
problems throughout life 315
psychological aspects of 309; psychosexual stages of development 309; sex instinct 309
sexual therapy 324
see also positive conditioning
sociocultural aspects of sexuality 311; and religion 312; sex stereotypes 311
sexual health, elements of 308
shaping 85
Skinner 77
social skills training 104-9
an illustrative case 107
components of 106-7
modelling in 106
the procedure 106
sociopath 212
specialling 162
stages of dying 263
suggestion 164
suicide 145-8
high risk periods 146
prevention of 149, 151
Sundeen 28

terminally ill
children 266
information to 268
psychological care 267
requirement of 267
the elderly patient 266
transsexualism 323
transvestism 323
token economy 86

unconditional positive regard 25-6
unemployment, as a bereavement 278

values 31, 71
learned 71
uniqueness of the individual 31

warmth 30-1
acceptance 30
conveyance of 30
non-verbal communication of 31
Warren 333
Watzlawick 35
Wolfe 79